Documenta Ophthalmologica Proceedings Series

VOLUME 51

Ultrasonography in Ophthalmology 11

Proceedings of the 11th SIDUO
Congress, Capri, Italy, 1986

Edited by
J. M. Thijssen, J. S. Hilman, P. E. Gallenga
and G. Cennamo

Kluwer Academic Publishers
DORDRECHT / BOSTON / LONDON

Library of Congress Cataloging in Publication Data

SIDUO Congress (11th : 1986 : Capri, Italy)
    Ultrasonography in ophthalmology 11 : proceedings of the 11th
  SIDUO Congress, Capri, 1986 / edited by J.M. Thijssen ... [et al.].
      p.   cm. -- (Documenta ophthalmologica. Proceedings series ;
  51)
    Includes index.

    1. Ultrasonics in ophthalmology--Congresses. 2. Eye--Diseases and
  defects--Diagnosis--Congresses.   I. Thijssen, J. M.   II. Societas
  Internationalis pro Diagnostica Ultrasonica in Ophthalmologia.
  III. Title.   IV. Series.
  RE79.U4S5 1986
  617.7'1543--dc19
                                                            88-7284
                                                            CIP

ISBN-13: 978-94-010-7083-6   e-ISBN-13: 978-94-009-1311-0
DOI: 10.1007/978-94-009-1311-0

Published by Kluwer Academic Publishers,
P.O. Box 17, 3300 AA Dordrecht, The Netherlands.

Kluwer Academic Publishers incorporates
the publishing programmes of
Martinus Nijhoff, Dr W. Junk, D. Reidel and MTP Press.

Sold and distributed in the U.S.A. and Canada
by Kluwer Academic Publishers,
101 Philip Drive, Norwell, MA 02061, U.S.A.

In all other countries, sold and distributed
by Kluwer Academic Publishers Group,
P.O. Box 322, 3300 AH Dordrecht, The Netherlands.

Contents

SECTION III. VITREORETINAL AND CHOROIDAL DISEASES

SECTION IV. INTRAOCULAR TUMOURS AND LEUKOKORIA

SECTION V. ORBITAL AND PERIORBITAL TUMOURS

SECTION VI. EXTRAOCULAR MUSCLES AND OPTIC NERVE

SECTION VII. BIOMETRY

Preface

The 11th Congress of SIDUO took place in the beautiful setting of Capri in springtime and was held in the impressive and stimulating atmosphere of the 'Certosa di S. Giacomo'.

The organisation was sponsored by the SIEO, the 'Società Italiana di Eco-Oftalmologia'. The Honorary President was Professor Antonio Rossi, Head of the University Department of Ophthalmology in Ferrara and one of the pioneers of Italy in this field.

The organizing committee further consisted of:

President: Prof. P. E. Gallenga, University Department of Ophthalmology, Chieti

Vice President: Dr. G. Cennamo, University Department of Ophthalmology, Napels

Scientific Secretary: Dr. J. M. Thijssen, University Department of Ophthalmology, Nijmegen

Treasurer: Dr. A. Reibaldi, University Department of Ophthalmology, Bari

The organizing Committee was supported by an International Scientific Programme Committee:

Regional Representatives:

G. Bellone (Torino)
A. Bertényi (Budapest)
D. J. Coleman (New York)
K. C. Ossoinig (Iowa City)
R. Sampaolesi (Buenos Aires)
A. W. Sawada (Miyazaki)
P. Till (Wien)

SIDUO Officers:

P. E. Gallenga (President)
J. S. Hillman (Treasurer)
B. L. Hodes (Vice-President)
J. M. Thijssen (Secretary)
H. G. Trier (Past-President)

As A Regional Advisory Committee served:
Honorary Chairmen:
A. Oksala (Turka), A. Alajmo (Venezia), A. Bonovolontà (Napoli)

In this volume of the Documenta Ophthalmologica Proceedings Series the topics of the sessions at the Congress have been maintained. The abstracts of the lectures from which no manuscript was received for publication have not been included in this volume. The reader is referred to the abstracts book for a complete overview of the abstracts. Due to some unfortunate political problems and the recent occurrence of an accident in a nuclear power plant in Eastern-Europe the participation of our North-American members was almost reduced to zero. This incidence of course has limited the final programme to a great extent.

P. E. Gallenga

Instrumentation and technology

Clinical performance measurements on ultrasonic transducers

W. HAIGIS AND W. BUSCHMANN

Summary

Clinical performance measurements on single-element transducers for ophthalmic ultrasound systems again stress the necessity to carry out such measurements. The results of the determination of different frequency parameters suggest that the use of "working frequency" according to IEC recommendations gives a better description of transducer frequency behaviour than the nominal frequency.

Introduction

One of the most important parts of diagnostic ultrasonic systems is the transducer. Forming the front end of the data acquisition chain, its performance essentially influences the quality of ultrasonic diagnosis — no matter how sophisticated subsequent signal processing may be.

Among the parameters describing transducer performance are frequency, bandwidth and sensitivity. Using the nominal frequency of a transducer as stated by the manufacturer has often turned out to be insufficient or even erroneous (Haigis, 1985). Therefore, in accordance with the INTERNATIONAL ELECTROTECHNICAL COMMISSION (IEC, 1986; Brendel, 1976), the use of "working frequency" is preferable to characterize the acoustical frequency behaviour of a transducer. Various approaches are recommended by the IEC to assess this parameter.

In a comparative study of several single-element transducers frequency parameters as well as transducer sensitivities were determined with different methods. The measurements were carried out on the basis of recommendations by the IEC (1986) and the AMERICAN INSTITUTE OF ULTRASOUND IN MEDICINE (AIUM, 1982).

University Eye Clinic, Schneiderstrassell, D-8700 Würzburg, FRG

J. M. Thijssen (ed.) Ultrasonography in ophthalmology.
© 1988, *Kluwer Academic Publishers, Dordrecht, ISBN 978-94-010-7083-6*

Measurement parameters and methods

For 9 single-element transducers of different make and kind, nominally ranging from 5 to 10 MHz, the following parameters were determined: working frequency, peak frequency, center frequency, bandwidth and transducer sensitivity.

Except for the working frequency, all frequency parameters were measured independently with two different methods (AIUM, 1982):

— spectrum analyzer method,
— tone burst method.

The block diagrams for the respective experimental set-ups are depicted in Fig. 1.

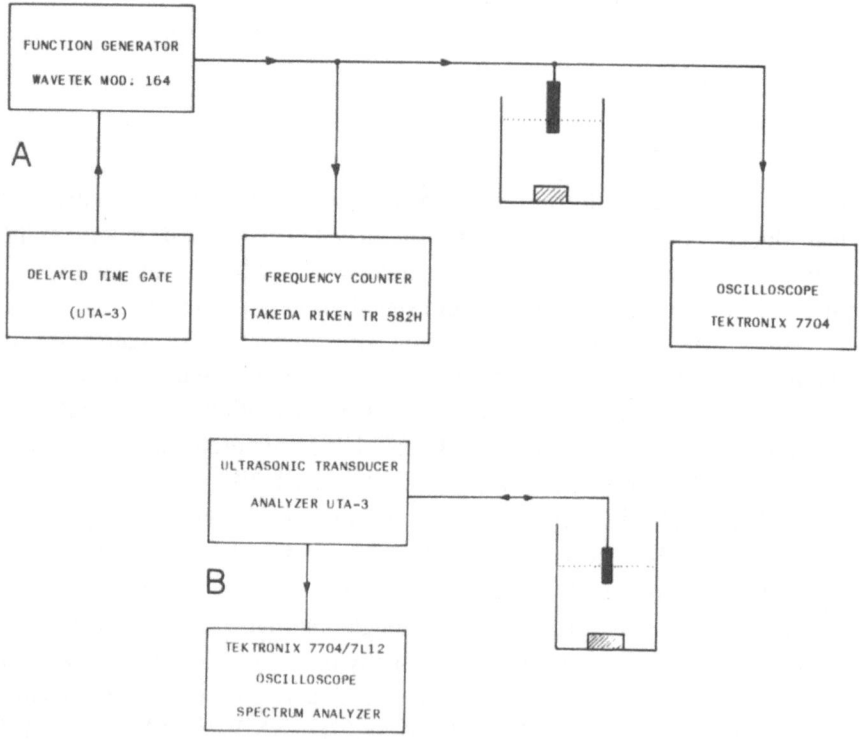

Fig. 1. Experimental set up for frequency measurements: (a) Block diagram for tone burst method. (b) Block diagram for spectrum analyzer method.

Spectrum analyzer method

The transducers were operated with the ULTRASONIC TRANSDUCER ANALYZER UTA-3 (KB Aerotech), which served as transmitter and calibrated broad-band receiver with adjustable time gate. As the target a plane W38-HEMA-reflector (Haigis, 1981; Haigis and Buschmann, 1985) acted as a "working standard plane echo interface" (IEC, 1986). For all transducers examined the distance to the reflector was kept constant and equivalent to a time of flight of 30 μsec. In diagnostic ophthalmic ultrasonography this reflector position would roughly coincide with the posterior pole of the human eye. On a broad-band TEKTRONIX 7704 oscilloscope with a 7L12 spectrum analyzer plug-in device the interface echo waveform as well as its amplitude spectrum were observed.

Tone burst method

A gated sine-wave oscillator (WAVETEK 30 MHz function generator Mod. 164) produced tone bursts of at least 15 cycles at all test frequencies. A TAKEDA RIKEN TR 582H counter was employed to accurately measure the frequency. Since the W38-HEMA-target causes rather low echoes, a plane glass plate served as a reflecting interface. Again, the transducer-reflector distance was equivalent to 30 μsec. On the TEKTRONIX 7704 oscilloscope the reflected tone burst was recorded.

Results of frequency measurements

Within the limits of measurement errors, both methods yielded comparable results. Whereas, with the electronic spectrum analyzer, the frequency spectrum is quickly available, the tone burst measurement is a time-consuming procedure. Typical amplitude spectra obtained with both methods are shown in Fig. 2. From these spectral data the frequency $f(p)$ of maximum pulse-echo response was determined for each transducer. Also, the center frequency $f(c)$ was calculated according to

$$f(c) = \frac{f(u) + f(l)}{2} \tag{1}$$

where $f(l)$ and $f(u)$ denote the lower and upper frequencies at which the pulse-response is one half (-6 dB) the peak response. The fractional bandwidth BW was obtained from

$$BW = \frac{f(u) - f(l)}{f(c)} \cdot 100\%. \tag{2}$$

Photographs of the echo waveforms as displayed on the oscilloscope screen (cf. Fig. 3) served to determine the working frequency. With the exception of transducer #9, which produced the waveform of Fig. 3a, all transducers showed waveforms similar to Fig. 3b. Therefore, the working frequencies $f(w)$ could be calculated from the zero crossings according to (IEC, 1986)

$$f(w) = \frac{n}{2t} \tag{3}$$

where n is the number of consecutive half-cycles with amplitudes not less than 30% of maximum amplitude and t is the time between commencement of the 1st half-cycle and end of the nth half-cycle (cf. Fig. 3b).

For the waveform of transducer #9 another approach to assess the working frequency was chosen. An "effective frequency" $f(eff)$ was calculated by sampling the waveform $A(t)$ at times $t_i = i \cdot T$ (T = sampling interval) from (IEC, 1986)

$$f(eff) = \frac{1}{2\pi T} \cdot \left\{ \frac{\Sigma_i B_i^2}{\Sigma_i A_i^2} \right\}^{1/2} \tag{4}$$

with $A_i = A(t_i)$: sample of the waveform at time $t_i = i \cdot T$ and $B_i = A_i - A_{i-1}$.

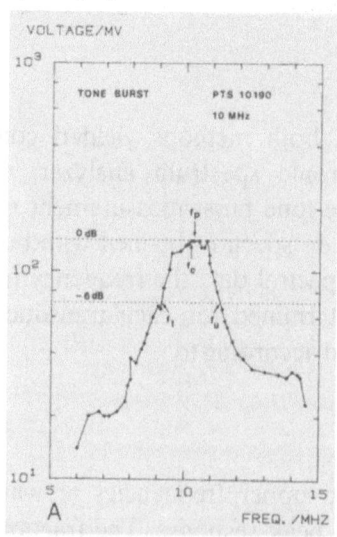

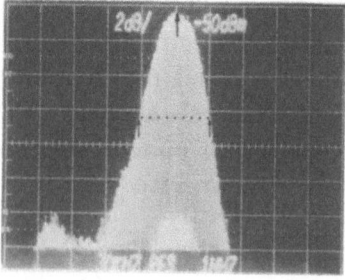

Fig. 2. Amplitude spectra: (a) Plot of log (amplitude) vs frequency as obtained by tone burst method. (b) Amplitude spectrum of interface echo measured by spectrum analyzer.

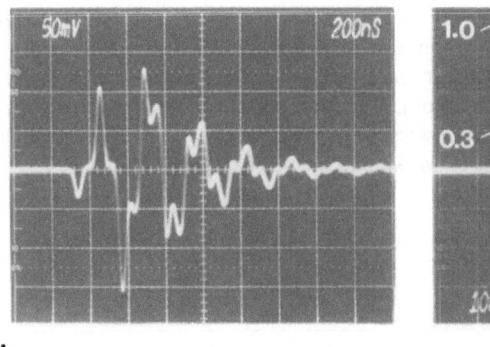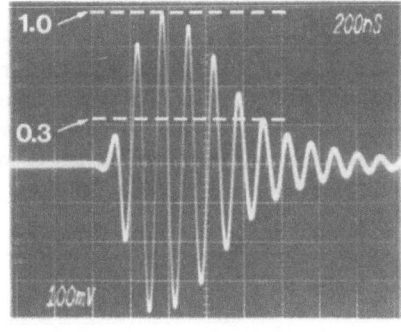

A   B

Fig. 3. Real-time waveforms of W38-interface echo of two different transducers: (a) High frequency ripple on dominant low frequency signal. Working frequency according to (3): f(w) = 3.8 MHz. Effective frequency according to (4): f(eff) = 6.5 MHz. (b) Typical waveform allowing calculation of working frequency by counting zero-crossings: f(w) = 7.4 MHz.

The frequency parameters thus obtained for all transducers are compiled in Table 1. Furthermore, the percentage deviations of peak, center and working frequency from nominal frequency as well as the deviation of working frequency from center frequency are also given. These values were calculated from

$$f(xy) = \frac{f(x) - f(y)}{f(y)} \cdot 100\% \qquad (5)$$

with x = p, c, w and y = n, c standing for the respective frequency values.

The waveform of transducer #9 (Fig. 3a) was evaluated according to (4) with a sample interval of T = 10 nsec (ensuring adequate sampling). Computation yielded f(eff) = 6.5 MHz. From the amplitude spectrum, a peak and center frequency of 3.9 MHz was derived. Another spectral peak 9 dB below the 3.9 MHz maximum showed up at 13 MHz, well separated from the dominant peak (by 40 dB). Comparison of these values with the effective frequency of 6.5 MHz gives no apparent relationship.

Therefore, the working frequency of transducer #9 was calculated from (3) ignoring the high frequency ripple. A value of f(w) = 3.8 MHz was obtained and listed in Table 1. This result seems to be a better characterization for the frequency behaviour of transducer #9 than the use of the "effective frequency" according to (4).

From the results of Table 1 it can be seen that with respect to nominal frequency considerable deviations of up to 67% were found for peak, center as well as for working frequency. This holds especially for heavily damped transducers with bandwidths ≳ 30%. On the other hand, the smallest deviations occur in all cases when working frequency is compared to center frequency. Irrespective of bandwidth they range from −4% to

Table 1. Transducer frequency data: f(n): nominal frequency; f(p): frequency of maximum pulse-echo response; f(l) and f(u): lower and upper frequencies at which pulse-echo response is one half (−6 dB) the maximum response; f(c): center frequency; f(w): working frequency; BW: fractional bandwidth. Δf(pn), Δf(cn) and Δf(wn): percentage deviations of peak, center, and working frequency, respectively, from nominal frequency relative to nominal frequency. Δf(wc): deviation of working frequency from center frequency relative to center frequency. (*): Determination of effective frequency according to (4) yields f(eff) = 6.5 MHz.

Transducer #		1	2	3	4	5	6	7	8	9
f(n)	(MHz)	10	10	8	10	5	10	6	10	10
f(p)	(MHz)	10.0	10.9	7.7	9.8	5.1	8.8	10.0	9.2	3.9
f(l)	(MHz)	8.9	10.1	6.6	8.4	4.3	7.7	6.2	7.1	3.2
f(u)	(MHz)	11.2	12.6	8.5	11.2	5.7	9.8	12.2	11.8	4.6
f(c)	(MHz)	10.0	11.3	7.6	9.8	5.0	8.8	9.2	9.5	3.9
f(w)	(MHz)	10.0	11.0	7.6	10.0	4.8	8.8	9.5	9.4	3.8 (*)
BW	(%)	23	22	25	29	28	24	65	49	36
Δf(pn)	(%)	0	9	−4	−2	2	−12	67	−8	−61
Δf(cn)	(%)	0	13	−5	−2	0	−12	53	−5	−61
Δf(wn)	(%)	0	10	−5	0	−4	−12	58	−6	−62
Δf(wc)	(%)	0	−3	0	2	−4	0	3	−1	−3

+3%, which is slightly above the margins of measurement errors. Therefore, if a whole set of frequency data (spectrum) is to be described by one single parameter, the use of "working frequency" according to IEC seems to be an acceptable choice — at least clinically.

Results of sensitivity measurements

Three different measurement techniques were employed to assess transducer sensitivity, the results of which are listed in Table 2:

1. With a HEMA-W38-reflector in saline placed 30 μsec away from the transducer, the necessary gain setting to produce a 10 mm interface echo on a KRETZ 7200 MA apparatus was measured. This value, denoted by S(7200), is determined by the transducer itself, but also by the system characteristics of the 7200 MA instrument (impedance matching, amplifier frequency response, transmitting pulse etc.).
2. The experimental set-up of Fig. 1b was used to measure the necessary UTA-3-attenuation, which produces a 100 mV (peak-peak) W38-interface echo (time of flight: 30 μsec). This value, denoted by S(UTA),

Table 2. Transducer sensitivity data: S(7200), S(UTA) and S(Burst): Transducer sensitivities measured with KRETZ 7200 MA, UTA-3, and tone burst method, respectively. For each line sensitivity data are normalized with respect to transducer #3, i.e. sensitivity of transducer #3 is set to be 0 dB.

Transducer #	1	2	3	4	5	6	7	8	9
S(7200) (dB)	−19	−22	0	−9	−11	−12	−6	−14	−
S(UTA) (dB)	−8	−15	0	−5	−11	−12	+5	−10	−7
S(Burst) (dB)	−2	−20	0	−7	−10	−14	−	−17	−

is mainly determined by the sensitivity of the transducer. It may be affected by impedance mismatches, but less by the (broad-band) amplifier frequency response of the UTA-3.

3. With the set-up of Fig. 1a the amplitude V(r) of the reflected tone burst at center frequency f(c) as well as the peak voltage of the transmitted burst V(0) were measured. The relative pulse-echo sensitivity S(burst) was calculated from (AIUM, 1982)

$$S(burst) = 20 \log \frac{V(r)}{V(0)} \, dB \qquad (6)$$

giving the best estimate for transducer sensitivity. The data of Table 2 are normalized with respect to transducer #3, i.e. for each line of the table the sensitivity differences are given relative to the sensitivity of transducer #3. Making allowance for the above mentioned effects influencing the measured data, the agreement of S(UTA) and S(burst) — which is to be expected — may be considered acceptable. The values of S(7200), on the other hand, are strongly influenced by the narrow band frequency characteristic of this instrument. On the whole, these measurements reveal clear differences in sensitivities of transducers used in ophthalmic ultrasonography.

Further measurements were carried out regarding correction curves for the diffraction effect, the results of which will be reported elsewhere.

Acknowledgement

This study was carried out within the framework of the Concerted Action Program on Ultrasonic Tissue Characterization of the European Community.

10

References

AIUM, American Institute of Ultrasound in Medicine. 1982. Standard methods for testing single-element pulse-echo ultrasonic transducers, Interim Standard, J Ultrasound Med, 7 (Suppl. 1).

Brendel K, Filpczynski LS, Gerstner R, Hill CR, Kossoff G, Quentin G, Reid JM, Saneyoshi J, Somer JC, Tchevnenko AA, Wells PNT. 1976. Methods of measuring the performance of ultrasonic pulse-echo diagnostic equipment, Ultrasound Med Biol 2: 343—000.

Haigis W, Reuter R, Lepper R-D. 1981. Comparative measurements on different pulse-echo systems using test reflectors. In: JM Thijssen and AM Verbeek (eds) Ultrasonography in Ophthalmology 8, Doc Ophthal Proc Series, Vol. 29, Junk, Den Haag, pp. 445—456.

Haigis W, Buschmann W. 1985. Echo reference standards in ophthalmic ultrasonography, Ultrasound Med Biol 11: 149—000.

Haigis W. 1985. Performance measurements in ophthalmic ultrasonography with respect to IEC-recommendations. In: RW Gill and MJ Dadd (eds) WFUMB'85, Proc of the 4th Meeting of the World Fed for Ultrasound in Med Biol, Pergamon Press, Sidney, New York, p. 433.

IEC, International Electrotechnical Commission, IEC Report. 1986. Methods of measuring the performance of ultrasonic pulse-echo diagnostic equipment, Publication 854, Bureau Central de la Commission Electrotechnique Internationale; 3, rue de Varembe, Geneve, Suisse.

Three dimensional ultrasonography of ocular region

Y. YAMAMOTO[1,2], M. KUBOTA[2], Y. SUGATA[2], S. MATSUI[2] AND
M. ITO[3]

Summary

A spiral scan is introduced to collect three dimensional (3D) data of the
ocular region so that it may give uniformly-spaced echo data with enough
resolution and that the cross-sectional image of any specified plane can be
reconstructed. The system consists of a 3D-Scanning unit, an image processing unit with memories of 2M bytes, and a ultrasound pulser and
receiver unit. The obtained 3D-data are stored on a floppy disk or directly
in the large memory for fast processing. A conventional probe of 10 MHz
is used to scan the total tissue and is driven spirally under the control
of the 3D-Scanning unit. The developed system can supply black and
white 3D-images with or without the pseudo-color cross-section, gradated
according to the echo levels, to allow quantitative and qualitative evaluation of the intraocular pathology. The shape and the contour image from
the desired viewing angle can be implemented by the built-in microcomputer. The present system was assessed by case studies to be qualified
as to contain more information as compared with the ordinary B-mode
echography and the rapid image processing to be useful in clinical routine
activities. Measurement of the volume is another function of the 3D
echography which is not obtainable by the conventional B-mode. The
precision was experimented by the measurement of the lens volume.

Introduction

Three dimensional information of ocular region is a useful diagnostic aid
for tracing the clinical course of ocular diseases, for determining opera-
tional access, and for giving quantitative data to the clinical study. The
method of piling up the sectional echogram was used to realize the idea of
3D imaging by the aid of microcomputer (Hirano et al., 1982; Yamamoto

[1] Metropolitan Tama Gerontology Center, Tokyo, Japan; [2] Department of Ophthalmology,
Metropolitan Komagome Hospital, Honkomagome 3-18-22, Bunkyo-ku, Tokyo 113, Japan;
[3] University of Agriculture and Technology, Tokyo, Japan.

J. M. Thijssen (ed.) Ultrasonography in ophthalmology.
© 1988, *Kluwer Academic Publishers, Dordrecht, ISBN 978-94-010-7083-6*

et al., 1983). The main problem of the method is rather time consuming for examination, which requires greater physical efforts of patients and naturally it resulted in a decreased quality of the ocular image compared with the higher quality of demand. We constructed the echograms obtained in a shorter examination time, giving a 3D image together with a sectional view seen from any desired direction, and colored by specified hue and luminance (Ito et al., 1985). The extraction of the contour of a line allows us to calculate the area or the volume of the closed area or space (Yamamoto et al., 1983). This is the new aspect of the echography, which is not fully developed at conventional B-mode echography.

Method

Conventional echography with a 10 MHz polymer transducer (Toray) (Sugata et al., 1982) was performed by the immersing method. The custom designed driving unit for the spiral scanning (Fig. 1) and an image processing unit are connected to the echograph (Hill et al., 1976; Ito et al., 1985).

System

The recently developed system is currently applied in ophthalmology to observe three dimensional relations between the shape and specified sections and to measure physical quantities such as length, area, and volume. The block diagram of the 3D system is shown in Fig. 2 and the system is composed of seven units such as ultrasound interfacing unit,

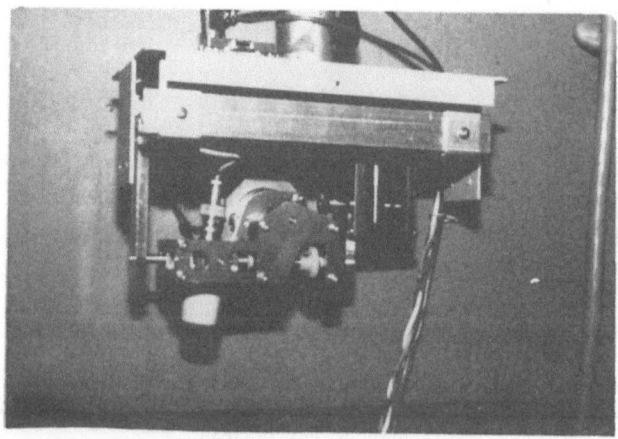

Fig. 1. The driving unit for the spiral scanning.

memory unit, and other units necessary for image processing and controls. The ultrasound interfacing unit (Fig. 3) manipulates the total data handling from the movement of a probe to the sampling and this unit interfaces the system with the ultrasound diagnostic equipment (or ultrasound pulser and receiver) through the A/D converter and buffer memory. The bank-selected memory stores all the digitized echo data, which are collected from the region of interest by a series of B-mode sector scans or spirally scanned A-mode signals, and is synchronized to the ultrasound interface unit. It takes about one minute and twenty seconds to scan the whole region in a spiral fashion. For most cases twenty to thirty seconds are enough for scanning. All the 3D image processing is carried out on this bank-selected memory of 2M bytes and the main memory of 512K bytes. The processing includes coordinate conversion to reconstruct sectional images, binarization of gray-scale images, gradation of the obtained contours, rotation of 3D images according to the viewing angle and others. Fig. 4 depicts the total process employed in this system.

Block Diagram of the 3D System

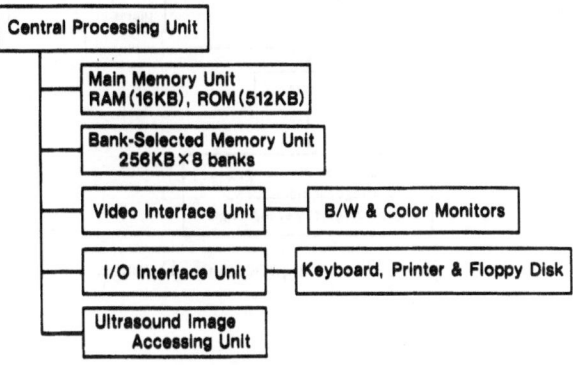

Fig. 2. The block diagram of the 3D system.

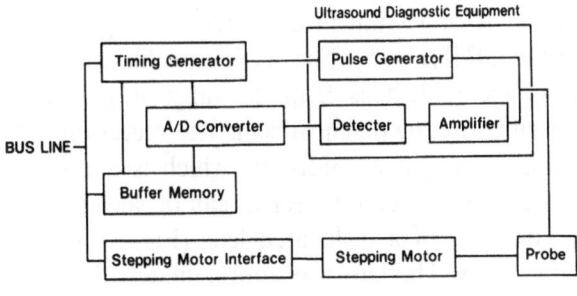

Ultrasound Image Accessing Unit

Fig. 3. The ultrasound interfacing unit.

14

Construction process of 3D image

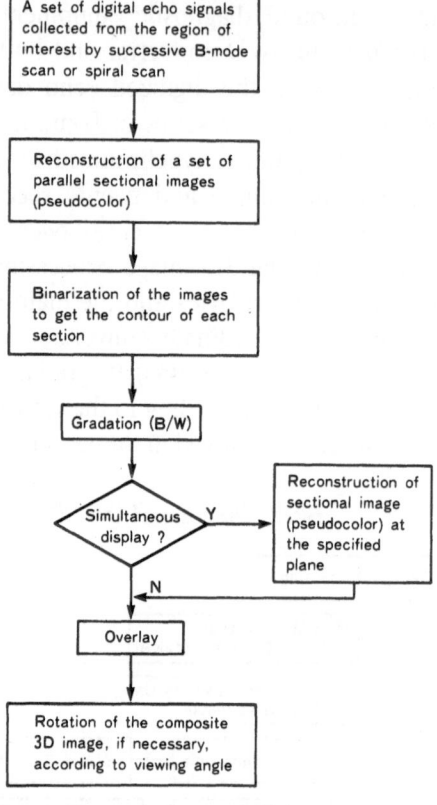

Fig. 4. The total process of 3D image.

Results

A soft contact lens of 13 mm in diameter on a sponge phantom is well displayed on the CRT (Fig. 5). The section profile is also depicted, on the side of the sponge fold. This B-mode image is gradated by color and luminance specified by the diagnostician. The recession of the disc area in a case of the morning-glory syndrome, which is approximately 5 mm in diameter, is clearly displayed on CRT as can be seen by comparing Figs. 6 and 7. The side view of a dislocated lens (Fig. 8) and its oblique view (Fig. 9) are quit clear. The lens was approximately 8 mm in diameter. For the purpose of calculating the lens volume, a series of sections of the lens was collected to count their inner pixels as shown in Fig. 10. The count from three different directions gave similar results.

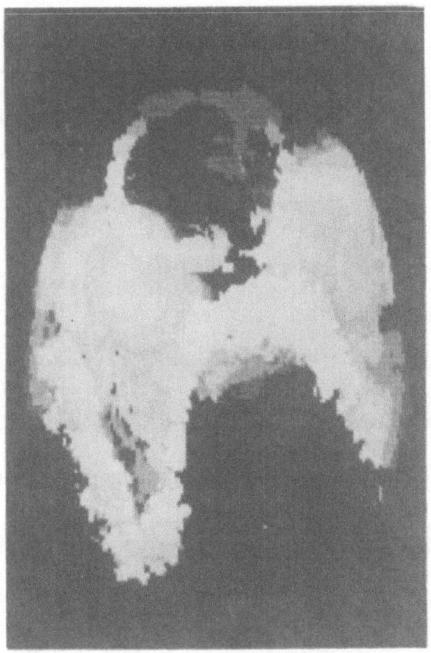

Fig. 5. The 3D image of a sponge phantom with a soft contact lens (oblique).

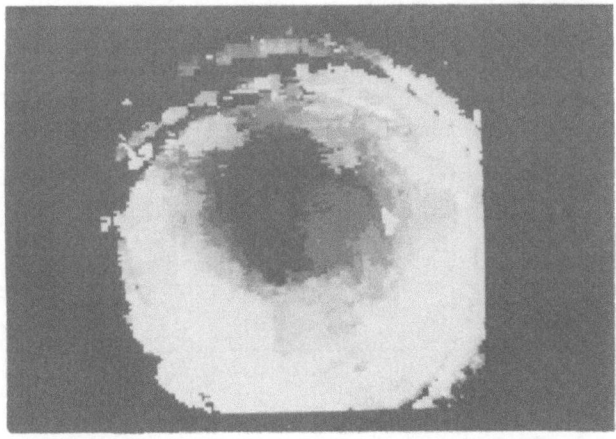

Fig. 6. Frontal view of the 3D image of a morning-glory syndrome.

16

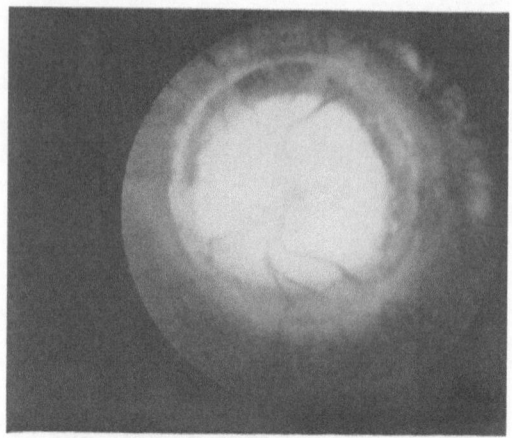

Fig. 7. Fundus photograph of a morning-glory syndrome.

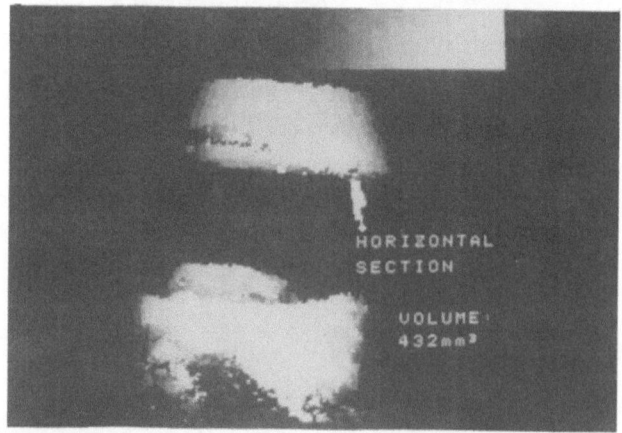

Fig. 8. Side view of the 3D image of a dislocated lens.

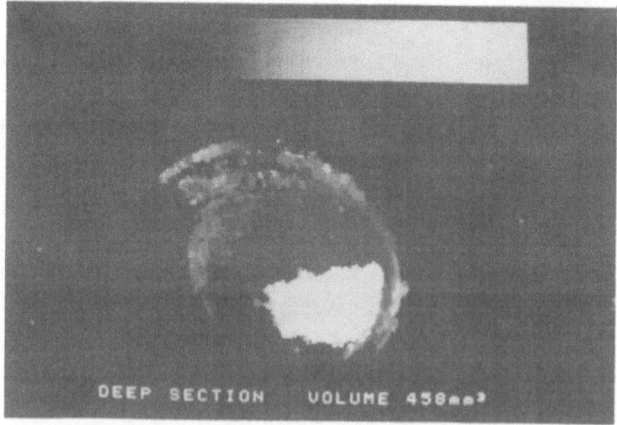

Fig. 9. Oblique view of the 3D image of a dislocated lens.

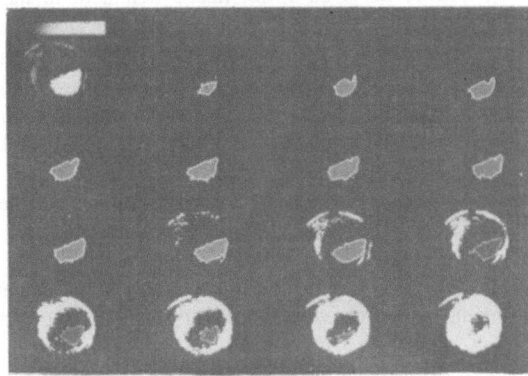

Fig. 10. A series of sectional views of the dislocated lens for calculating the lens volume.

Discussion

This three dimensional display system equipped with the rotation of the image section and with specific color scales incorporates all functions of conventional B-mode echography. The function of volume measurement is the additional function to allow a quantitative assessment in the clinical diagnosis (Yamamoto et al., 1983). The faster processing of a large volume of data is the clinical motivation to expand this function for the daily diagnostic use. From this motivation, electronic scanning is also proposed to obtain easier and faster scanning (Ito et al., 1985; Yanashima et al., 1985), but the homogeneous distribution of the spatial information must be guaranteed so that any desired section may be extracted with enough gradation.

References

Hill CR, Carpenter DA. 1976. Ultrasonic echo imaging of tissues: instrumentation. Brit J Radiol 49: 238—243.

Hirano S, Yamamoto Y, Sugata Y et al. 1982. Image treatment in the eye in ultrasound diagnosis and clinical significance. X. Contour line extraction and three dimensional display. Jpn J Clin Ophthalmol 36: 475—480.

Ito M, Yamamoto Y, Sugata Y. 1985. On highly-gradated ultrasonography by color and luminance specifications. In: RW Gill and MJ Dadd (eds) Proc of 4th meeting of the World Federation for Ultrasound in Medicine and Biology. Pergamon, Sydney, p. 555.

Ito M, Yamamoto Y, Sugata Y. 1985. Three-dimensional display with a specified-plane ultrasonogram by a spiral scanning. In: RW Gill and MJ Dadd (eds) Proc of the 4th meeting of the World Federation for Ultrasound in Medicine and Biology. Pergamon, Sydney, p. 558.

18

Sugata Y, Hirano S, Tomita M et al. 1982. Image treatment in the eye in ultrasound diagnosis and clinical significance. XI. Improvements of images on cathode ray tube by new polymer transducer and new color grading. Acta Soc Ophthalmol Jpn 86: 1004—1011.

Yamamoto Y, Hirano S, Sugata Y et al. 1983. Microcomputer aided imaging techniques in ophthalmic B-mode. In: JS Hillman and MM May (eds) Ophthalmic Ultrasonography, Junk, The Hague, pp. 467—477.

Yamamoto Y, Hirano S, Sugata Y et al. 1983. Image treatment in the eye in ultrasound diagnosis and clinical significance. XIV. Measurements of vitreous volume. Folia Ophthalmol Jpn 34: 2473—2477.

Yanashima K, Akeo Y, Okade Y, Ishiguro M, Fukuma H. 1985. 3-Dimensional echography using a linear acanning tomography..Jpn J Med Ultrasonics 12 (suppl 1): 839—840.

A mechanical sector scanner for ophthalmic ultrasonic diagnosis

A. SAWADA[1], H. TORII, T. HAYASHIDA AND S. YOSHIDA

Summary

1. Using Santesonic SSD-121, distinct B-mode images can be displayed easily and constantly. Specific skill of the examiner is not required.
2. Of intraocular membranous lesions, kinetic analysis in real time can be done. The shape, extent, mobility and connection to the posterior wall are clearly shown. Of orbital space-occupying lesions, the shape, size as well as consistency are shown.
3. Minute observation after images freezing is available. And the equipment can be connected to a video-recorder and hard copy devices.
4. Measurement of the size of ocular and orbital lesions, as well as of axial length can be done with incorporated electronic calipers. Distance in two directions on a frozen image can be measured at the same time and the result is displayed on the monitor.
5. In A-mode display the area of displaying is very small and the top of spikes is prone to be rectangular. Further improvement is required for precise ultrasonic tissue characterization.

Introduction

Many kinds of B-mode ultrasonic diagnostic equipments have been introduced. Recently a new equipment specific to ophthalmic ultrasonography, Santesonic SSD-121, has been on sale in Japan. We studied clinically the usefulness of this equipment in several ocular and orbital disorders.

Equipment

Santesonic SSD-121 is a mechanical scanning ultrasonic diagnostic equipment (Fig. 1) A-mode and B/A-mode are available at the same time. The

---

[1] Department of Ophthalmology, Miyazaki Medical College, 5200 Kihara, Kiyotake, Miyazaki 889-16, Japan.

J. M. Thijssen (ed.) Ultrasonography in ophthalmology.
© 1988, *Kluwer Academic Publishers, Dordrecht, ISBN 978-94-010-7083-6*

frequency of the transducer is 7.5 MHz. The major and minor axes of the contact surface of the probe are 4.9 cm and 1.4 cm. The probe has a water chamber on the front of it. The horizontal and vertical range for diagnosis is 6.0 cm each. Lateral and axial resolution is within 1.0 mm, respectively. The frame rate is 15 per second. The number of scan lines is 128 per frame. The image is displayed on 5.5 inch-wide TV-monitor. Sensitivity control operates from 0 to 100 dB, which is shown as the scale of 0 to 10. The transducer is 13 mm in diameter and focus-typed. The angle of scanning is about 40 degrees. The images can be frozen at any time. After freezing the image distances can be measured in two directions on the same image. The measured values are displayed on the monitor with a precision of 0.1 mm. Date, ID-number, and reference number can be displayed on the screen as well. The size of Santesonic SSD-121 is 37 (W) × 45 (D) × 27 (H) cm. The weight is 19 kg. The equipment can be connected

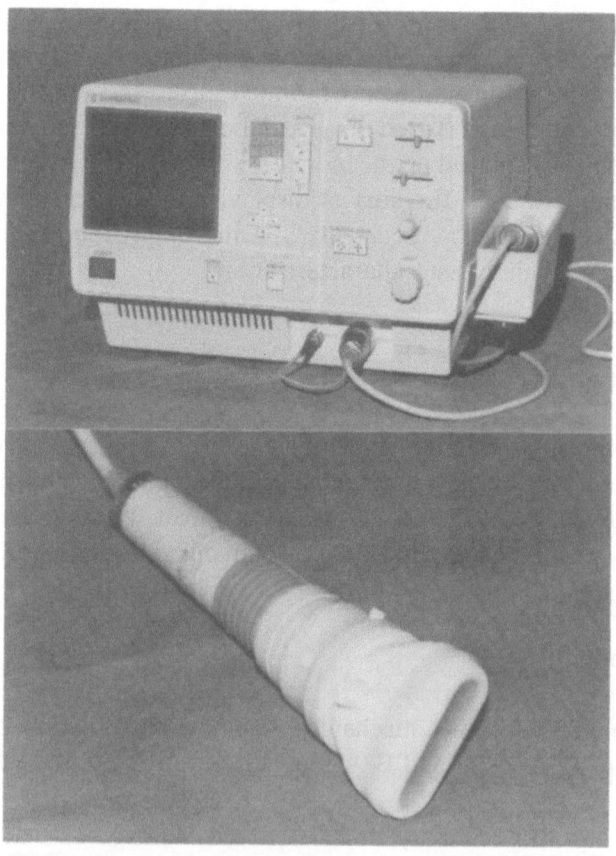

Fig. 1. Santesonic SSD-121.

directly to videorecorder. Ultrasonography can be done either by the contact method or by the immersion method using surgical drape.

Results and discussion

Anterior lesions

In those superficial cases as squamous cell carcinoma of the lid and dermoid cyst in the orbit, the immersion method should be employed. The size and thickness of the lesion are easily measured and the result is displayed on the screen. It is very efficient is recording. Santesonic SSD-121 has the function of A-mode display and B/A-mode display as well as B-mode display. B/A-mode display reveals the level of ultrasonic reflectivity inside of the target tissue, which is poorly shown in B-mode display only. However, the pulse repetition rate of the A-mode is not fast enough so that it is difficult to freeze the A-mode image exactly as desired. The display height of A-mode spikes is very small and the top of the spike is sometimes rectangular. Further improvement is required if precise evaluation is wanted for ultrasonic tissue characterization.

Intraocular lesions

In asteroid hyalosis a large ball-like, highly reflective mass is displayed in the center of the vitreous. With reduced sensitivity, mobile granules of high reflectivity remain. The mass is distinctly separated from the posterior wall of the eye with definite distance. With induced movement of the eye the mass shows a quick rotatory motion like a decoration ball.

Vitreous membrane formation from vitreous hemorrhage is one of the most common vitreous disorders. It should be strictly differentiated from retinal detachment. On the echograms poorly continuous membranes with coarse surface and irregular thickness, are displayed in the center of the vitreous. Ultrasonic reflectivity is relatively strong. Topographic findings, one of which is the connection of membrane formation to the posterior wall of the eye, are clearly shown with the equipment. As the equipment is a high-speed mechanical scanner, movement of membranous structure is clearly observed in real time. However, finer kinetic analysis using digitizer and computer can not be performed, as with electronic scanning equipment can be done.

The next common membrane-like lesion in the eye is retinal detachment. Detached retina is shown as a continuous membrane of higher reflectivity and of constant thickness. Elevation of detached retina can be clearly displayed with little distortion. The degree of elevation is measured with incorporated electronic calipers. The results are shown on the monitor. A flat retinal detachment can be displayed also, though slightly inferior to Ophthascan B (Biophysique Medical Inc.). Like in vitreous membrane formation, movement of a detached retina can be evaluated.

The third membrane-like structure in the eye is proliferative diabetic retinopathy. In such a case retinal detachment possibly due to traction of fibrous proliferative tissue formation is frequently developed (Fig. 2). Discrimination between detached retina and proliferative tissue in front of the fundus is frequently requested. Although Santesonic SSD-121 can afford sufficient topographic information, quantitative information based on reflectivity is not satisfactory.

The luxated lens, or a foreign body can be displayed very easily. Mobility of a luxated lens is shown by eye movement or postural change.

In retinoblastoma the shape, the connection to the optic nerve and other complicated changes are clearly displayed. Information on reflectivity such as acoustic shadow is satisfactorily given.

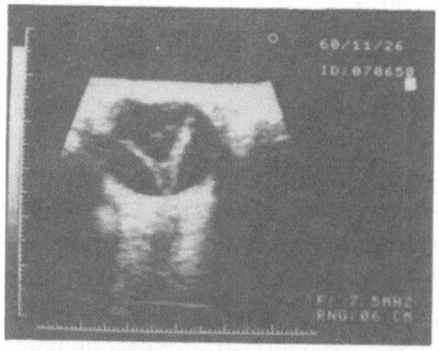

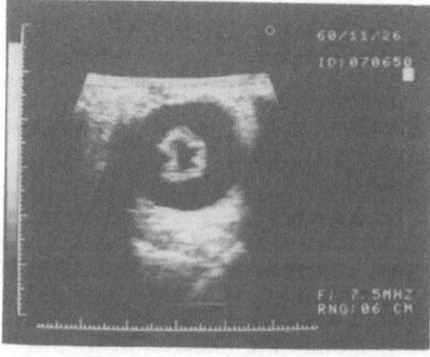

Fig. 2. A case of proliferative vitreoretinopathy.

Orbital and periorbital lesions

Hematoma from traffic accident, swelling of extraocular muscles, mucocele from the frontal and ethmoidal sinuses, orbital cellulitis due to invasion from paranasal inflammation, postsurgical buccal cyst were examined with Santesonic SSD-121. Internal reflectivity inside the lesion can be fairly estimated by reducing the sensitivity setting. In those cases oblique scanning is sometimes needed as well as horizontal and vertical scanning. The equipment has a probe of more convenient shape and size than electronic scanning equipment.

Acknowledgement

This study was supported in part by a grant-in-aid for scientific research (59480349) from the Japanese Ministry of Education.

References

Sawada A, Baba Y, Torii H, Yamamoto A, Harada K. 1984. Electronic linear scanning ultrasonic diagnostic device for use in ophthalmology, Folia Ophthalmol Jpn 35: 2377—2385.

The Ophthascan B: a new A/B-Scan unit

L. FALCO,[1] C. MAZZINI[2] AND F. PASSANI[2]

Summary

The authors refer their 6 months experience of diagnostic echography using a relatively new ophthalmic echographic unit: the Ophthascan A/B produced by Biophysic Medical.

The characteristics of the unit are evaluated; normal and pathologic echographs which demonstrate the advantages and the disadvantages of this diagnostic machine are evaluated.

Introduction

A presentation of a new echographic device is usually carried out by an opinion leader who has contact with the manufacturer.

Instead we are presenting here, on the basis of six months of our own personal experience, a new diagnostic echographic device, Ophthascan B, produced by Biophysic Medical in France. The more common kinds of eyeball pathology have been examined with this apparatus. Some patients were also examined with other instruments in order to be able to compare the images obtained.

The following is an evaluation of this machines' capacity for evaluating pathological and normal structures.

Material and methods

The apparatus used is the Ophthascan B produced by the French company Biophysic Medical in Clermont-Ferrand Cedex. It is a new type of echo-ophthalmoscope for A/B and Vector Scan.

The principal characteristics as listed by the company are as follows:

[1] U.S.L. 18, H. S. Guiseppe. Div. Oculistica, Empoli, Firenze, Italy.
[2] University Eye Clinics of Florence, Italy.

J. M. Thijssen (ed.) Ultrasonography in ophthalmology.

— Cathode-ray tubes of the television type and an 18 cm screen.
— Examinations at two depth levels, 40 and 60 mm, for each of four possible presentations: B-Scan, B-Scan and Vector Scan, Vector Scan and A-Scan.
— Using an incorporated keyboard, it is possible to display on the screen a thirty character description of the patient and/or the conditions of the examination.
— The B-Scan has 90 dB logarithmic amplification. It has an ample memory capacity: 256 lines and 512 points × 6 bites. The grey scale is composed of 64 levels enabling us to differentiate the structures examined according to their reflectiveness. It is possible to retain the image on the screen by using a pedal-operated control. We made use of two different types of B-Scan probes.

Type I probe, as described by the company, has the following characteristics:

— incorporated water bath;
— fixed transducer;
— mobile mirror locator;
— frequency: 10 MHz;
— scanning angle 40°;
— scanning velocity 22 images per second.

Type II probe with modification, again as described by the company:

— a new mirror is used for clearer definition of the focal point;
— the motor has been constructed with more resistent materials;
— the transducer has been redesigned in order to obtain greater sensitivity;
— one ball bearing has been used instead of two so that motor blockage can be avoided;
— the connection circuitry has been completely redesigned so that grounding is more precise and longlasting.

The diagnostic A-Scan can be carried out either with logarithmic amplification with volume range adjustable from 0—50 dB, or with an S curve with a fixed volume range of 33 dB from 5 to 95% of the screen, or with linear amplification with fixed volume range at 15 dB.

The A-Scan which we selected from among those available, is a pencil probe with a diameter of 6 mm, not focused, and with 8 MHz frequency.

Aside from purely biometric functions such as IOL calculations and the measurement of thickness, the biometrics option enables us to evaluate the difference between the amplitude of two echoes by displaying them in dB (ΔdB) on the screen. We thereby have a more practical and precise quantitative echo (Ossoinig, 1979).

We have used the well known American Ocuscan 400 (Sonometrics) with a 10 MHz contact probe, to compare some ocular pathologies (Lizzi and Feleppa, 1979). We have examined the following pathology:

— Pathology of the tear gland particularly regarding the follow-up of treated neoplasms.
— Simple or complicated cataracts.
— Vitreal haemorrhage associated or not with retinal detachment.
— Detached vitreous associated with retinal detachment.
— Tractional retinal detachment.
— Rhegmatogenous retinal detachment.
— Degenerative pathologies of the posterior pole.
— Neoplasia in the eyeball.

Results

In examining the characteristics of the new apparatus, we think it is useful to subdivide the pathologies which we examined by using topographic criteria: diseases of the anterior segment and diseases of the vitreous/retinal interfaces. The resolution of the anterior segment using the contact B-Scan technique has been excellent.

In a normal eyeball (Fig. 1), it is possible to clearly visualize the anterior and posterior lens capsule both at high (Fig. 1a) and low amplification (Fig. 1b) using either probe.

Using the water bath technique, it is possible to distinguish clearly the anterior and posterior surface of the cornea and the interface of the iris. In Fig. 1c, aside from the above structures, a small cystic formation can be noted in the ciliary body. In Fig. 1d the same pathology is presented but another apparatus has been used in order to make a comparison.

The definition of the anatomical-pathological structures (interfaces) at the vitreous level was different in the two probes used.

The first type of probe displayed little capacity for defining subtle vitreous pathology or for following vitreous/retinal profiles, particularly those not perpendicular to the ultrasonic beams (Fig. 2a).

Instead, there was a good resolution of the interfaces perpendicular to the ultrasonic beams which could be clearly distinguished owing to the grey scale. The ambit of reflectiveness of the grey scale proved very useful in differential diagnosis.

In the second, modified type of probe, we observed better lateral

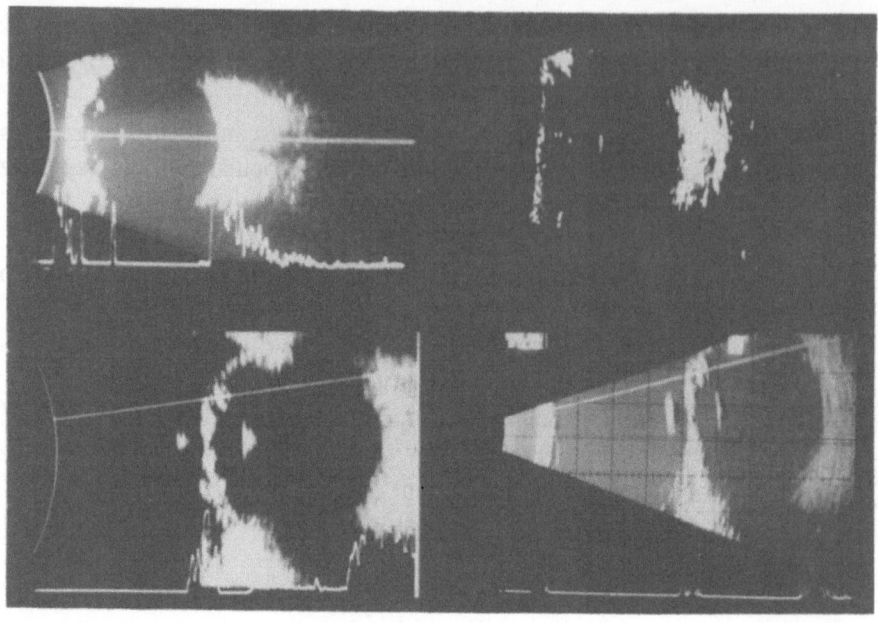

a　b

c　d

Fig. 1. A. Echogram obtained with Ophthascan B at high sensitivity. B. Same as A at low sensitivity. C. Echogram obtained with Ophthascan B with immersion technique. D. Same as C obtained with Ocuscan 400.

resolution in vitreous/retinal pathology and we obtained better resolution in the structures with major axis perpendicular to the ultrasonic beams. Less obvious pathologies were more easily displayed and the outline of pathological alterations of the vitreous/retinal better followed (Fig. 2b).

As far as the A-Scan method is concerned, we have found better evidence of vitreal alterations in vitreous/retinal pathology than in the B-Scan method using the first type of probe.

In choosing option "ΔdB", which based on the amplitude of the echo measures the reflectiveness of different tissues and visualizes them numerically off the screen, we have found it is possible to carry out a quantitative examination in differential diagnosis through the membrane.

The A-Scan examinations were done with "S" amplification curve (Fig. 2b).

Comments

Our experience with this apparatus allows us to draw the following conclusions:

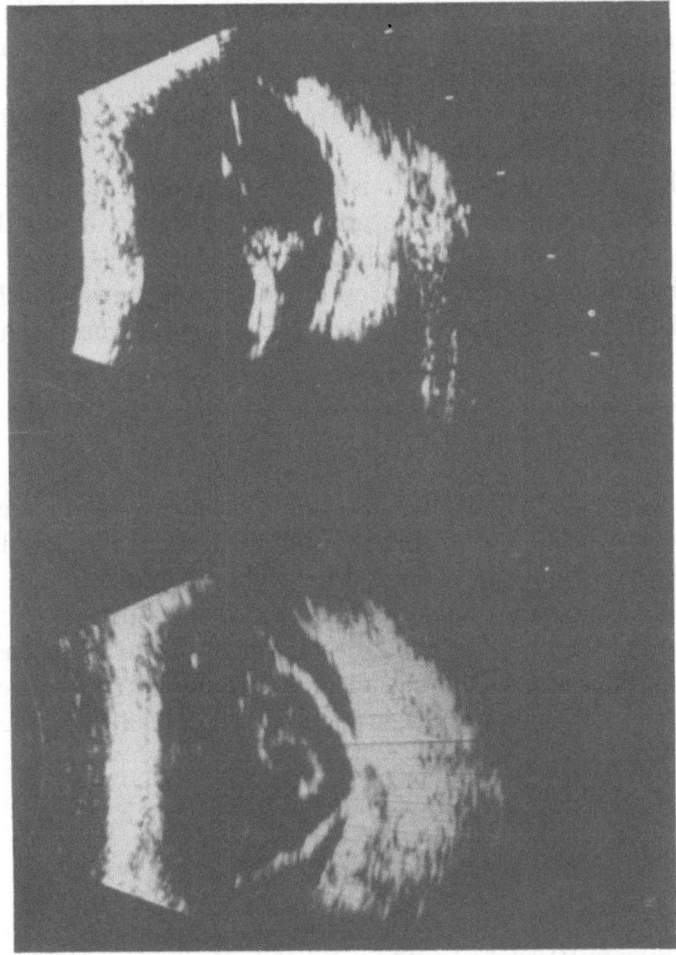

Fig. 2. A. Echogram of eye with vitreous pathology, Ophthascan B, old probe. B. Same as A, new probe.

— Excellent axial and lateral resolution of the anterior segment and therefore good definition of pathological structures also in contact method.
— Regarding vitreous/retinal structures, the resolution is different depending on which probe is used.
— With the first type of probe, the less obvious vitreous pathology and the vitreous/retinal membrane structures not perpendicular to the ultrasonic beams are seen with a certain difficulty thereby making a precise diagnosis difficult.

— In the second modified type of probe this problem has been partly eliminated, resulting in better lateral resolution and therefore a more precise vitreous/retinal diagnosis.
— A valid grey scale which allows us to differentiate the structures clearly according to their luminosity.
— In the A-Scan method, there is the advantage of a pencil probe which can be used with linear or logarithmic amplification or with the special "S" curve. The possibility in choosing amplification system of the curve enables us to vary sensitivity levels and dynamic ranges which, in turn, facilitate tissue diagnosis. The "ΔdB" system can also be used here.

Conclusions

Having ascertained the differences of the machine's performance capacity after the modification of the B-Scan probe, we can understand the importance of the design and its realization if it is to be efficient.

We are also convinced that the probe's characteristics must correspond to those furnished by the manufacturer. Indeed, it often happens that the frequencies declared by the manufacturer do not correspond to the real ones thereby causing considerable interpretative difficulties for the operator (Buschmann).

References

Lizzi FL, Feleppo EJ. 1979. Practical physics and Electronics of Ultrasound. In: R Dallow (ed) International Ophthalmology Clinics, Vol. 19, No. 4.
Buschmann W, Haigis W, Linnert D. 1981. Influence of equipment parameters on results in ophthalmic ultrasonography. In: JM Thijssen and AM Verbeek (eds) Ultrasonography in Ophthalmology. Doc Ophthal Proc Series, Vol. 29, Junk, The Hague, pp. 487—498.
Ossoinig KC. 1979. Standardized Echography: Basic Principles, Clinical Applications and Results. In: R Dallow (ed) International Ophthalmology Clinics, Vol. 19, No. 4, pp. 127—210.
Shammas HJ. 1984. Atlante di Ultrasonografia e biometria oftalmologica. Medical Books.

A system for computer controlled Doppler waveform analysis

V. J. MARMION[1] AND C. P. E. BARRAN

KEY WORDS: Doppler pulse waveforms: Analysis programmes (time and frequency domain): Carotid stenosis.

Summary

A computer controlled system has been developed which permits the averaging of Doppler wave form signals. The electrocardiograph standardises the recordings. Five forms of analysis have been applied to the data obtained. Comment is made about further developments that can be incorporated into the system.

Introduction

The averaging of Doppler pulse waveforms eliminates pulse to pulse variability and observer error. The use of the electrocardiograph (Craxford and Chamberlain, 1977) provides a fixed point of reference for each cardiac cycle. The Doppler Waveform shape can then be quantified in terms of its Pulsatility Index (Gosling and King, 1975), Pourcelot Index (Planiol and Pourcelot, 1971) and principal components (Evans et al., 1985). Such indices of waveform shape may provide diagnostic information which is more applicable to one disease than another. If this is correct, then variant analysis using the Chebychev Polynomials should indicate differences in disease state. A micro-processor Doppler system was therefore developed which allows feature extraction from the Doppler pulse waveforms.

[1] 73 Pembroke Road, Clifton, Bristol BS8, United Kingdom.

J. M. Thijssen (ed.) Ultrasonography in ophthalmology.
© 1988, *Kluwer Academic Publishers, Dordrecht, ISBN 978-94-010-7083-6*

Materials and methods

A computer based system has been designed which incorporates a simple micro-computer (BBC B+) and twin floppy disk drive system (Fig. 1). The computer system is integrated with an ecg system and a two-channel recorder which allows simultaneous display of ecg and the Doppler maximum velocity signals. Ultrasound Doppler signals are obtained using a specially designed focussed 10 MHz Doppler probe, and processed using phase quadrature techniques allowing directional discrimination between forward and reverse flow signals. A maximum frequency estimator provides an analog signal which is proportional to the maximum velocity

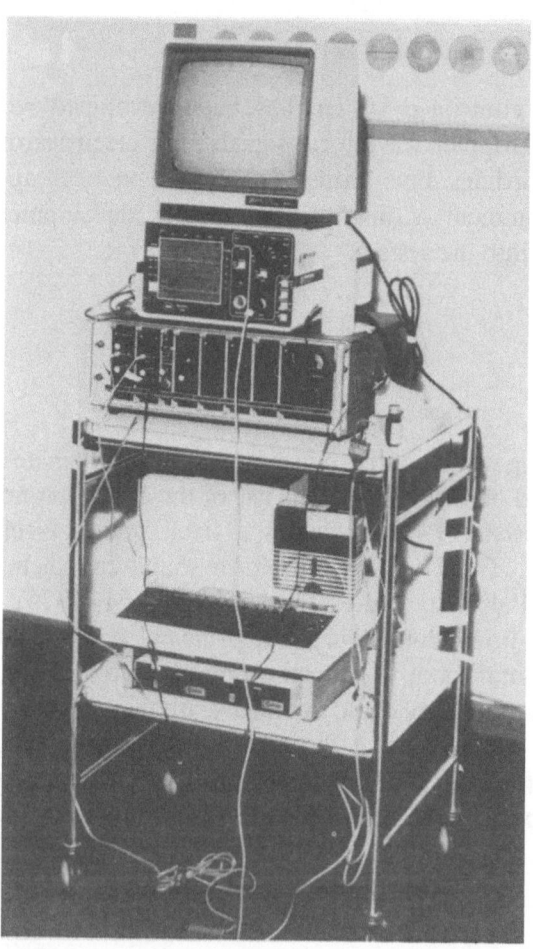

Fig. 1. Computer controlled system for Doppler waveform analysis.

present in either the forward flow or reverse flow channel. The computer is run on three different programmes.

1. The data base
2. Data acquisition
3. Data analysis

Eight test sites are routinely examined in strict sequence and space is allocated for a further four examinations, thus enabling repeat examinations of some of the sites.

Results

The analysis programmes

The principal features extracted from the maximum velocity process include Pulsatility Index and Pourcelot Index, the time to start (TS) and principal component analysis. The results from 100 patients in relation to the disease categories are shown in Table 1. The Pulsatility Index showed variation between 0.56 to 4.0 falling to 1.25 and 3.0. In the supraorbital signals, 31% of normals had a Pulsatility Index greater than 2.5. The Pourcelot Index for all four test sites gave values in the range 0.6—0.95, whereas the normal range is 0.55—0.75. The time to start using the signals from the superficial temporal artery showed a value of greater than 110 milliseconds in 83% of patients. The time to peak values and time to half peak values were also calculated, showing a considerable degree of scatter ranging between 75 and 140 milliseconds.

Table 1. Categories and numbers of subjects employed in the study.

100 patients Category	Disease description		No.
1.	Normals	(age matched)	45
2.	Amaurosis Fugax	AF	36
3.	Controls	aged (35—45)	13
4.	Glaucoma	(1OP <= 21 mmHg)	2
5.		(1OP = 22 mmHg)	85
6.	Ischaemic neuropathy	(AION)	6
7.	Central Vein Occlusion		6
8.	Diabetes		4
9.	Others		3

Fourier transform analysis

The Fourier Transform converts the original data to a series of sine and cosine waves of known frequency. The amplitudes of these are given by the values of Fourier coefficients. There is a Fast Fourier Transform available for the computer used on a ROM Chip (Structured Software, Limited). It was found that 15 to 20 terms produced a reasonable fit to the original waveform (Fig. 2). The efficacy of transform in terms of data reduction was not especially high, at best a factor of five.

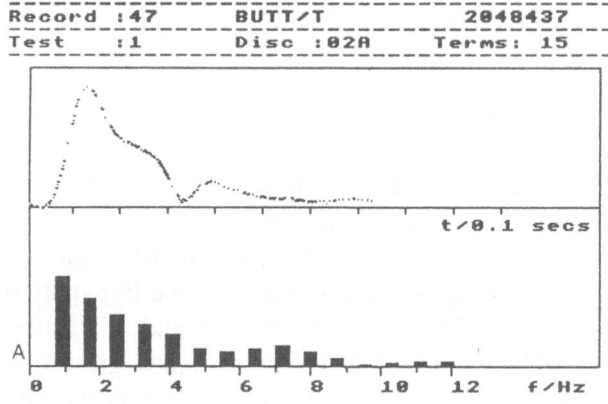

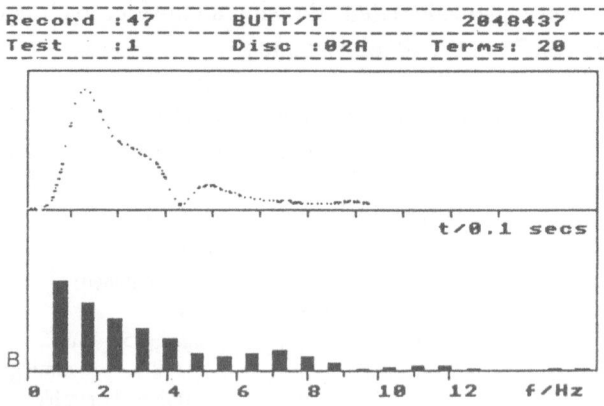

Fig. 2. Doppler waveform (dotted curves) and corresponding spectra, estimated by 15 (A) and 20 Fourier terms as shown in block diagrams (B).

Principal component analysis

It was found that the main features of the waveforms examined could be constructed using the first, second or third principal components; whereas the maximum features seems to be reflected in the second and third principal components. (Fig. 3). A particular feature which has become apparent during the review of the data is the increase in velocity within the superficial temporal artery in the presence of ipsilateral internal carotid stenosis. (Fig. 4).

Discussion

Averaging is an important concept in signal analysis. The present system as developed permits the averaging of a number of waveforms and once

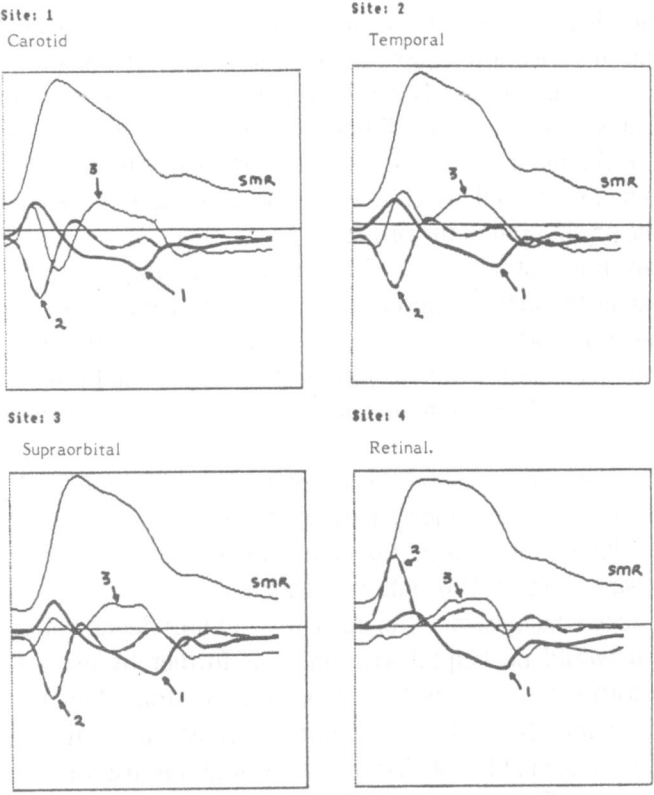

Fig. 3. Results of principal component analysis for Doppler waveforms (SMR) obtained from four different blood vessels, first three components indicated by 1 through 3.

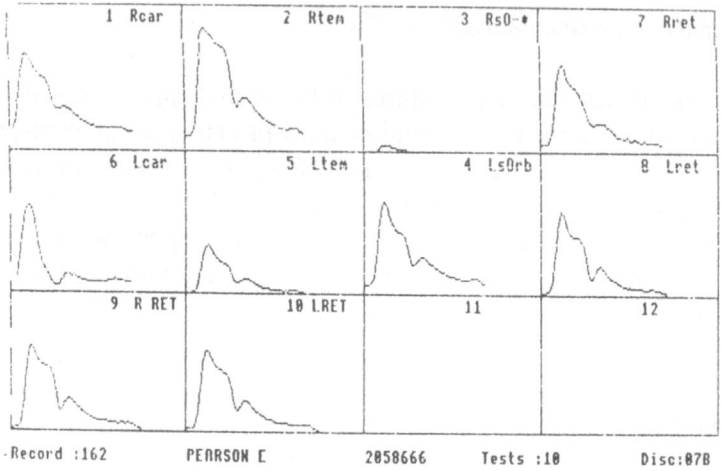

Fig. 4. Doppler waveforms at various sites, showing increased velocity in superficial temporal artery caused by stenosis in internal carotid (ipsilateral).

consistency has been obtained, the data can be stored for analysis at the end of the investigation. Averaging of a large number of waveforms from superficial and larger vessels is relatively easy, however, it is more difficult in the smaller vessels. The difficulty with smaller vessels lies with the inability to maintain alignment. This is particularly true in relation to the supraorbital and retinal arteries, where the movement of the eye or lid may disturb the orientation of the probe.

The accuracy obtained by the use of averaging and standardisation in time using the ecg has permitted expansion of the analysis programme to routinely include analysis both in the time and frequency domain, for example, Pulsatility Index, Pourcelot Index, Fast Fourier Transform Analysis, principal component analysis and time to peak and half peak time.

The Pulsatility Index varies accordingly with heart rate and it has been observed that in many elderly patients there is a considerable degree of heart rate fluctuations during the course of the examination. By normalising each waveform to 100 data points, such variations can be accounted for. A marked tachycardia can lead to a minor degree of stretching in diastole. It would be helpful to refine this further by using the ecg and Kubicek formula to segregate systole and diastole. The resynthesis of waveform shapes from the Fast Fourier Transform in this investigation seems to be reasonably satisfactory, as well as the use of principal component analysis. The use of statistical methods to correlate the Pulsatility Index, principal components and timings with various diseases opens up an interesting prospect for a future investigation.

While the Pulsatility Index has been shown to correlate well with changes in peripheral resistance, its limitations lie in the poor correlation with the degree of aterosclerosis and in particular with minor degrees of stenosis within a vessel. Scatter of the results in this investigation, however, was disappointing and only a small proportion of patients in Group 4 showed a trend different to the other groups. The Pourcelot Index, surprisingly, showed quite high values in the control subjects and no significant difference between the controls and any of the other groups, other than a trend between the controls and Group 5. The value of recording the Pulsatility Index and Pourcelot Indices along vessels, as performed in this study, is the ability to infer the presence of increasing peripheral vascular resistance along the arterial tree.

The time-to-peak and half-peak measurements were very encouraging. Recent developments in increased computer cycle speed has improved this measurement along with the prediction of systolic slope which provides another parameter whereby the evaluation of peripheral vascular disease can be assessed.

References

Craxford AD, Chamberlain J. 1977. Pulse wave form transit ratios in the assessment of peripheral vascular disease. Brit J Surg 64: pp. 449—452.

Evans DH, Archer LNJ, Levene MI. 1985. The detection of abnormal neonatal cerebral haemodynamics using principal component analysis of the Doppler ultrasound waveform. Ultrasound Med Biol 11: 441—449.

Gosling RG, King DH. 1975. Ultrasonic angiography. In: AW Hascus and L Adamson (eds) Arteries and Veins, Churchill Livingstone, Edinburgh, pp. 61—98.

Kubicek WG, Karnegis JN, Patterson RP, Witnes DA, Mattson RH. 1966. Development and Evaluation of an impedance cardiac output system. Aerosp Med 37: 1208.

Planiol T, Pourcelot L. 1971. Etude de la circulation carotidienne au moyen l'effect Doppler. In: Traites de Radiodiagnostique, Vol. 17, Masson, Paris.

Standards in ophthalmic ultrasonography

W. BUSCHMANN[1] AND W. HAIGIS

Summary

Different standards have been recommended in the literature for equipment checks, data declaration, examination techniques and echogram evaluation. The different background is elucidated and the correlation to internationally accepted recommendations of standardization authorities is shown. An equipment check program was developed which can be applied by trained technicians under hospital conditions. It provides comparable data which can be presented in generally accepted units, like dB or MHz. Use of these methods allowed measurement-based studies on the influence of selected changes of technical parameters on diagnostic criteria in the echograms. The results are shown using intraocular melanoblastoma echograms and orbital echograms (especially endocrine orbitopathy) taken with A- and B-scan techniques. Further development of apparatus and transducers for ophthalmic ultrasonography should be based on such studies. Empirical ultrasonography without data check, however, or with inadequate data checks, yields ultrasonographic results which neither can be compared nor reliably be evaluated.

Introduction

In the past the empirical approach has dominated. To get more uniform results, various reference echo sources were recommended, like sclera echo, vitreous echoes, (Oksala, 1978) a plain steel reflector in calibrated paraffin oil (Buschmann, 1966), fresh liver tissue, formalin-treated tissue, citrated blood or Till's tissue model (Till and Ossoinig, 1977). These are not acceptable as international standards.

The clinical use of ophthalmic A-scan ultrasonography was promoted by Ossoinig's attempt to offer a series of equal apparatuses and to use a

[1] University Eye Clinic, Schneiderstraße, D-8700 Würzburg, FRG.

J. M. Thijssen (ed.) Ultrasonography in ophthalmology.
© 1988, *Kluwer Academic Publishers, Dordrecht, ISBN 978-94-010-7083-6*

uniform examination and evaluation technique, which he called "standardized A-scan" (Ossoinig, 1984). The aim was great; however, it proved impossible for the Kretz Technik Company to produce a series of ultrasonic A-scan apparatuses with identical technical parameters. Furthermore, the test program recommended by Ossoinig did not yield sufficient information.

Recommended measurements of equipment parameters

Nowadays, we are facing a variety of ophthalmic A-scan and B-scan ultrasonoscopes with different amplifier characteristics, frequencies, and transducer probes. It is mandatory to warrant reliable diagnostic results in our own laboratory and to compare our results with those of other groups.

The International Electrotechnical Commission (IEC), as standardization authority, issued a document on performance tests (IEC, 1979). Simultaneously, Dr. Trier's and our group developed a set of simple measurement procedures which are adapted to ophthalmic clinical use, but are in accordance with the IEC recommendations.

Sensitivity

dB-scale readings can be compared only if the dB-difference to a generally accepted standard test echo is given. The IEC document recommends steel or glass reflectors, but their strong echo is usually out of the range of our built-in dB-attenuators.

Therefore, we use the W38 test reflector made from soft Hema contact lens material (Haigis et al., 1981, Haigis and Buschmann, 1985). It is well defined, reproducible and generally available; its echo amplitude is 17 dB below the ideal reflector as defined in the IEC document.

Using it, we found that the maximum sensitivity available is remarkably different even in the apparatuses of one type and series delivered by one manufacturer (Haigis et al., 1981). Nevertheless, all echo amplitudes found in tissues can be made comparable by their amplitude difference to the W38 test echo. Additionally, B-scan distortions can be shown using the W38 reflector.

Frequency

The nominal frequency given by the manufacturers is often incorrect. We have to measure at least the working frequency as defined by the IEC document. This working frequency remains practically unchanged when we replace the water-bath by silicon oil AP 500, if the transducer probe has a narrow frequency spectrum. However, if there are powerful low frequency components, these may dominate in the pulse after a few millimeters of oil or tissue. Orbital examination is then actually performed not at the nominal 8 or 10 MHz, but at a lower frequency. The complete frequency spectrum can be analyzed with the Echosimulator, developed by Reuter and Trier (Reuter et al., 1980).

Meaningful comparable data on resolution must include information on the reflector used, the probe distance, the amplifier adjustment, and the criteria used (e.g. the −6 dB criterion). IEC recommends a steel ball reflector with micrometer drives in three coordinates. For clinical purposes, a nylon thread (10.0 monofilament) provides sufficient results. A row of filaments with increasing distances between each other is used for B-scan resolution measurements. A test cage, for example, the AIUM model, adapted to ophthalmic size, can be used to have simultaneous information on resolution and geometric distortions. Electronic measurements with the Echosimulator enable us to analyze in addition the amplifier dynamics and the accuracy of the dB-scale and of the time-scale. The gray scale in B-scan can be calibrated as well.

This measurement program can be done by a trained technician and provides a reasonable basis for comparable and reproducible echogram evaluations. It is not available just for a single type of apparatus, but it can be applied generally.

Clinical examples

The interaction of working frequency and sensitivity is shown in an echogram series from an intraocular melanoblastoma. At corresponding sensitivity levels (related to the W38 test reflector echo) the solid nature of the tumour tissue is well shown at 5 as well as at 10 MHz working frequency. The surface echo remains visible, and the structure echoes disappear, if sensitivity is reduced by about 10 dB, giving a cyst-like appearance. The tumour echogram is similar with 5, 10, and 15 MHz, but its structure appears coarse with 5 MHz, and the orbital fat is shown at greater depth even at reduced sensitivity.

A retinoblastoma echogram appeared to be quite typical at a sensitivity of 68 dB above test echo, but after reduction to 53 dB above test echo, we noticed that the high amplitude echoes typical for calcifications were missing. A choroidal naevus could not be shown at 9.7 MHz working frequency and a sensitivity of 52 dB above test echo. However, after reduction to 39 dB above test echo, the intensive naevus echo became visible clearly.

550 measurements with three different transducers yielded typical foreign body echo amplitudes six times more often with 10.5 than with 5.5 MHz working frequency.

Orbital problems

Is it a solid orbital tumour or a cyst, possibly a mucocele? A reflectivity of 52 dB above test echo is insufficient at a working frequency of 9.7 MHz to answer this question reliably. At 64 dB and 6 MHz, the tumourous nature of a skin melanoma metastasis in the orbit is clearly shown.

Another patient had a tremendous mass lesion of his left orbit, and it appeared cystic at 9.3 MHz and 66 dB; actually, it was a mucocele of the frontal sinus. 66 dB above test echo, however, are not sufficient for safe differentiation from tumours of homogeneous structure. We examined another mass lesion at 10 MHz working frequency and 68 dB above test echo, and we nearly missed the internal structure echoes of this solitary neurofibroma (histopathologic diagnosis).

The swollen muscles in endocrine orbitopathy can well be shown if there is only a low-grade fibrosis. If marked fibrotic changes have developed, it may become difficult to detect the muscle at all, because the structure echoes are approaching the intensity of orbital fat echoes. However, at reduced sensitivity (45 dB above test echo) we can show the muscle contours.

Fibrosis of the orbital fat in endocrine orbitopathy is more difficult to evaluate in the echograms, but it has clinical importance in connection with decompression surgery. Surgery proved that fat fibrosis was minimal in a patient whose echograms are shown in the upper line (Fig. 1A). On the contrary, extensive fibrosis was found in the patient whose echograms are shown below (Fig. 1A). No safe differentiation could be made at 8.6 MHz and 60 dB above test echo; however, with the same probe and 10 dB reduction of sensitivity, some differences in the fat echo pattern could be detected in A-scan (Fig. 1B) and were also shown in the B-scan echograms (Fig. 1C) (above, patient without fat fibrosis; below, with extensive fat fibrosis; 10 MHz, $\Delta W38 = 48$ dB).

Conclusion

Equipment performance measurements according to the IEC document are indispensable. They are the precondition for reproducible, reliable and comparable echographic results.

CT and MRI machines are getting monthly checks and recalibrations lasting one to three days. Without such checks, disastrous failures could happen.

Ultrasonography can and will play an important role in diagnosis and follow-up of intraocular and orbital tumours also in the future, but we have got to work on safe ground and at a similarly sophisticated technological level as other imaging techniques.

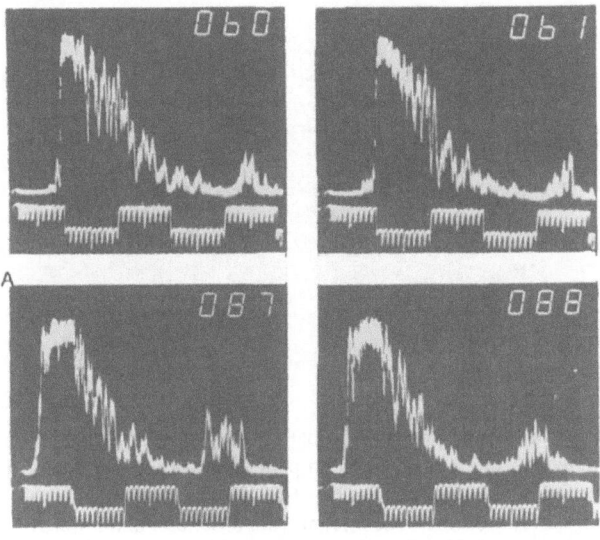

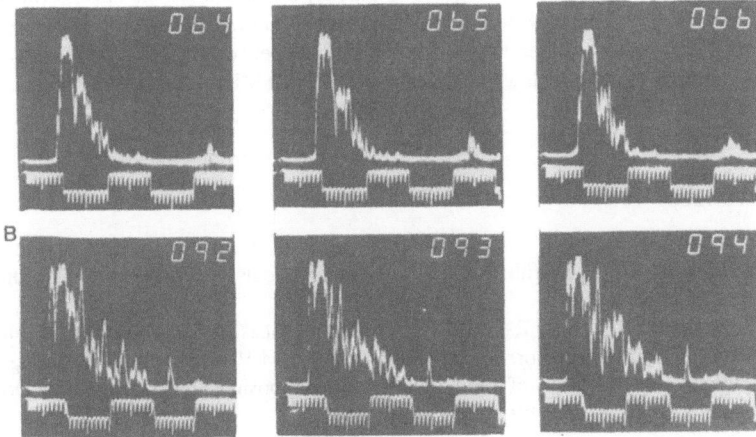

44

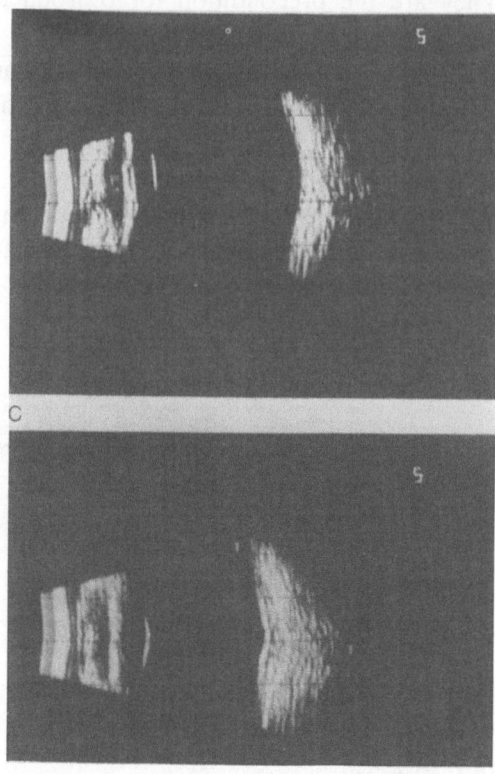

Fig. 1. Fat fibrosis in endocrine orbitopathy, influence of examination parameters on echographic detection of fat fibrosis. Echo-patterns of orbital fat behind posterior pole of the eye. Upper line of echograms (no. 060—066 and B-scan): Patient with surgically proven minimal fat fibrosis. Lower line of echograms (no. 087—094 and lower B-scan): Patient with surgically proven extensive fat fibrosis. (A) No safe differentiation possible between echograms from low-grade fibrosis (above) and extensive fibrosis (below) at 8.6 MHz and a sensitivity 60 dB above W38 test reflector echo. (B) Noteworthy differences detectable in the same patient between minimal fibrosis (above) and extensive fat fibrosis (below) at a sensitivity 50 dB above W38 test echo; apparatus 7200 MA. (C) Same patients as in Figs. 1A and 1B; detectable differences in B-scan pattern between minimal fat fibrosis (above) and extensive fat fibrosis (below); Ocuscan 400, WF = 10 MHz, ΔW38 = 48 dB.

References

Buschmann W. 1966. Einführung in die ophthalmologische Ultraschalldiagnostik. VEB Georg Thieme, Leipzig.
Haigis W, Reuter R, Lepper R-D. 1981. Comparative measurements on different pulse-echo systems using test reflectors. In: JM Thijssen and AM Verbeek (eds) Ultrasonography in Ophthalmology 8, Proc of the SIDUO VIII Symposium. Nijmegen 1980. Doc Ophthalmol Proc Series, Vol. 29, Junk, Den Haag, p. 445.

Haigis W, Buschmann W. 1985. Echo reference standards in ophthalmic ultrasonography, Ultrasound in Med Biol 11: 149.

IEC International Electrotechnical Commission, Technical Comm 29 Electroacoustics, Subcommittee 29D: Ultrasonics, WG 4: Draft. 1979. Methods of measuring the performance of ultrasonic pulse-echo diagnostic equipment.

Oksala A. 1978. Ultraschalluntersuchung des Glaskörperraumes bei idiopathischer Netzhautablösung. Klin Monatsbl Augenheilk 173: 150—155.

Ossoinig K. 1984. How to obtain maximum measuring accuracy with standardized A-scan. In: JS Hillman and M LeMay, Ophthalmic Ultrasonography, Junk, The Hague, pp. 197—216.

Reuter R, Trier HG, Lepper R-D. 1980. Ein elektrisches Prüfverfahren und Prüfgerät für Ultraschalldiagnostik-Anlagen. In: Medizinalmarkt/Acta Medicotechnica, 28: 58.

Reuter R, Lepper R-D, Haigis W. 1981. Comparative measurements on ultrasonic pulse-echo equipment with the ECHOSIMULATOR. In: JM Thijssen and AM Verbeek (eds) Ultrasonography in Ophthalmology 8, Proc of the SIDUO VIII Symposium. Nijmegen 1980. Doc Ophthalmol Proc Series, Vol. 29, Junk, Den Haag, pp. 463.

Till P, Ossoinig KC. 1977. First experience with a solid tissue model for the standardization of A- and B-scan instruments in tissue diagnosis. In: D White and RE Brown (eds) Ultrasound in Medicine, Vol. 3B, Plenum Publ Corp, New York, pp. 2167.

A new instrument for axial length measurement

A. SAWADA, H. SHIBATA, A. YAMAMOTO, A. NAKAMURA
AND S. DEMIZU

Summary

A simple and low-cost A-mode device for ocular biometry is described. The A-mode echogram is visible at a liquid crystal display for reference, whereas the intrinsic measuring accuracy is 0.01 mm. The sound velocity in the various ocular media can be adjusted independently. Averaging is automatically performed over 128 successive A-lines and after insertion of keratometric data the power of a lens implant is calculated with either of the four installed algorithms.

Introduction

Up to date many kinds of equipment for measurement of the axial length of the eye have been used in refraction research and IOL implantation. We describe a new Japanese equipment, Santesonic SSZ-48, for ultrasonic measurement of axial length of the eye and calculation of the diopter of IOL, spectacles and CL (Fig. 1).

Equipment

Santesonic SSZ-48 is an A-mode ultrasonic diagnostic equipment made specially for measurement of axial length of the eye and calculation of refractive power of IOL. Santesonic SSZ-48 is equipped with 10 MHz transducer. The probe has the tip full of water in front of it, and a red internal fixation light. With designated velocity of ultrasound, axial length, anterior chamber depth, lens thickness and vitreous length are measured promptly with accuracy of ± 0.01 mm. The velocity of ultrasound in the eye can be selected. Usually the sound velocity in the anterior chamber,

Department of Ophthalmology, Miyazaki Medical College, 5200 Kihara, Kiyotake, Miyazaki 889-16, Japan.

J. M. Thijssen (ed.) Ultrasonography in ophthalmology.
© 1988, *Kluwer Academic Publishers, Dordrecht, ISBN 978-94-010-7083-6*

48

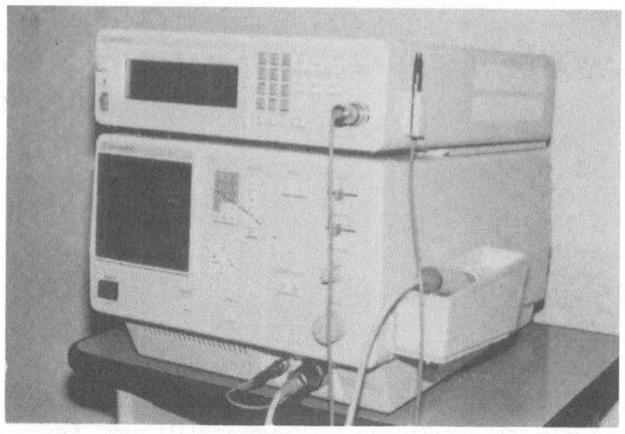

Fig. 1. Santesonic Inc. SSZ-48 equipment (A-mode, biometry) on top coupled to SSD-121 B-mode equipment of same brand (bottom).

the lens and the vitreous is set as 1532 m/sec, 1641 m/sec and 1532 m/sec, respectively. The measurement of the axial length can be adopted in aphakic eyes as well as in phakic eyes. In case of aphakic eyes, the sound velocity is set as 1532 m/sec. Four different kinds of calculation formulae are used. They are S.R.K., Binkhorst, Colenbrander-Hoffer and Regression formulae. Adding the values of corneal curvature or connecting to the designated keratometer, refractive power of IOL, spectacles and CL are simultaneously and promptly calculated and displayed. Regression formula provides IOL-power only. The results are printed out.

Measurement and calculation

When the power switch is on, the green pilot lamp is turned on and WAIT-mode is automatically set. On the display of liquid crystal, date, time, the selected formula and buzzer's state are shown.

Next, when "MEAS" button is pressed, buzzer starts to make an intermittent sound. Using the button of 1 or 2, "PHAKIC" or "APHAKIC" is indicated. Also the side of the examined eye is set using upward and downward arrow button.

The probe is put on the center of the locally anesthesized cornea so gently that the total axial length, particularly anterior chamber depth is not influenced. When the ultrasonic wave is aligned with the line of the axial length, buzzer sound changes from the intermittent to the continuous. At the same time, a simple A-mode pattern is displayed on the liquid crystal screen and the monitor screen of the connected B-mode equipment, Santesonic SSD-121. While buzzer continues to sound, the measurement is

49

repeated again and again. After enough data are gained, the probe is taken off and "MEAS" button is again pushed.

The equipment collects the data 150 times in about 0.5 seconds. When the data in coincidence become more than 128, the mean and the standard deviation are displayed. When the data measured so far, is needed, they are printed out by pressing "PRINT" button. When the results are satisfied, "CALCU" button is pushed for the process of calculation. However, when the data measured, particularly the standard deviation is not satisfied, the measurements can be repeated by pushing "MEAS" button. Then the values of corneal curvature, horizontal and vertical, are put in, using "ENTER" and number button. The unit of corneal curvature can be either diopter or mm. They are converted each other according to the selected formulae. Selection of formula is done by "SELECT" button and the cursor. And "CALCU" button is again pushed. Refractive power can be calculated and displayed of IOL, spectacles and CL. By pushing "PRINT" button, the selected formula, the used parameters and the results are printed out (Fig. 2).

```
ID :  5 6 C C 8
      --------------------
EYE : LEFT  (PHAKIA )
DATE : 86.04.14 17:25
    EXAMINER : YAIIA

    < CALCULATED VALUE >

FORMULA : BINKHORST
RESULT :
    IOL-POWER = 13.88D
    SP-POWER  =  8.78D
    CL-POWER  =  9.78D
PARAMETER :
        DIOPTER =- 1.00D
        R1      =  7.85mm
        R2      =  7.50mm
        LENGTH  = 25.01mm
        ACDEPTH =  3.53mm
        VDIS    = 12.00mm
```

Fig. 2. Print-out of biometry data together with calculated lens results.

50

Conclusion

As a biometric equipment we introduce is able to calculate the power of IOL, spectacles and CL, wide application will be expected.

References

Hoffer KJ. 1980. Biometry of 7,500 cataractous eyes. Am J Ophthalmol 90: 360—368.
Jaffe NS. 1984. Cataract surgery and its complications, Mosby, St Louis.

Tissue characterization

Improvements to computer assisted echography

A. REIBALDI[1], S. GUERRIERO[2], T. AVITABILE[1], N. VENEZIANI[3],
G. PASQUARIELLO[3] AND F. PASQUALI[3]

Summary

The authors report their continuing research aimed at computer aided echography by processing B-scan videofrequency images with SGLD method. They find a reduction of subjectivity of diagnosis of pathology.

Introduction

Continuing our researches, aimed at computer aided ocular echography (Reibaldi et al., 1985) through a texture analysis of B-scan videofrequency images, we find a reduction of subjectivity of interpretation and the achievement of a more objective diagnosis of pathology.

Procedures and instrumentation

We used videofrequency B-scan images resulting from Renaissance STORZ echograph equipped with a probe of 7.5 MHz frequency having electronic scanning option.

The images were videorecorded and the most interesting ones stored in digital form in the two-dimensional memory of a TESAK VDC 501 graphic-pictorial system and from this later recorded on the magnetic mass storage of a PDP 11/24 minicomputer used for the image and signal processing.

The echographic image under examination was analyzed under direct medical control by isolating diagnostic areas with closed polygonal lines; on these areas texture parameters calculations, together with average value and standard deviation were later performed. The data acquisition took place at Bari University in the Eye Clinic, while the digital elaboration

[1] Clinica Oculista, University of Catania, Catania, Italy; [2] Clinica Oculistica University of Bari, Bari, Italy; [3] Signals and image processing institute C.N.R., Bari, Italy.

J. M. Thijssen (ed.) Ultrasonography in ophthalmology.
© 1988, Kluwer Academic Publishers, Dordrecht, ISBN 978-94-010-7083-6

54

phase was performed at I.E.S.I. (Signals and Images Processing Institute) of C.N.R.

Our case report considers 14 cases of melanoma, 3 cases of metastatic carcinoma and 7 of choroidal haematoma (see Table 1).

All the neoplastic pathologies have been histologically confirmed, whereas for haematoma we report our survey according to the clinical course or to the surgical outcome.

Texture measurements

Tone and texture are two components of vision; they are correlated and are present with different weights within an image.

More specifically we can say that texture is related to the grey levels of an image i.e. to the roughness or to the smoothness created by the variation in tone or by the repetition of visual schemes, or due to the spatial distribution of grey levels.

The tone and texture measurement procedures, in the analysis of digital images, require a quantitative characterization of these two quantities.

Image tone variations constitute a kind of information directly obtainable through digital electronic optical devices.

Conversely, the qualitative texture information is not directly perceptible through the acquisition system and has to be drawn from the data of the digital image.

The procedure reported in the literature to quantify an image texture are different and are normally based on the measurement of spatial correlation among the image grey levels, in oriented directions (d, θ).

The 4 most frequently used are:

— PSM: (Fourier) Power Spectrum Method, based on the subdivision of spectrum in annular and sectoral regions for examining the roughness of the area and the direction of structures.
— SGLDM: Spatial Grey Level Dependance Method, or Second Order Grey Level Statistic, is based on a M (d, θ) matrix calculation, of the grey level spatial dependences.

Table 1.

Examined pathologies	N. cases
Choroidal haematoma	7
Metastatic carcinoma	3
Choroidal melanoma	14

— GLDM: Grey Level Difference Method, in which the analysis is made with First Order statistics on local frequencies vector defined by: $f_{\vec{d}}(x,y) = |f(x,y) - f(x+\Delta x, y+\Delta y)|$ with

$$d = (\Delta x, \Delta y)$$

— GLRM: Grey Level Run Length Method based on "run length" statistics i.e. on values $P(i,j)$ = length "i" runs number (in a prefixed direction), related to couples of grey levels belonging to a range "i".

Conners and Harlow showed, both theoretically and experimentally, in case of synthetically produced textures, the better resolution given by GLCM compared with the other methods.

The superiority has been confirmed by the empirical studies which have been made in the remote sensing field, where this kind of measurement is used successfully for texture classification.

The texture was estimated on 64 × 64 pixels image parts. For this procedure, which we used, we present now a more detailed description.

SGDLM

Consider a rectangular image with Nx elements along each line and Ny elements along each column, and take NL as the highest brightness value to be given to a pixel. If we indicate with Lx = 1, 2, ..., Nx the horizontal spatial field, with LY = 1, 2, ..., NY the vertical spatial field and with G = 0, 1, ..., NI, the grey levels as a whole, we can represent our image by a function I, defined in the LxXLy field with values in G, which assigns to every couple (i, j), with elements in LxXLY field, a tone value GK so that $I(i, J) = GK$.

Now suppose that all information concerning the image texture be in the co-occurrence "M" matrix, which is also defined second order calculated probability matrix, built according to the spatial distribution of the grey levels on the image. Each element (i, j) of the matrix represents the frequency $P(i, j)$ wherewith transition (i, j) occurs between the grey levels "i" and "j" comparing two pixels at distance "d" in "θ" direction.

Matrices of these kinds which contain level coupling frequencies, depend on the chosen direction and on distance between the pixels with which we make the comparison.

In our investigation we took into consideration only direction θ = 0, shiftings along the lines, whereas for distances between the pixels we took values from 1 to 10. In "low frequencies" images, pixels presenting a slight spatial division show similar grey levels; that implies the most meaningful values in the co-occurrence "M" matrix will be concentrated along the main diagonal and next to it.

Conversely for the "high frequencies" fine texture, in which at a great difference in the grey levels pixels a greater meaningfullness will correspond, then in "M" matrix the values which are spaced outside the main diagonal become important.

In our investigation we used 4 different texture parameters, calculated on the co-occurrence matrix and defined as follows:

— Contrast

$$\text{Con.} = \sum_{i=0}^{NL} \sum_{j=0}^{NL} (i - j)^2 P(i, j)$$

which represent a measurement on M matrix dispersion value with the main diagonal: it is null if it results $P(i, j) = 0$ only for $i = j$; or its value is low if concentration occurs next to the principal diagonal.

— Entropy

$$\text{Ent} = - \sum_{i=0}^{NL} \sum_{j=0}^{NL} (i, j) \log[P(i, j)]$$

which has very low levels when $P(i, j)$ have, quite unequal values.

— Second angular moment

$$\text{ASM} = \sum_{i=0}^{NL} \sum_{j=0}^{NL} P(i, j)^2$$

whose values are inversely proportional to the number of the $P(i, j) = 0$ in the matrix.

— Inverse difference moment

$$\text{IDM} = \sum_{i=0}^{NL} \sum_{j=0}^{NL} \frac{P(i, j)}{(i - j)^2 + 1}$$

which shows the presence of $P(i, j) \neq 0$, in which $i \sim j$.

None of these parameters singularly taken into consideration can show the whole content of co-occurrence matrix information; it is clear that for a good estimate of a texture in the image they are used together.

In our investigation texture parameters have been calculated for various value of "d" distance, among pixels couples in θ direction (along the lines).

Besides before calculating $M(d, \theta)$ matrix, we "normalized the contrast" of the image through the histogram equalization in order to stress the structures contained in it.

Results

Histologically our case report involved 14 cases of melanoma:

— 1 case proved atypical presenting large necrotic areas,
— 2 cases of spindle cell melanomas,
— 1 case of mixed cell 1st type,
— 8 cases of mixed cell 2nd type,
— 1 case in which the hepatic biopsy gave the spindle cell melanoma diagnosis (the eye was not enucleated because of the presence of orbital and general metastases).

For the metastatical carcinoma we had:

— 1 case of breast carcinoma,
— 2 cases of pulmonary metastatic carcinoma.

As stated before, in the case of choroideal haematomas we can refer to the clinical course.

We have some difficulties concerning:

— the low case report, in particular for the metastatic pathology,
— the fluctuation of texture parameters piked out by single videorecorded sequence which can be found in different images of the same clinical case.

As to this second point we have lessened the problem by equalising single image histogram.

Nevertheless, there still exist fluctuations of texture parameters which can be ascribed to variation in the relative position between the probe and the eye, and that is therefore difficult to eliminate.

However some improvement have been achieved by averaging the textural parameters of 5 echographic images taken randomly from the sequence of every single case.

Histogram equalization, on the other hand, showed different grey levels

58

images (16) more easily visible to the eye. The dependence of Con and Con/ASM on the pixels distance (varying in the range d = 1, d = 10) has been proved to be meaningful.

Only 0 degrees measurements have been considered, because the instrument resolution has a maximum along this direction, corresponding to the ultrasonic beam propagation. Moreover, the textural parameters reach an acceptable stability for distance values in the range d = 3, d = 10.

The Con/ASM and ASM/IDM proved to be very meaningful as in homogeneous areas the contrast tends towards 0 and ASM towards 1; whereas in non-homogeneous area the contrast tends to 0 and ASM to 0.

We also calculated the texture parameters both considering the whole pathological area (concerning normal eye structures, such as retina, which acted as covering of the neoplastic tissue or a haematoma) and considering the area occupied by the pathological material only. This procedure shows the different behaviour of the 3 groups of pathologies.

The higher contrast and Con/ASM values related to metastatic carcinoma, the medium to haematoma, and the lower to melanoma (see the following Tables 2—4).

Table 2. Metastatic carcinoma.

Cases	Histopathological type	Contrast	Con/ASM
1	pulmonary carcinoma	12	35
2	" "	10	40
3	breast carcinoma	15	35
Average:		12.33	36.67
S.D.		+2.055	+2.357

Table 3. Choroidal haematoma.

Cases	Contrast	Con/ASM
1	7.0	22
2	7.5	23
3	8.0	25
4	10.0	27
5	10.0	27
6	7.5	22
7	6.0	16
Average:	8.0	23.4
S.D.	+1.39	+2,97

Table 4. Choroidal melanoma.

Cases	Histopathological type	Contrast	Con/ASM
1	mixed 2nd type	4.5	8
2	" "	4.5	10
3	" "	4.5	10
4	" "	15.0	5
5	" "	4.5	10
6	" "	6.0	15
7	" "	3.5	6
8	" "	5.0	8
9	" "	6.0	15
10	" "	5.0	13
11	mixed 1st type	3.0	6
12	spindle cell	6.0	15
13	" "	3.0	7
14	" "	5.0	10
Average:		5.39	11.64
S.D.		+2.83	+5.95

However, it should be noticed that the present values of textural parameters are different from the ones quoted in our previous work (Reibaldi et al., 1985) due to variation of instrumental parameters. Nevertheless the separation among carcinoma, haematoma and melanoma were distinct.

In the metastatic carcinoma group we found a similar behaviour both in pulmonary and breast carcinoma. This was confirmed from the histological report of a pseudo-glandular structure in both cases examined. As for haematomas as there is no histological verification, we cannot explain the variation found in the different cases without assuming different stages of haematoma organization, proved by the different clinical course (spontaneous resolution or surgical drainage).

As for melanomas we observed a variability of texture parameters; that can be explained only in one case with the aid of a histological report of undifferentiated epitelioid melanoma, heavily pigmented and vascularized, with necrotic areas; in this case, the contrast and Con/ASM values proved to be high and laid upon those of the metastatic carcinoma.

In the 13 cases left, in which diagnosis was mixed melanoma for 10 and spindle cells for 3, unfortunately we did not observe variation in the texture parameters correlated to the above mentioned melanoma categories.

We believe the differences between the various cases and different images of the same case to depend on the different areas of the neoplasm scanned by the ultrasound beam.

We confirm again that, even in presence of these numerical variations, the values of texture parameters which characterize melanoma, are separate from those of haematoma and particularly from those of carcinoma.

The ultrasonic diagnostic accuracy is higher when measurements are limited to the pathological area only.

We did notice that in cases of melanomas we have even lower contrast and Con/ASM values, than those obtained by making the textural analysis of the entire area of neoplasm.

This effect is less evident in metastatic carcinoma in which we have high contrast values apart from the choice of the measured area probably because of the carcinoma reflectivity.

The retinal influence on the texture parameters is more evident when the neoplasm extension is smaller. Besides, in small neoplasms the texture values, which are statistical values, were of little account because of the limited number of pixels on which the measurement of the values was made.

Conclusions

This approach has been completed only recently, and for this reason only a limited number of cases have been processed. It is not yet possible, therefore, to evaluate the diagnostic significance of such a procedure.

According to our results we think that it is possibly a useful objective differentiation among metastatic carcinoma, haematoma and melanoma (see the following resuming Table 5).

Table 5. Experimental averages of textural parameters for different choroidal pathologies.

	n. cases	Contrast	Con/ASM
Metastatic carcinoma:	3	$12.3 + 2.06$	$36.6 + 2.37$
Haematoma:	7	$8.0 + 1.39$	$23.4 + 2.97$
Melanoma:	14	$5.4 + 2.83$	$11.6 + 5.95$

Student's t test:

Melanoma vs. haematoma[1]

Contrast:	2.19	$(P < 0.05)$
Con/ASM:	4.703	$(P < 0.001)$

[1] Fr. degrees = 19

Haematoma vs. carcinoma[2]

Contrast:	3.473	$(P < 0.01)$
Con/ASM:	6.128	$(P < 0.001)$

[2] Fr. degrees = 8

However, it is important to stress the role played by an experienced operator in the choice of the echographic images to be processed and in the choice of the pathological area on which texture analysis has to be made.

This procedure is still at an experimental stage which, however, is susceptible of improvements if it is applied to the radiofrequency survey.

References

Baum G, Greenwood I. 1958. The Application of Ultrasonic Locating Techniques to Ophthalmology: II Ultrasonic slit lamp in the ultrasonic visualization of soft tissue. Arch Ophtal 60: 263–279.

Baum G. 1972. Quantized ultrasonography. Ultrasonics 10: 14–15.

Cardia L, Reibaldi A, Avitabile T, Guerriero S, Veneziani N, Distante A. 1984. First results about echographical ocular tissue differentiation by false colours. Poster VII Cong European Society of Ophthal, Helsinky.

Colemann DJ, Lizzi FL, Jack RL. 1977. Ultrasonography of the eye and the orbit. Lea and Febiger, Philadelphia.

Colemann DJ, Katz L. 1974. Color Coding of B-scan Ultrasonograms. Arch Ophthalmol 91: 429–431.

Conners RW, Harlow CA. 1978. Equal Probability Quantizing and Texture Analysis of Radiographic Images. Computer Graphics and Image Processing 8: 447.

Conners RW, Harlow CA. 1980. A Theoretical Comparison of Texture Algorithms. IEEE Trans on Pattern Analysis and Mach Intell PAMI-2: 204.

Davis LS, Johns SA, Aggarwal JK. 1979. Texture Analysis Using Generalized Co-Occurrence Matrices. IEEE Trans on Pattern Analysis and Mach Intell PAMI-1: 251.

Haralick RM, Shanmugam K, Its'Hak Dinstein. 1973. Textural Features for Image Classification. IEE Trans Syst, Man, Cybern SMC-3: 610.

Haralick RM. 1979. Statistical and Structural Approaches to Textures. Proceedings of the IEEE 67: 768.

Pasquali F, Pasquariello G, Veneziani N, Selvaggi F, Martino P, Reibaldi A, Guerriero S. 1985. Texture analysis di immagini ultrasoniche in medicina. Cong G.N.B.C./S.I.P.B.A., Lipari.

Reibaldi A, Avitabile T, Guerriero S, Distante A, Veneziani N. 1983. Primi risultati sulla possibilita' di differenziazione ecografica tissutale mediante tecniche di falso colore. Atti VIII Cong Naz S.I.S.U.M., Bologna.

Reibaldi A, Avitabile T, Guerriero S, Uva MG. 1984. Possibility of ocular tissue differentiation by means of false colour assisted echography. Atti X Cong Int S.I.D.U.O., St Petersburg Florida.

Reibaldi A, Guerriero S, Avitabile T, Uva MG, Veneziani N, Pasquariello G, Pasquali F. 1985. La caratterizzazione dei tessuti con l'ecografia assistita. Atti I Congr Naz SIEO, Ferrara.

Weska JS, Dyer CR, Rosenfeld A. 1976. A Comparative Study of Texture Measures for Terrain Classification. IEEE Trans on Syst, Man, Cybern SCM-6: 269.

Wyszecki, Judd. 1975. Color in Business, Science and Industry J Wiley, New York.

Ultrasonographic observations of ocular walls

Y. SUGATA[1], Y. YAMAMOTO[1,2], M. YANO[1], N. SHIBUYA[3] AND
K. ITO[3]

Summary

The radiofrequency signals from the posterior ocular walls were studied
with the purpose of detecting the pulsating sites and computing impedance
distribution in the ocular walls for the basic studies of measuring the thickness of retina, choroid and sclera. Recording of the stable radiofrequency
signals necessary for analysis was attained by separating the head-rest from
the body bed to minimize irregular movements of the wave from various
origins. The reflected signals from the fundus were lead to a storage-scope
and onto video tape. The trace of serial pictures from the frame on CRT
fixed every one fifteenth second was taken by a photo camera. Additionally, a single trace of reflected signals was stored on magnetic disc
through the storage-scope. The signals were then subjected to the further
analysis, such as spectral analysis, cepstrum analysis, and computing the
impedance distribution. Each wave was compared with the synthetic wave
simulated to the posterior walls of the three layer-model. The specific locus
was interpreted as relating to the pulsation of the second layer, implying
the choroid. The thickness of the retina and choroid cannot be determined
as proposed earlier in a fixed model, but must be considered in their
dynamic nature.

Introduction

It is valuable to know the thickness of retina and choroid in living state,
which are inaccessible by the ordinary diagnostic media, since the quantitative assessment can be introduced to ocular pathology whether the fundus
is visible or not. Regarding the computer analysis of RF signals obtained
from the retina and choroid, several methods have been introduced by
various authors: spectrum analysis by Coleman (1979), deconvolution by

[1] Tokyo Metropolitan Komagome Hospital; [2] Tama Geriatric Hospital of Tokyo; [3] Tokyo
University of Agriculture and Technology, Tokyo, Japan.

J. M. Thijssen (ed.) Ultrasonography in ophthalmology.
© 1988, *Kluwer Academic Publishers, Dordrecht, ISBN 978-94-010-7083-6*

64

Bayer and Thijssen (1981), M-mode method by Lepper et al. (1987) and Trier et al. (1987), wave pulsation method by Purnell (1987) and Sugata (1985), Cepstrum analysis by Sugata (1985), and impedance synthesis by Shibuya (1985). The form of the RF signals, which are the complex of pulse wave reflected from many layers, is so mobile by pulsation according to heart beats and involuntary ocular movements.

It is not directly justifiable to take out one voluntary wave-form for analysing the thickness of layers because of indeterminate nature. The thickness of anatomical layers is thinner compared with the pulse length of approximately 400 n seconds. And also sonographic reflections may not conform to the anatomical boundaries. Notches on the reflected wave-form might not be the anatomical boundary but might be simply a recession by interference in time domain. From the above considerations successive recording of mobile wave-forms was practiced to start with.

Methods

RF signals collected by the ultrasonographic equipment (ZD-252, General Co.) with a concave synthetic transducer of polyvinylidene fluoride (10 MHz, focal depth of 44 mm, diameter of 10 mm, Toray), were lead to a storage-scope (TS-8123, Iwatsu), monitoring pulsation by finger sphygmograph (Fig. 1).

The signals were stored on video tape. Then the serial pictures of frozen images were taken by photo-camera every one fifteenth second for detecting pulsation. The picture was traced by a digitizer and stored on a floppy disc to be subjected to a further analysis of power spectra, cepstrum and impedance distribution. Examination was carried out by immersion method and RF signals were collected through the pupil from a phakic eye

Block Diagram of the Experimental System

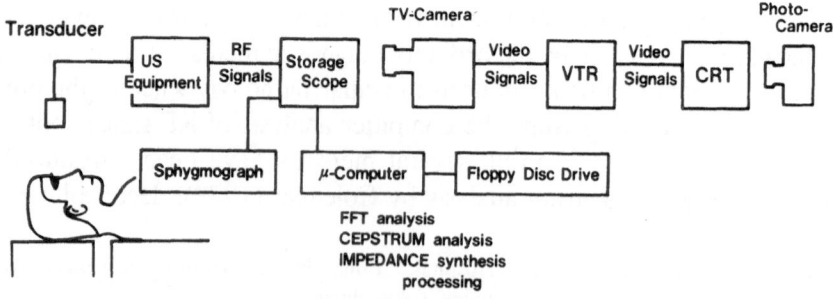

Fig. 1. Block diagram of the experimental system.

of a supine subject. Specific attention was paid to holding the transducer firmly by using a holder of operation microscope (Fig. 2) and the head-rest was separated from the bed to minimize the undesirable involuntary movements of the body. An echowave reflected from silicone rubber was used for an incident wave for cepstrum or impedance analysis (Fig. 3).

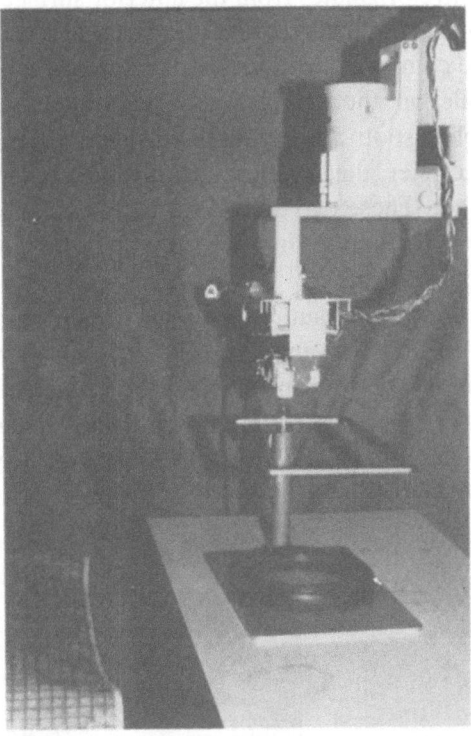

Fig. 2. The separated head-rest and the transducer held by the holder of operation microscope.

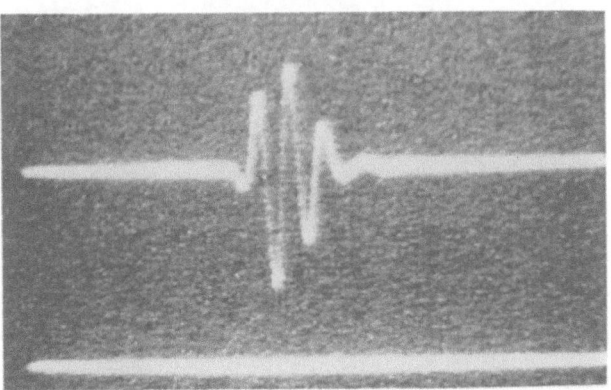

Fig. 3. An incident wave taken from the surface of silicone rubber.

Results and discussion

There are several types of echowave structure taken perpendicularly against the posterior wall of a phakic eye by a sound beam introduced through the pupil and monitored by B-mode (Figs. 4 and 5). The major cluster of echowave originates from the anterior surface of the sclera. Then the echowave from the posterior scleral surface shows the spindle shape of lower amplitude compared with that of the anterior cluster. There are two hot spots mobile on the serially taken echowaves every one fifteenth second. The mobile spots are seen in the major troughs of both sides of the anterior scleral cluster, that is, the third to fourth peak and the 7th to 8th peak in every trace. These two different traces of echowaves from the same person differ in gross shape from each other, but the mobile spots regularly appear in the different traces.

There is no established authority to select out which waveform is the authentic scan for further analysis. The first smaller cluster might be composed of the reflection from the anterior surface of the retina and the following layers. The nature of the anterior part of the wave is complex because it includes many cell layers, and the approximate duration is almost the length of one incident wave. If the earlier part of the echowave

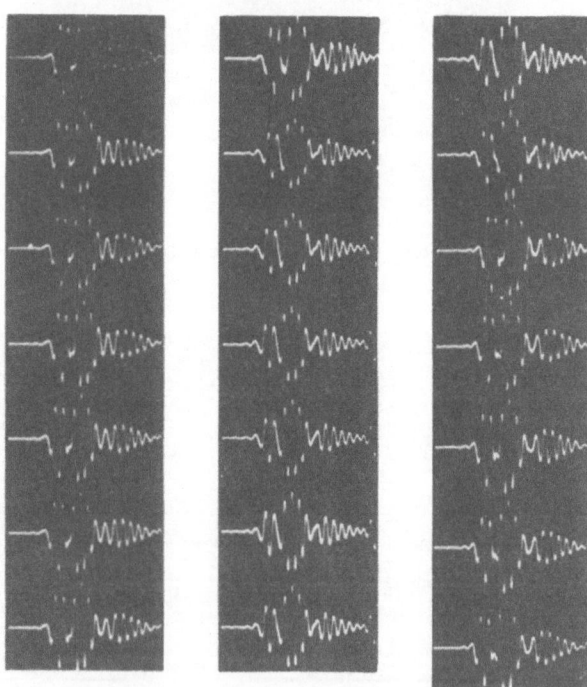

Fig. 4. Echowave taken serially from the posterior ocular wall every one fifteenth second.

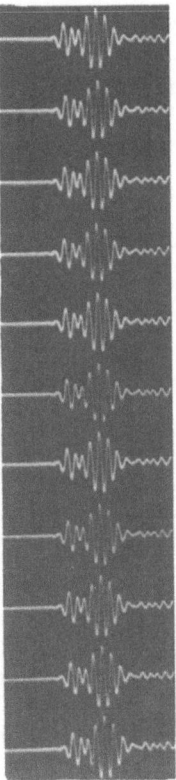

Fig. 5. Echowave taken serially from the person same as the Fig. 4.

is subjected to Fourier analysis, it is difficult to separate two layers from the obtained power spectra, because its complex nature of inconsistent appearance of the peak to peak or the trough to trough distance (Fig. 6, middle).

It is therefore impossible to separate two layers within the wave before the reflection of anterior scleral surface. There is no justification to assume that the boundaries of retina and choroid make echo-reflection, nor to assume that an anatomical boundary makes an echographic boundary. The possibility must be equally considered that pulse waves receive continuous modification whilst traversing tissues as well as expecting layer to layer separation. The cepstrum of the first one microsecond shows the several frequency peaks from the multiple layers (Fig. 6, bottom), but the complex nature of the membrane structure does not allow one to identify which peak of frequency corresponds to the specific boundary of adjacent layers. It is also still uncertain if retina and choroid produce sonographical boundaries, because the close observation of RF signals at time domain helps more the biological understanding of the nature of membrane struc-

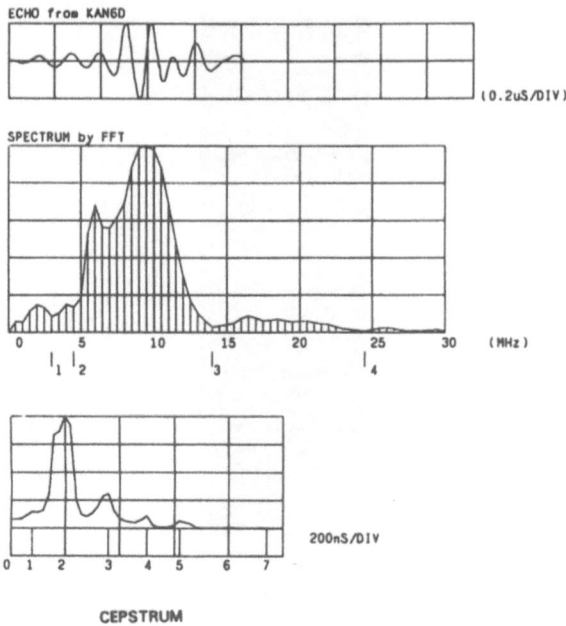

ECHO from KAN6D

(0.2uS/DIV)

SPECTRUM by FFT

0   5   10   15   20   25   30   (MHz)

$|_1$ $|_2$ $|_3$ $|_4$

CEPSTRUM

200nS/DIV

0 1 2 3 4 5 6 7

Fig. 6. Power spectrum and cepstrum of one echowave.

ture. The mobile spots seem to recur to the similar shape lightly pulsating according to the heart beat (Figs. 4 and 5). To prove if the mobility really relates to the pulsation of heart beats, the echowave was collected simultaneously with finger sphygmogram. The moving parts were seen in three parts in this trace including pulsating amplitude on the major cluster corresponding to the anterior scleral reflex (Fig. 7). The largest change in a wave form is seen synchronously in the sphygmogram of which the largest change in amplitude occurs. From these fact, we can assume the anterior scleral reflex is indeed pulsating according to heart beats. Then the simulation study of three layer model assuming retina, choroid and sclera, corresponding thickness of these layers were assumed 80 n sec, varing 280 to 310 n sec, 550 n sec respectively by time domain traversing the sound through the layers (Fig. 8). The arbitrary impedance ratios relative to the vitreous body are 1.3, 0.9, 1.2 respectively and 1.3 for retrobubar tissues.

The change in the thickness of the second layer, the third boundary is subjected to be modified in its shape nearly at the start and the end part. By the simulation study, it is possible to interpret the anterior scleral reflex of the living trace is pushed backward according to the choroidal pulsation. The comparison of synthetic echowaves and the traces of living ocular wall implies the lower impedance ratio and the thinner thickness of the second layer than arbitrally assumed.

Then the impedance of plastic membrane in the saline was studied

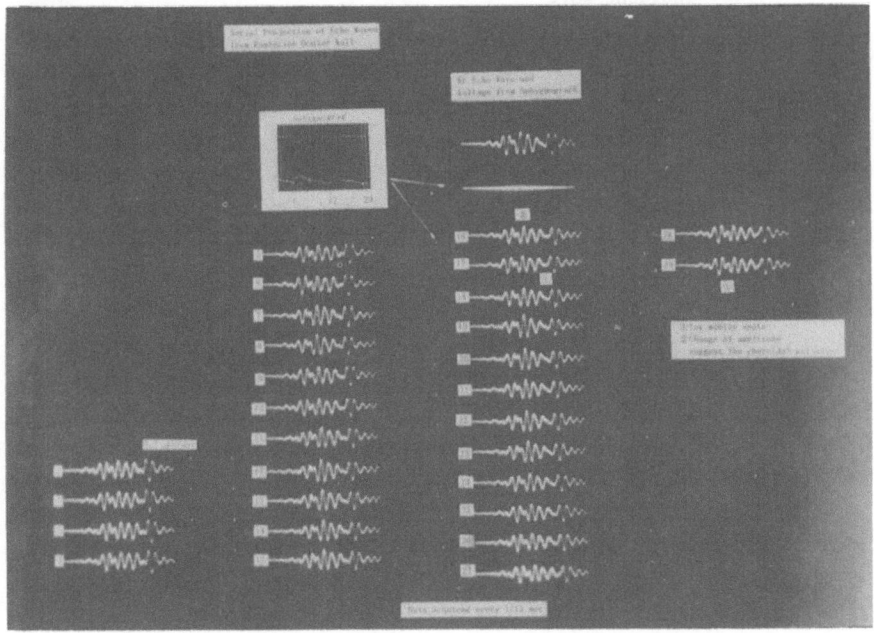

Fig. 7. Synchronously taken serial echowaves with sphygmogram from the posterior ocular wall.

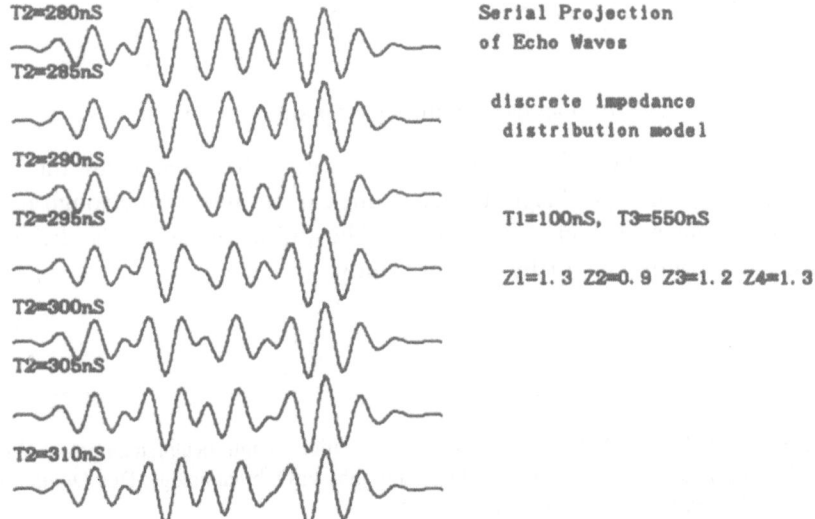

Fig. 8. Simulation of pulsating echo structure by three layer model.

preliminarily. The fairly stable plateau was achieved for impedance distribution (Fig. 9). The impedance distribution of the posterior wall of human eye shows a more complex characteristic (Fig. 10). There seems to be a step at the 200 n sec from the start which corresponds to the anterior

70

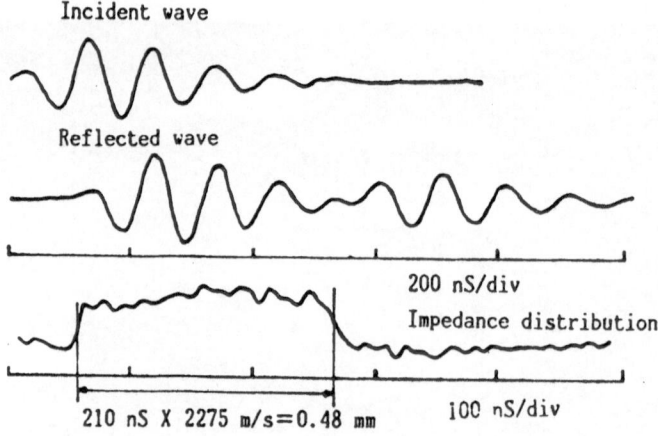

Incident wave

Reflected wave

200 nS/div

Impedance distribution

210 nS X 2275 m/s=0.48 mm   100 nS/div

Fig. 9. Impedance distribution of a plastic membrane.

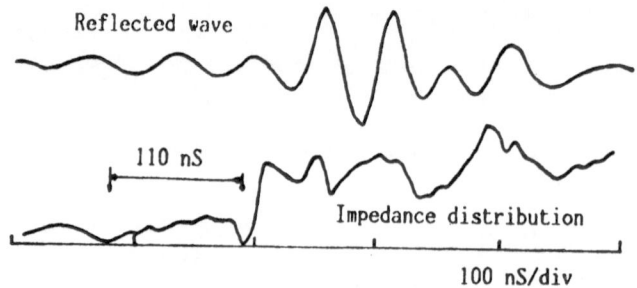

Reflected wave

110 nS

Impedance distribution

100 nS/div

Fig. 10. Impedance distribution of posterior ocular wall.

scleral reflex. There is a small step before 100 n sec from the start. However, its biological significance is unclear because of the rough nature of the whole impedance distribution. The pulsating nature of the impedance distribution is worthy of future study.

References

Bayer AL, Thijssen JM. 1981. In vivo characterization of intraocular membranes. In: JM Thijssen and AM Verbeek (eds) Ultrasonography in Ophthalmology, Doc Ophthal Proc Ser, Vol. 29, Junk, The Hague, pp. 411—418.

Coleman DJ, Lizzi FL. 1979. In vivo choroidal thickness measurement. Am J Ophthalmol 88: 369—375.

Lepper RD, Trier HG, Reinert S, Reuter R. 1987. In vivo study of the human retinochoroidal layers by RF signal analysis. I. visual echogram interpretation. Part I: Techniques. In: KC Ossoinig (ed) Ophthalmic Echography. Martinus Nijhoff/Dr W Junk Publishers, Dordrecht, pp. 139—143.

Purnell EW, Frank KE, Holasek E, Jennings WD. 1987. Ultrasonic microbiometry of the eye. In: KC Ossoinig (ed) Ophthalmic Echography. Martinus Nijhoff/Dr W Junk Publishers, Dordrecht, pp. 123—130.

Sugata Y et al. 1985. Measurement of thickness of living ocular walls by ultrasound-wave pulsation method. In: RW Gill and MJ Dadd (eds) Proceedings of the fourth meeting of the World Federation for Ultrasound in Medicine and Biology. Pergamon Press, Sydney, p. 431.

Sugata Y et al. 1985. Ultrasound measurement of the thickness of living ocular walls-cepstrum method. In: RW Gill and MJ Dadd (eds) Proceedings of the fourth meeting of the World Federation for Ultrasound in Medicine and Biology. Pergamon Press, Sydney, p. 431.

Shibuya N et al. 1985. Measurement of accoustic characteristic impedance of tissue by ultrasound. In: RW Gill and MJ Dadd (eds) Proceedings of the fourth meeting of the World Federation for Ultrasound in Medicine and Biology. Pergamon Press, Sydney, p. 504.

Trier HG, Reinert S. 1987. In vivo study of the human retino-choroidal layers by RF-signal analysis. I. Visual echogram interpretation. Part 2: Results on choroidal thickness and pulsation under physiological conditions and under tonometry. In: KC Ossoinig (ed) Ophthalmic Echography. Martinus Nijhoff/Dr W Junk Publishers, Dordrecht, pp. 144.

Spectral analysis for ultrasonic tissue characterization

S. TANE, Y. KIMURA AND M. KANO

Summary

The authors developed a computerized ultrasonic tissue characterization system for clinical ophthalmology. In animal experiments and clinical trials, it was possible to differentiate retinal detachment from various intraocular haemorrhagic membrane.

Mathematical evaluation techniques to determine the calibrated power spectrum of reflected ultrasonic echoes from tissue involved by various ocular diseases could be used with a clinical computer system to objectively classify retinal detachment and vitreous haemorrhagic membrane. Tissue structures could be acoustically stained in B-mode images to define the specific anatomic and structural properties that provide the acoustic differentiations. These data were obtained under in vivo conditions and allowed a non-invasive differentiation of intraocular membranes in a way not previously possible, aiding in the definitive diagnosis of intraocular diseases, as well as in the planning and monitoring of treatment.

Introduction

Ultrasonic spectral analysis of the ultrasonic A-mode (A-scan) wave form by computed wave form analysis makes it possible to perform tissue differentiation in living eyes. In addition to the conventional macroscopic morphologic diagnosis (according to wave form, attenuation, morphology, etc.) by A- and B-scan, microscopic analytic diagnosis of ophthalmic disorders has become easy.

Methods

In the present study, B-scan images of ophthalmic disorders were pictured

Dept. of Ophthalmology, St. Marianna University, School of Medicine 2-16-1 Sugao, Miyamae-ku, Kawasaki-shi, Japan.

J. M. Thijssen (ed.) Ultrasonography in ophthalmology.
© 1988, Kluwer Academic Publishers, Dordrecht, ISBN 978-94-010-7083-6

by the immersion method, and the A-mode wave was set to the part (a 5 × 5 cm box) representing the most marked characteristic of the ophthalmic disorder. Ultrasonic spectral analysis was conducted by Fourier analysis of the image [pictured by a V-650 type oscilloscope (HITACHI) at the radio-frequency signal of this part] by means of a DATA-6000 computer wave form analyzer. A PZT focused transducer at 10 MHz or 15 MHz was attached to a St. Marianna's high-resolution ophthalmic ultrasonic diagnostic equipment for collecting ultrasonic images. These images were pictured on the V-650 type oscilloscope, and ultrasonic spectral analysis was performed with the DATA-6000 analyzer.

Ultrasonic spectral analytic diagnosis was preliminarily made in living rabbit eyes: eight eyes with experimental vitreous haemorrhage, two with retinal detachment, and six with uveitis due to albumin sensitization. The eyeballs were then excised and the findings were compared with histopathological findings.

Results

In the present experiment, the usual A- and B-mode images and findings of the fundus oculi were compared with findings obtained by ultrasonic spectral analytic diagnosis in 44 human eyes consisting of 12 with retinal detachment, 14 with vitreous haemorrhage, 2 with retinoblastoma and 16 with other ophthalmic diseases.

The eyes with retinal detachment showed a peak spectral reflex in the frequency range of the reflex echo around 10 MHz or 15 MHz of the transducer used, showing a convex pattern. In the subsequent range, 20–50 MHz, they showed a weak and relatively flat spectral reflex of less than −30 dB. (Fig. 1) The eyes with vitreous haemorrhage showed an approximately fixed and flat spectral reflex around −30 dB over the entire area in the frequency range of the reflex echo. By contrast, the eyes with intravitreal membrane formation after absorption of the vitreous haemorrhage were found by spectral analysis of the reflex waves to give small convex or flat continuous waves of about −20 dB. (Fig. 2)

References

Coleman DJ, Lizzi FL. 1981. Computerized ultrasonic tissue characterization of ocular tumour. Am J Ophthalmol 96: 165–175.

Tane S, Kohno J, Komatsu A, Horikoshi J. 1984. Tissue characterization by computerized ultrasonic spectral analysis of ocular diseases. Folia Ophthalmol Jpn 35: 2361–2365.

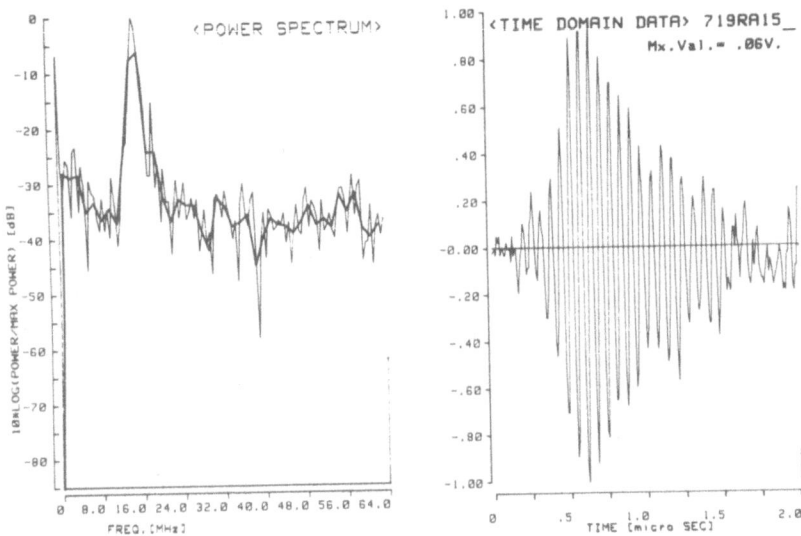

Fig. 1. Spectrum analysis of RF echogram (right) of retinal detachment. The power spectrum (left) shows a convex pattern with a maximum at 15 MHz.

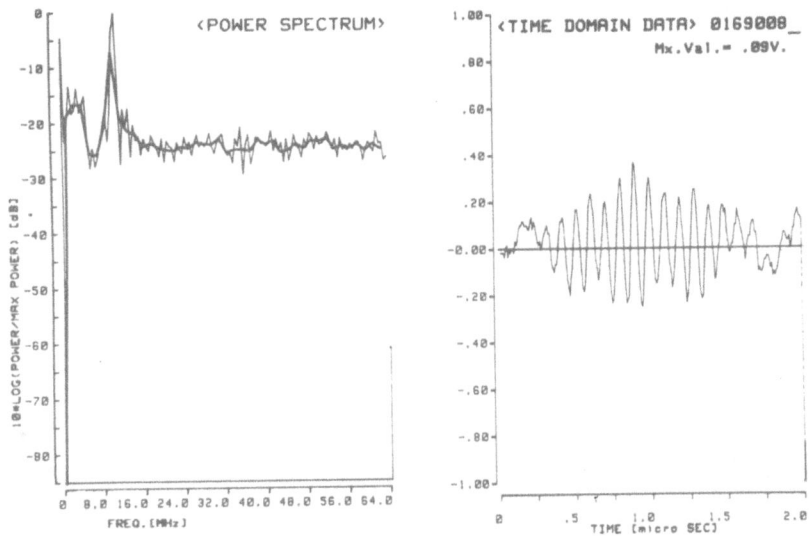

Fig. 2. Spectral analysis of RF echogram of intravitreal membrane (right). The power spectrum (left) displays scalloping at frequencies from 0—15 MHz.

Thijssen JM, Cloostermans M, Bayer AL. 1981. Measurement of ultrasound attenuation in tissues from scattered reflections. In: JM Thijssen and AM Verbeek (eds) Ultrasound in Ophthalmology. Proceedings of the 8th SIDUO Congress, Junk, The Hague, pp. 431—439.

Trier HG, Lepper RD. 1982. Tissue characterization in ophthalmology. In: JM Thijssen (ed) Ultrasonic Tissue characterization, Nijhoff, The Hague, pp. 74—86.

Texture of echographic B-mode images

J. M. THIJSSEN AND B. J. OOSTERVELD

Summary

The influences of the properties of the sound field and of the effective density of scatterers within a tissue were investigated by a realistic simulation study. The results indicate a great dependence of the texture parameters on the depth of the insonated tissue volume. The density of the scatterers is revealed by the texture up to a limit set by the transducer characteristics. For ophthalmic transducers this limit is still far above the cellular dimensions. It is concluded, that for quantitative analysis of B-mode images correction for the effects on the texture caused by the sound field is a prerequisite.

Introduction

The introduction of digitized systems for A- and B-mode echography has enhanced the interest of ophthalmologists, as well as of physicists, in the quantitative evaluation of the images. The B-mode systems are at present able to display the reflectivity of the tissues in eight to thirty two gray levels. Better transducers have improved the resolution both in axial and lateral direction. The question to be answered in this paper is whether it is possible, and if so to what extent, to characterize tissues by quantitative analysis of the so-called texture of B-mode images. Texture can be defined as the spatial distribution of gray levels in a picture, in other words the pattern of white "blobs" with which a tissue, is displayed.

This kind of analysis has been employed subjectively in A-mode echography for many years in echo-ophthalmology. Terms like relative, or absolute, reflectivity (echogenicity), attenuation (either expressing the decrease in echo-amplitude, within a tissue, or the decrease of the echo from a structure distal to a process and the irregularity of a tissue echo-

Biophysics Laboratory of the Institute of Ophthalmology and Centre for Eye Research, University of Nijmegen, 6500 HB Nijmegen, The Netherlands.

J. M. Thijssen (ed.) Ultrasonography in ophthalmology.
© 1988, *Kluwer Academic Publishers, Dordrecht, ISBN 978-94-010-7083-6*

gram were proposed (Oksala, 1962, 1979; Buschmann, 1964; Ossoinig, 1965; Poujol, 1971, 1975). An effort to quantify the A-mode echopattern of tumours objectively, i.e. by employing a computer, was described by Thijssen and colleagues (Thijssen et al., 1981; Thijssen and Verbeek, 1981). The quantitative evaluation of B-mode echograms is still at a preliminary stage.

The authors recently undertook a systematic study by a computer simulation of the whole process of ultrasonic beam formation, backscattering by tissues and image construction (Thijssen and Oosterveld, 1985; Oosterveld et al., 1985). This study was inspired by the work published by Burckhardt (1978) and Abbott and Thurstone (1979), who demonstrated the analogy between the "speckle" pattern caused by coherent light sources (laser light) and the texture of B-mode echograms from parenchymal tissues. From theory it emerges, that the average reflectivity level of B-mode images is proportional to the square root of the number (i.e. density) of effective scatterers in the insonated volume of tissue. At the limit of a very high density the texture is just a speckle pattern which is independent of the tissue microstructure and merely reflects the acoustic field properties brought about by the employed transducer.

More recently Wagner et al. (1983) derived a set of parameters describing the average first and second order statistical properties of the B-mode texture. These parameters have been employed in the simulation study by the authors. The effects on the texture caused by the diffractive nature of the sound beam and the focussing by the transducer were investigated by positioning the simulated tissue at different distances to the transducer surface. The question whether it is possible to find any correlation between tissue microstructure and the texture was investigated by systematically increasing the density of scatterers from 1 per cubic centimeter to 20,000 per cubic centimeter.

The generation of texture in B-mode echograms

The tissue is simply modelled by a homogeneous base medium, either or not with frequency dependent attenuation, which contains randomly distributed pointlike scatterers. An even more simple situation is drawn in Fig. 1: only four scatterers are present. When an ultrasound pulse is transmitted into the medium these scatterers are hit at slightly different times. According to the Huygens' principle the scatterers act as secondary sources of ultrasound and the spherical wavefronts will propagate back towards the transducer. Since the transducer is a phase sensitive receiver the incoming waveforms of the echoes will be linearly added at every point of the transducer surface. This is shown in Fig. 2. Due to the small time differences the waveforms will interfere, which results in a rather complex RF-echowaveform. This process occurs at every point of the surface so that even for four scatterers it will be evident that the overall echopattern does not reveal the position, nor the reflectivity of the individual scatterers. The RF-waveform is then demodulated by the receiver electronics and employed to display one A-line of the B-mode echogram. The next A-line is obtained after a slight displacement of the sound beam and so on (Fig. 3a).

As is also shown in Fig. 3 (a and b), the simulations were restricted to eight rectangular parts of the total depth of the scan: three in front of the focus (8 cm), one in focus and four beyond the focus. The simulations concerning the effect of the density on the B-mode texture were confined to the focal zone.

Influence of depth on the texture of B-mode echograms (diffraction effects)

Before showing the effects of beam diffraction on the texture the B-mode

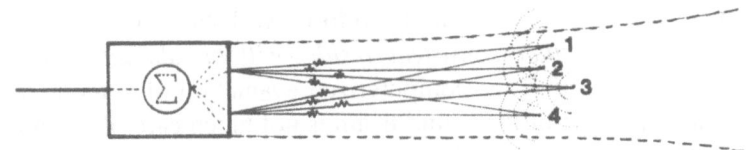

Fig. 1. Scheme of insonation of "tissue" containing four scattering structures. The scatterers act like secondary sources and produce spherical wave fronts. At reception the echo waveforms are summated at each point of the transducer, and over the whole surface.

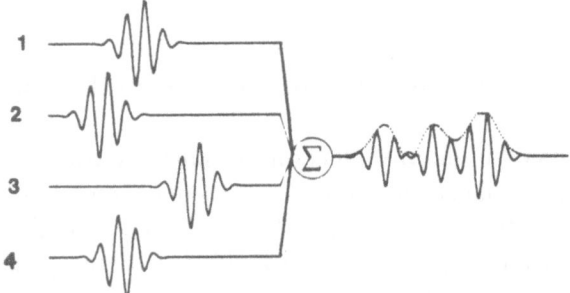

Fig. 2. Summation of echowaveforms at a single point of the transducer, note the irregular interference pattern after the summation. Dashed line: envelope (i.e. video A-line) after demodulation.

display of a linear scan of a single point-like reflector should first be considered. It is evident that such a display as is shown in Fig. 4, bottom row, yields the effective beam diameter vs. depth. This effective diameter is commonly used as an indication of the lateral resolution. It can be seen that the axial resolution, i.e. the dimension in axial (= depth) direction of the reflector images is almost independent of depth, whereas the lateral size follows the focussing of the simulated transducer and the sound field it produces (5 MHz, 13 mm diameter, 8 cm focal distance).

If we now consider the situation of 1000 scattering structures per cubic centimeter and simulate B-scans vs. depth as schematized in Fig. 3 a rather striking phenomenon becomes evident: the lateral (i.e. vertical in the top row in Fig. 4) size of the texture "blobs" is smallest near to the transducer and then increases monotonously till beyond the focus. A similar picture would have been obtained with a non-focused transducer. The explanation for this phenomenon is that the interference of the echoes from the individual scatterers is highest near to the transducer (cf. Fig. 2) and low beyond the focus, or in the far field.

Since the B-mode echograms in Fig. 4 were normalized to the mean gray level, the effects of beam diffraction on the gray level do not show-up. It was found by Thijssen and colleagues (Thijssen and Oosterveld, 1985, Oosterveld et al., 1985), that the mean level increases with depth till the focus and decreased beyond it. Therefore, we have to conclude that it is *highly improbable that consistent results will be obtained* from either subjective, or objective, i.e. computerized evaluation of B-mode images if the diffraction effect of the sound beam is not taken care of. A simple way to do this is always to place the focus of the transducer in the centre of the region of interest and employ a limited depth range (cf. Lizzi et al., 1983), which is possible by employing an immersion technique. A second possibility is to use a transducer with a relatively long focal zone (Thijssen, 1981), so that diffraction effects can be neglected to a first approximation.

Influence of the tissue on the texture of B-mode echograms

As is mentioned in the Introduction, the characteristics of the texture (1st and 2nd order statistical parameters) are independent of the density of scattering structures at very high densities. One exception must be mentioned: the mean gray level is proportional to the square root of the density, as well as to the mean reflectivity of the scatterers. The interesting question then remains: what happens at low scatterer densities?

Our simulations revealed, that the mean gray level is proportional to the square root of the density of the scatterers over a long range, i.e. also at

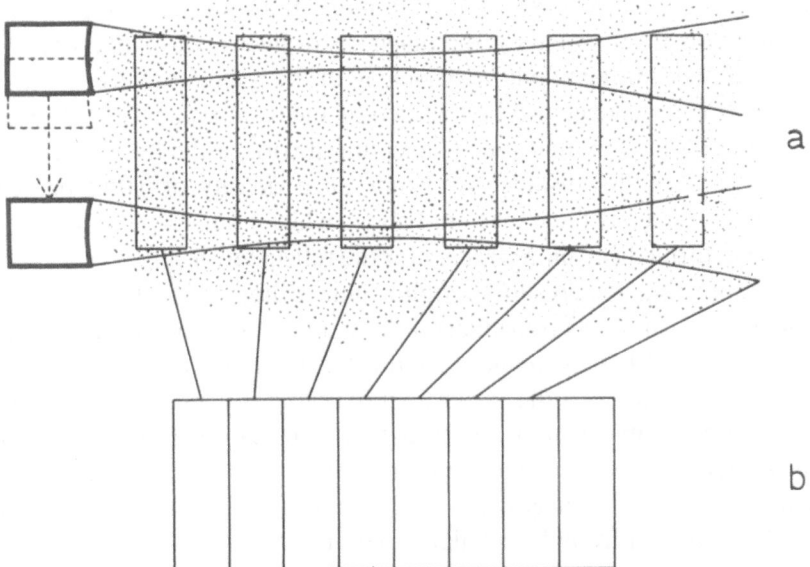

Fig. 3. (a) Generation of B-mode echogram with linear scanning. (b) The rectangular boxes indicate the parts calculated in the computer simulation study.

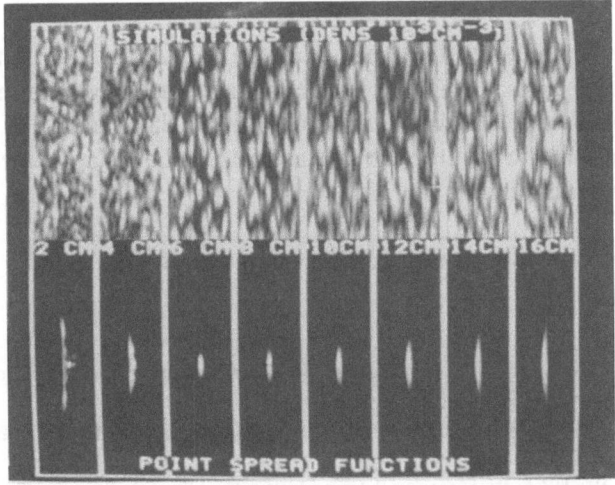

Fig. 4. Top row: B-mode display of simulated tissue (containing 1000 scatterers per cm^3) with increasing distance to the transducer (cf. Fig. 3). Bottom row: B-mode display of single point-like reflector at increasing distance to the transducer. Centre spot coincides with focus.

relatively low densities. The axial and lateral sizes of the texture "blobs" monotonously decrease when going from low to high scatterer densities. The axial dimension decreases to 2/3 and the lateral dimension to 1/2 of the size obtained for a single scatterer in focus. So, there is a range of scatterer densities in which the coarseness of the texture bears information about the tissue microstructure. Since the simulations discussed till now were concerned with a 3.5 MHz abdominal transducer the impact of this conclusion is for instance for the diagnosis of liver disease, that only if the diffuse changes bring about a coarsening of the microstructure of the liver tissue this latter change will be revealed by the texture pattern. This is to be explained by the fact that the collagen meshwork of the liver parenchyma has a characteristic distance of 1 mm, so a density of 1000 per cubic centimeter, which is the limit found above which no tissue characterization can be performed any more (except for the reflectivity level).

Extrapolating this result to ophthalmic echography (10 MHz, 5 mm diameter, 2.5 cm focus transducers) the sampling volume at focus is of the order of 10 to 30 times smaller than for the abdominal transducers. Hence, it may be expected that the upper limit of scatterer densities is of the order of 30,000 per cubic centimeter, or higher. So it follows from our study that much finer structural changes in tissues will be revealed in the texture of ophthalmic B-mode images, but at the same time it has to be concluded that the limit is far from the cellular dimensions.

Acknowledgements

This work is supported by grants from the Netherlands' Technology Foundation (S.T.W.) and from the Netherlands' Cancer Foundation (Koningin Wilhelmina Fonds), and is carried out within the framework of the Concerted Action Programme on Ultrasonic Tissue Characterization of the European Community.

References

Abbott JG, Thurstone FL. 1979. Acoustic speckle: theory and experimental analysis. Ultrasonic Imag 1: 303—324.

Burckhardt CB. 1978. Speckle in ultrasound B-mode scans. IEEE Trans Sonics and Ultrasonics SU-25: 1—6.

Buschmann W. 1964. Probleme und Fortschritte der Ultraschalldiagnostik am Auge. Klin Mbl Augenhk 144: 321—347.

Lizzi FL, Greenebaum M, Feleppa EJ, Elbaum M, Coleman DJ. 1983. Theoretical framework for spectrum analysis in ultrasonic tissue characterization. J Acoust Soc Am 73: 1366—1373.

Oksala A. 1962. About selective echography in some eye diseases. Acta Ophthal (Kbh) 40: 466—474.

Oosterveld BJ, Thijssen JM. 1985. Texture of B-mode echograms: 3-D simulations and experiments of the effects of diffraction and scatterer density. Ultrasonic Imag 7: 142—160.

Ossoinig KC. 1965. Zum Problem der akustischen Tumordiagnostik von Auge und Orbita. In: Diagnostica Ultrasonica in Ophthalmologia. Wiss. Z. Humboldt Univ Berlin Math-Nat R. XIV, pp. 185—191.

Ossoinig KC. 1979. Standardized echography: basic principles, clinical applications and results. Intl Ophthal Clinics 19: 127—210.

Poujol, J. 1971. L'echographie clinique des tumeurs intra-oculaires. In: J Böck and KC Ossoinig (eds) Ultrasonographia Medica, Verlag Wiener Med Akad, Part II, pp. 275—290.

Poujol J. 1975. Calculations entre la réflectivité et l'atténuation ultrasonique des tumeurs intra-oculaires et leur structure histologique. In: J François and F Goes (eds) Ultra-sonography in Ophthalmology, Karger, Basel, pp. 172—177.

Thijssen JM, Verbeek AM. 1981. Computer analysis of A-mode echograms from choroidal melanomas. In: JM Thijssen and AM Verbeek (eds) Ultrasonography in Ophthalmology, Doc Ophthalm Proc Series, Vol. 29, Junk, Den Haag, pp. 123—130.

Thijssen, J. M. 1981. Functional realization of a SAB scanner. In: JM Thijssen and AM Verbeek (eds) Ultrasonography in Ophthalmology. Doc Ophthal Proc Series, Vol. 29, Junk, Den Haag, pp. 515—520.

Thijssen JM, Bayer AL, Cloostermans MJ. 1981. Computer assisted echography: statistical analysis of A-mode video echograms obtained by tissue sampling. Med Biol Eng & Comp 19: 437—442.

Thijssen JM, Oosterveld BJ. 1985. Texture in B-mode echograms: a simulation study of the effects of diffraction and of scatterer density on gray scale statistics. In: AJ Berkhout, J Ridder, and LF van der Wal (eds), Acoustical Imaging, Vol. 14, Plenum, New York, pp. 481—485.

Wagner RF, Smith SW, Sandrik JM, Lopez H. 1983. Statistics of speckle in ultrasound B-scans. IEEE Trans Sonics and Ultrasonics SU-30: 156—163.

Numerical expression in kinetic echography

A. SAWADA, H. TORII, A. NAKAMURA AND A. YAMAMOTO

Summary

We tried to analyze quantitatively the movement of membrane-like lesions in the eye. We made the analyzing system and verified it in the specially prepared phantom. Mobility of a membrane in the phantom was strongly influenced by the surroundings. Afterwards some cases of membrane in the eye were analyzed. The results suggest strongly the necessity of standardization in kinetic ultrasonography. To get to the final goal further improvement is needed.

Introduction

Significance of ultrasonographic investigation on mobility of intraocular lesions was first noticed by Baum and his co-worker in 1960. Since then many workers have been engaged in studying the mobility of intraocular and orbital lesions. In 1964 Ossoinig described the new examination method to evaluate the mobility of A-mode spikes using Kretztechnik 7200 MA and named kinetic echography. After development of high-speed mechanical sector scanning and electronic linear scanning ultrasonic diagnostic equipment, many investigators observed many aspects of mobility of ocular lesions, particularly membranous structures (McLeod et al., 1977; Restori et al., 1977 and others). However, the description has been subjective and qualitative. Sometimes the expression was too prosaic to be used in the follow-up or in the comparison. In 1982, Susal and his collaborators described ultrasonographic images using electronic linear scanning equipment and attracted our intense attention. They analyzed echo patterns of asteroid hyalosis and mobile retinal detachment which were recorded on video-tapes. It was the first trial to express the mobility of intraocular lesions as numeral. However, the changes of echo patterns

Department of Ophthalmology, Miyazaki Medical College, 5200 Kihara, Kiyotake, Miyazaki 889-16, Japan.

J. M. Thijssen (ed.) Ultrasonography in ophthalmology.
© 1988, Kluwer Academic Publishers, Dordrecht, ISBN 978-94-010-7083-6

by induced eye movement are superimposed on the movement of intra-ocular membranous structures. These two different kinds of movement which are displayed simultaneously should be separated and evaluated. The purpose of the present study is to analyze the independent mobility, which is not influenced by induced eye movement and expressed as numeral.

Methods and materials

Analyzing system

To evaluate the movement of membranous lesions in the eye quantitatively and numerically, velocity during the induced eye movement, and velocity and the duration time after the cessation of eye movement were studied. Velocity to be investigated can be divided into three components. They are angular velocity of eye movement (W), angular velocity of membrane (w) and polar velocity of membrane (v).

As shown in Fig. 1, when the eye is induced to rotate around the center (O) of the eye for the time from t_0 to t_1, a certain point in the eye moves from p_0 to p_1. If p_0 is fixed in the eye, p_0 moves to p_2 with rotation of the eye. The point of p_3 is imaginary, which has the same distance as Op_0 from the center of the eye (O) in the line of Op_1. Angular velocity of eye (W) was indicated as

$$\frac{\text{angle } p_1Op_0}{t_1 - t_0},$$

angular velocity of membrane (w) as

$$\frac{\text{angle } p_2Op_1}{t_1 - t_0},$$

and polar velocity of membrane (v) as

$$\frac{\overline{p_3p_1}}{t_1 - t_0}.$$

The parameter of max. $w \cdot v/W$ corresponds to the amount of motion of the target membrane with consideration of eye movement. The symbol of $\overline{W}$ means the averaged W.

To calculate the velocity components described above, an analyzing system was made. Echo patterns by an electronic linear scanning ultrasonic diagnostic equipment (Aloka 210 DX) and the lapsing time which was shown in 1/100 second by the timer, were displayed on the TV monitor and recorded successively on video-tapes. Using the video-writer FVW-

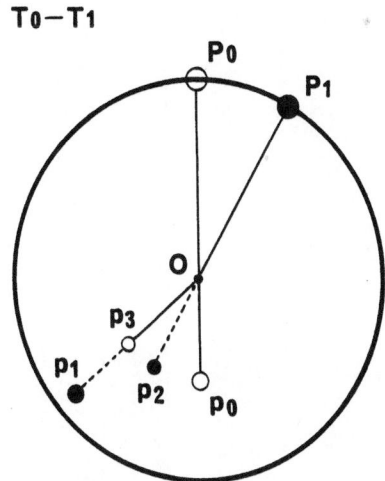

To−T1

Fig. 1. Scheme for the evaluation of movement of a point p_0 due to an eye movement (rotation from $p_0 \rightarrow p_1$). Explanation see text.

300 (FOR, A) and the microcomputer (PC-9801 F II NEC) with the analysis program composed by ourselves, the speed and the elapsed time of movement of intraocular membranous structures during eye movement and after its cessation, were calculated.

Phantom

Prior to the evaluation of experimental and clinical cases, basic experiments were done on a phantom to ascertain the reliability, efficiency and reproducibility. The phantom was made for experimental analysis of mobility of a thin membrane in water or another liquid. The phantom was composed of a plastic-made cylinder bottle and a thin membrane, film for dialysis of 0.01 mm thickness, which was set in the cylinder bottle. The one side, which was put in, was considered as the internal chamber and was filled with water or silicone oil. The other side, which received the stretched membrane, was considered as the external chamber and filled with water. The cylinder bottle was rotated by the converted power from a reciprocal shaker. The speed of rotation could be controlled. As a marker, a tiny piece of metal was sticked on the surface of the wall of the cylinder. The marker had intense reflectivity to ultrasound and produced multiple signals. The marker could be detected and followed on the echograms very easily (Fig. 2).

Clinical cases

Using the analyzing system mentioned above, mobility of membrane

88

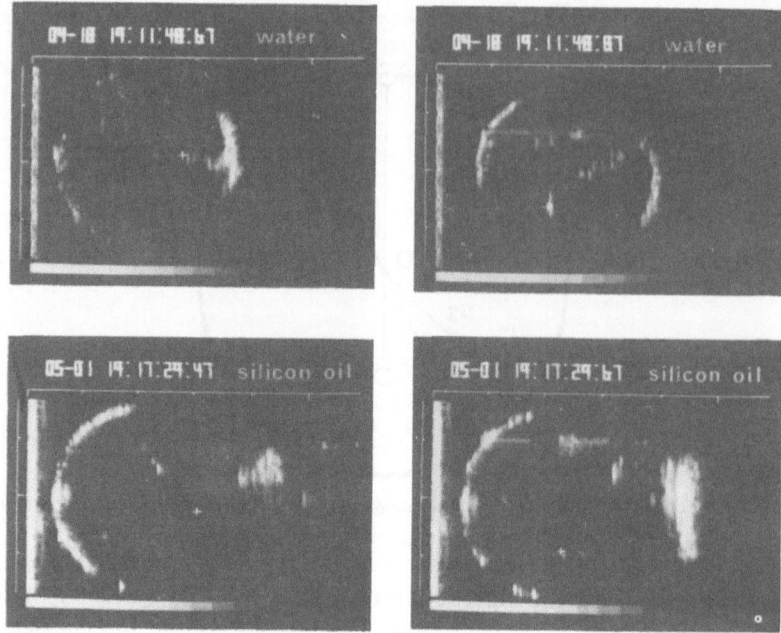

Fig. 2. Kinetic echography of a phantom filled with water (a) and with silicone oil (b). The marker, a small steel ball, can be seen from the accompanying reverberations and shadowing. The point of measurement is shown by the cursor (cross). Left pictures: before rotation, right pictures: after rotation.

structures in vitreous haemorrhage and retinal detachment was evaluated. The difference of direction of induced eye movement was also studied.

Results and discussion

Phantom

When the internal chamber is filled with water, the maximum velocity of the membrane, maximum $w \cdot v/W$ was 62.46 ± 26.6 mm/sec. In the case of silicone oil the maximum velocity was 24.12 ± 2.07 mm/sec. The maximum velocity after the cessation of cylinder motion, max. $w \cdot v/\overline{W}$ was 0.36 ± 0.12 mm/sec with water and 0.04 ± 0.02 mm/sec with silicone oil. The duration of aftermovement of the membrane was 0.41 ± 0.06 seconds with water and 0.13 ± 0.00 seconds with silicone oil. These results showed that the membrane with silicone oil was less mobile than with water and suggested that mobility of the membrane was strongly depended on the condition around the membrane.

Clinical cases

The values on velocity in a case of vitreous haemorrhage and in a case of retinal detachment were:

direction of eye movement	vitreous haemorrhage		retinal detachment	
	downward	upward	downward	upward
max. w · v/W (mm/sec)	22.48	67.07	10.17	21.30
max. w · v/$\overline{W}$ (mm/sec)	4.54	30.16	0.49	4.24
reach to max (sec)	0.00	0.00	0.14	0.26
aftermovement (sec)	1.17	2.04	0.54	0.67

The third line indicates the time of reaching to the maximum velocity after the cessation of the induced eye movement. The fourth line indicates the duration time of aftermovement. In both vitreous haemorrhage and retinal detachment, the eye downward movement was greater and continued longer. These results suggest that kinetic analysis should be done in a definite way.

Acknowledgement

This study was supported by a grant-in-aid for scientific research (59480349) from the Japanese Ministry of Education.

References

Baum G, Greenwood I. 1960. Ultrasound in ophthalmology. Am J Ophthalmol 49: 249—261.

McLeod D, Restori M, Wright JE. 1977. Rapid B-scanning of the vitreous. Br J Ophthalmol 61: 437—445.

Ossoinig K. 1965. Zur Ultraschalldiagnostik der Tumoren des Auges. Klin Monatsbl Augenheilkd 146: 321—337.

Restori M, McLeod D. 1977. Ultrasound in pre-vitrectomy assessment. Trans Ophthalmol Soc U.K. 97: 232—234.

Susal AL, Gaynon MW, Walker JT. 1983. Linear array multiple transducer ultrasonic examination of the eye. Ophthalmology 90: 266—271.

Susal AL, Walker JT. 1983. In-vivo measurement of vitreous and retinal acceleration. In: JS Hillman and MM LeMay (eds) Ophthalmic Ultrasonography, Junk, The Hague, pp. 163—168.

In vivo measurement of the thickness of the retino-choroidal layers by RF-signal analysis

S. TANE, J. HORIKOSHI, A. HARIGAYA AND M. MIYAKE

Summary

We have developed a system that permits exceptionally accurate measurements of human retinal, choroidal and scleral thickness in vivo by means of ultrasound and Fourier analysis.

With minicomputer techniques, the complementary functions of the time and spectral domains of reflected sound can be used to permit measurements accurate to less than 20 percent at 10 MHz center frequency.

Methods and techniques

The mid-posterior part between the temporal or nasal equator and macular region of the normal eyes were examined. In this investigation 81 normal eyes of 46 cases between 14 to 80 years old person were examined by using $10 \sim 20$ MHz center frequency transducer of St. Marianna Ophthalmic Ultrasonic Diagnostic Equipment model ZD-252. The A-mode echo signals from the retina, choroid and sclera were converted to radiofrequency echo signal through the oscilloscope Hitachi 610. (Fig. 1) These R.F. signal were digitized by the A—D converter and spectrally analyzed by the minicomputer in the Universal Waveform Analyzer DATA 6000. The retinal transit time was determined from the distance between the troughs around the spectral peak. (Fig. 2) Since the chorio-retinal transit time from the anterior retinal surface to the anterior scleral surface was obtained in the time domain by the digitized R.F. signal waves, the choroidal transit time was determined by subtracting the retinal transit time from the chorio-retinal transit time. The scleral transit time was obtained in the time domain by the digitized R.F. signals. To calculate each thickness of the retina, choroid and sclera, the ultrasonic propagation velocity in each tissue reported by Coleman was used.

Dept. of Ophthalmology, St. Marianna University, School of Medicine, 2-16-1 Sugao, Miyamae-ku, Kawasaki-Shi, Japan.

J. M. Thijssen (ed.) Ultrasonography in ophthalmology.
© 1988, *Kluwer Academic Publishers, Dordrecht, ISBN 978-94-010-7083-6*

92

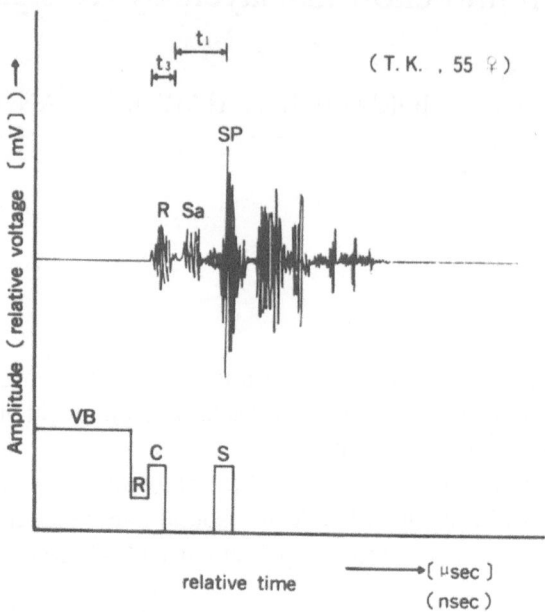

Fig. 1. Ultrasonic evaluation of the posterior eye wall. Top, RF echogram displaying retina (R), anterior (Sa) and posterior (SP) scleral echoes. C = choroid.

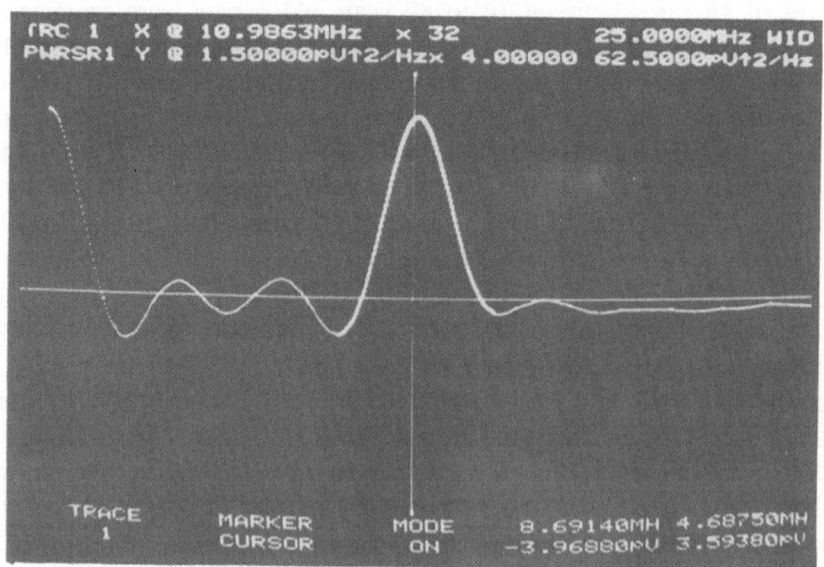

Fig. 2. Power spectrum corresponding to the RF echogram. The width of the oscillations (scalloping) is inversely proportional to the thickness of a layer.

Results

The average thicknesses of the retina, choroid and sclera in all age groups were 151.2 ± 28.03 μm, 370.0 ± 92.08 μm and 708.0 ± 11.34 μm respectively. The average value of the retinal thickness in the group older than 51 years old was significantly thicker than that in the group younger than 30 years old. Those results were almost equal to the anatomical and ultrasonic biometric data at the same region as examined (Table 1).

Next, the thickness of the eye wall was determined in morbid eyes. Twenty-two non-operated eyes of 11 patients with primary open angle glaucoma (consisting of 5 men and 6 women) between the age of 38 and 73 years were examined. The intraocular pressure was controlled within a range of 12 mmHg to 25 mmHg. These patients had early or middle stage disease. No patients in the late stage of disease were involved. If possible, any use of eye lotion or eye drops or internal medication was withdrawn for three days before measurement. The mean thickness was 144.4 ± 29.32 μm for the retina, 414.32 ± 114.94 μm for the choroid and 755.25 ± 102.34 μm for the sclera. There was no significant difference in the mean thickness of the retina or sclera between the normal subjects and the patients, but thickness of the choroid increased significantly in patients with glaucoma ($p < 0.05$).

There was no significant difference in thickness of the retina between the normal eyes and operated eyes with primary open angle glaucoma, although the number of the operated eyes was small (4 eyes of 4 patients).

Table 1. The mean values and standard deviations of the thickness of the ocular layers estimated in vivo.

The thickness of the retina, choroid and sclera in living normal human eyes by means of ultrasonic RF signal analysis.

age groups (cases)	Sclera		Retina		Retina + Choroid	Choroid	
	t_1	μm	t_2	μm	t_3	t_3-t_2	μm
30y ≥	848.6	700.1	175.4	135.5	670.8	500.0	392.5
(6 cases, 9 eyes)	±11.53	+95.23	±34.26	±26.56	±118.09	±97.82	±76.80
31 – 50y	854.3	+704.9	194.2	149.9	714.0	460.5	361.5
(14 cases, 23 eyes)	±14.19	±11.70	±34.68	±26.94	±202.11	±16.56	±13.01
51 – 70y	850.3	701.5	201.2	155.0	708.1	469.3	368.5
(21 cases, 39 eyes)	±13.53	±11.16	±40.06	±30.98	±14.12	±97.56	±76.57
71y ≤	904.0	745.8	201.8	155.4	677.1	478.9	376.0
(5 cases, 10 eyes)	±16.06	±13.25	±22.98	±17.93	±78.67	±84.16	±65.91
Average	858.1	708.0	196.1	151.2	702.8	471.3	370.0
(46 cases, 81 eyes)	±13.75	±11.34	±36.23	±28.03	±15.49	±11.73	±92.08

The thickness of the choroid and sclera increased significantly (P < 0.05) in the operated glaucomatous eyes.

Next, the thickness of the eye wall was determined in the eyes with retinal pigmentary degeneration.

Twenty-four eyes of 12 patients between the ages of 49 and 71 years were examined.

The mean thickness was 152.0 ± 18.04 µm for the retina, 382.2 ± 26.19 µm for the choroid and 767.1 ± 46.05 µm for the sclera. There was no significant difference in the mean thickness of the retina, choroid and sclera between the normal subjects and the patients.

References

Coleman DJ, Lizzi FL. 1979. In vivo choroidal thickness measurement. Am J Ophthalmol 88: 369—376.

Tane S et al. 1986. Total Imaging Diagnosis in Ophthalmology: New Experiments and Clinical Applications. Acta Soc Ophthalmol Jpn 90: 67—103.

Thijssen JM, Cloostermans MJTM, Verhoef WM. 1982. Ultrasonic tissue differentiation in Ophthalmology. In: JM Thijssen and D Nicholas (eds) Ultrasonic Tissue Characterization, Martinus Nijhoff, The Hague, pp. 146—158.

Trier HG, Decker D, Lepper RD, Irion KM, Reuter R, Kottow M, Müller-Breitenkamp R, Otto KJ. 1984. Ocular tissue characterization by RF-signal analysis. In: JS Hillman and MM LeMay (eds) Ophthalmic Ultrasonography Doc Ophthalmologica Proc Ser, Vol. 38, Junk, The Hague, pp. 455—466.

Retinal biometry by RF signal analysis

G. CENNAMO[1], P. DAPONTE[2] AND M. SAVASTANO[3]

Summary

Thin ocular layers can be characterized by analyzing RF echo signals in the time domain and/or in the frequency domain. In the first case the time interval between pulses reflected from anterior and posterior surfaces gives immediately the thickness measurement if the sound velocity is known. In the second case, by considering that the power spectrum can be interpreted as a plot of tissue reflectivity vs frequency, the above mentioned time interval is obtained as the inverse of the difference between two successive frequencies of the power spectrum.

The first results in a group of eyes are reported.

Introduction

Thin ocular layers can be characterized by analyzing RF echo signals in the time domain and/or in the frequency domain. In the first case the time interval between pulses reflected from anterior and posterior surfaces gives immediately the thickness measurement if the sound velocity is known. In the second case by considering that the power spectrum can be interpreted as a plot of tissue reflectivity versus frequency, the above mentioned time interval is obtained as the inverse of the difference between two successive frequencies of the power spectrum. See: Coleman and Lizzi (1979), Tane et al. (1984).

The aim of the present paper is to describe a system configuration developed at the Institute of Ophthalmology — 2nd School of Medicine — University of Naples, the measurement method and the first results obtained in a group of eyes.

[1] University Eye Clinic Naples, [2] University of Calabria, [3] C.N.R. Naples, Italy.

J. M. Thijssen (ed.) Ultrasonography in ophthalmology.
© 1988, *Kluwer Academic Publishers, Dordrecht, ISBN 978-94-010-7083-6*

System configuration

The proposed system shown in Fig. 1 consists of:

(a) an OPHTHALMOSCAN 200,
(b) a high precision RF signal pre-amplifier,
(c) a DATA 6000 Universal Waveform Analyzer with 100 MHz, 8 bit sampling plug-in,
(d) an IBM AT Personal Computer,
(e) a X—Y plotter and graphic printer.

The DATA 6000 is a Universal Waveform Analyzer (Cennamo et al., 1985) that with its high reconfigurability of both hardware and software, is useful for solving problems which arise in RF signals analysis. Modularly designed, the instrument mainframe accepts plug-in front-end modules with sampling rates of up to 100 MHz. The internal storage capability is 56 kwords and may be expanded with two 360 kbytes floppy disk drives. By means of software-programmed groups, it is possible to execute all functions, including integration, auto and cross-correlation, Fast Fourier Transforms and so on. For repetitive waveforms analysis, sweep-to-sweep weighted averages of the input signal may be generated. The instrument allows simultaneous display of present value and continuous maximum and minimum values of the envelope over any time period. Four overlaid traces can display complete signal excursion along with present value.

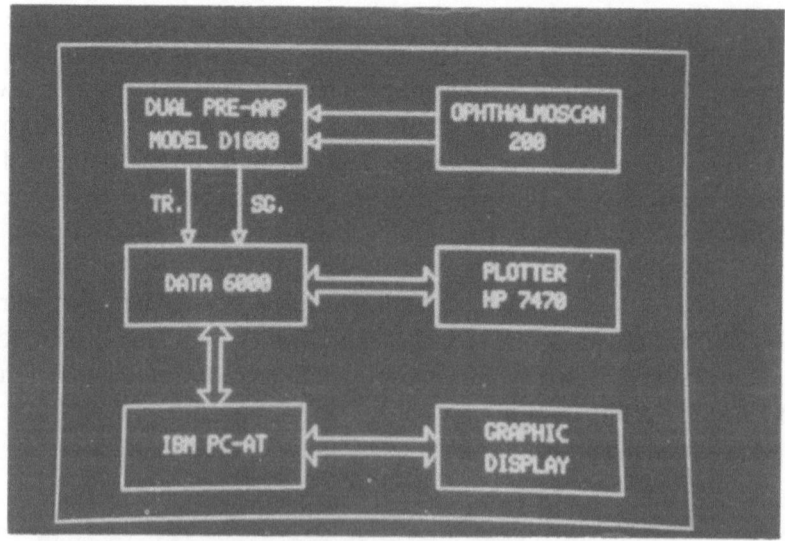

Fig. 1. Block diagram of RF data acquisition and processing system.

The DATA 6000 will accept connection to a number of appropriate plotter models at present on the market, such as the HP 7470 plotter. Because of the limited plug-in sensitivity (1 Vpp full scale), a high precision RF signal pre-amplifier is used for amplifying the trigger signal and the transducer output picked up before any analog conditioning from the OPHTHALMOSCAN 200.

To obtain a system utilizable by a medical operator and to overcome some limitations presented by the DATA 6000, of which the most important are: the keyboard is awkward to use, the graphic display is oscilloscope-oriented, programming flexibility is scanty, the Universal Waveforms Analyzer was interfaced with an IBM AT Personal Computer (Daponte and Landi 1986).

By means appropriate software, developed by the Authors, with the PC-AT it is possible to choose the gain of the pre-amplifier, as well as to send the control signals:

(a) of start and end acquisition at the DATA 6000,
(b) for storing on mass memories the RF signals acquired signals,
(c) to choose appropriately the time base. Besides the PC-AT is linked to a graphic printer.

Methods

A-scan standardized echography allows to identify by means of the KRETZTECHNIK 7200 MA only the thickness of the retina-choroid-sclera echocomplex. This method does not allow measurement of each of the ocular layers separately, therefore it is necessary to have recourse to other techniques, by using:

(a) probes with higher nominal frequencies,
(b) RF signals, appropriately drawn from the echograph,
(c) analysis in frequency domain of the RF signals.

To achieve greater accuracy the duration of the RF pulse must be as short as possible, i.e. the frequency bandwidth of the transducer must be as high as possible. The frequency response of the entire equipment is limited by the bandwidth of the RF pre-amplifier and by the highest sampling rate available (100 MHz). (Daponte and Savastano, 1986; Trier et al., 1984). In practice a focused probe at 15 MHz working frequency is used by the Authors. During the measurement the probe is placed with the direct contact method, under the careful observation of A-mode so that the beam

98

can be directed at a right angle to the posterior wall of the eye, as shown in Fig. 2. Thereby it is possible to obtain steeply rising slim high and "overloaded" echo-spikes. When human ocular tissues are examined, difficulties are due to:

(a) the tissues' multilayer structure with different sound velocities and non flat separation surfaces,
(b) scattering problems,
(c) frequency attenuation.

The RF signal coming from the posterior wall of the eye can be divided into three zones:

(a) an echo spike, produced from the interference of the echoes coming from the anterior and posterior surfaces of the retina,
(b) the echo due at the boundary surface between the choroid and the sclera,
(c) the echo from the posterior surface of the sclera.

For every eye, at each of the following positions (Cennamo et al., 1985):

h 12.00, 1.30, 3.00, 4.30, 6.00, 7.30, 9.00, 10.30

several acquisitions were carried out.

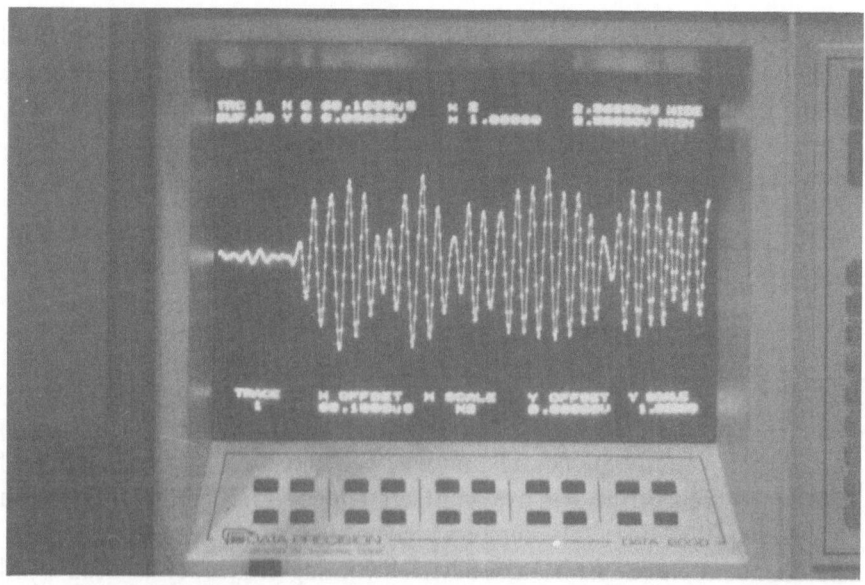

Fig. 2. RF echogram of posterior occular wall redisplayed after digitization.

Subsequently the stored data, at each position of the transducer, are averaged, after applying an alignment procedure as described by Bayer and Thijssen (1981). The result of this procedure on the echoes from the retinal area is shown in Fig. 3.

Since the retina is very thin, a direct measurement is not possible in the time domain, because of the interference of echoes coming from the anterior and posterior surfaces of the retina. Therefore, the RF signals produced from the retina are treated by Fast Fourier Transform; the power spectrum produced by this technique can be interpreted as a plot of tissue reflectivity versus frequency. By measuring the frequency interval Df (Fig. 4) an accurate retinal thickness measurement is obtained by the formula (Tane et al., 1984):

$$S = T * V * 1000 * 0.5 \ (\mu m)$$

where T is the reciprocal of the frequency interval obtained from the power spectrum. V is the sound velocity in the retina (1.54 mm/μsec) in accordance with Coleman and Lizzi (1979).

The thickness of the choroid is calculated in the time domain, by subtracting from the interval between the echo from the anterior surface of the retina and the echo from a boundary surface between the choroid and the sclera, the time thickness of the retina. From this time interval, the

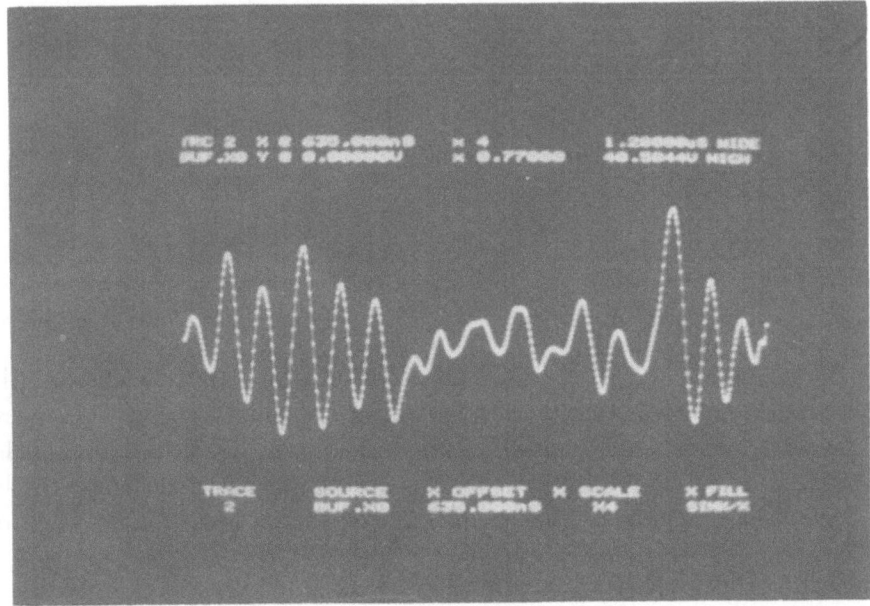

Fig. 3. Posterior wall echo complex (RF) after averaging as described by Bayer and Thijssen (1981).

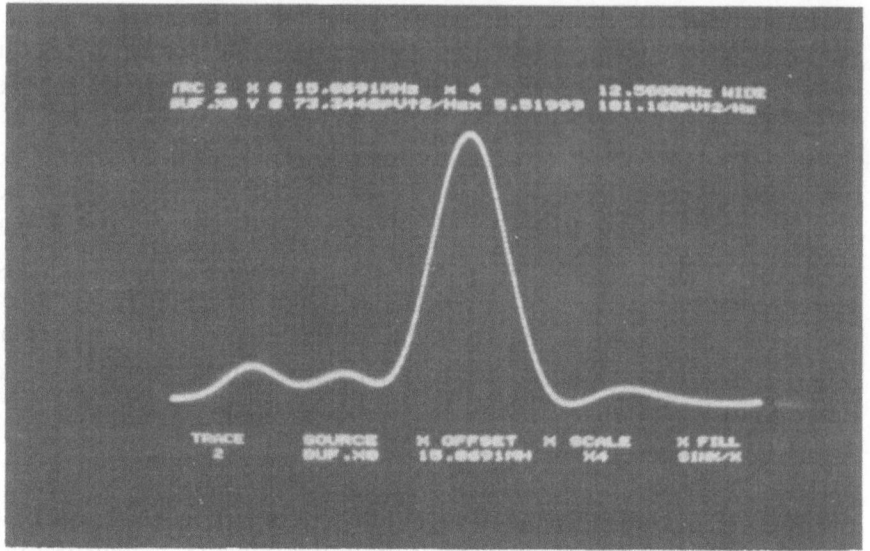

Fig. 4. Amplitude spectrum of retinal segment of the RF posterior wall echo complex (Fig. 3). Central frequency approximately 16 MHz.

thickness of the choroid is known, assuming that the sound velocity in the choroid is equal to 1.57 mm/μsec. Also the measurement of the sclera thickness is calculated in time domain, in according to the formula (Tane et al., 1984):

$$S = T * V * 1000 \times 1.2 \ (\mu m)$$

where T is the tissue interval and V is the sound velocity (1.65 mm/μsec) in the sclera.

Results

The Authors have carried out signal acquisition on 28 normal subjects (48 normal eyes) consisting of 17 men (25 eyes) and 11 women (19 eyes) between the ages of 18 and 81 years. In Fig. 5 the age-distribution of the subjects is presented. By using a statistical software package some results have been obtained. The mean thickness of the layers of the eye wall for the examined subjects is:

— 10(140 ± 11) μm for the retina;
— 10(390 ± 30) μm for the choroid;
— 10(860 ± 10) μm for the sclera.

As shown in Fig. 6 no appreciable difference has been found along some parallel at the equator site for the retinal thickness.

The authors have verified the increase of the retinal thickness versus age, and they found no variation in the thickness of choroid and sclera with age.

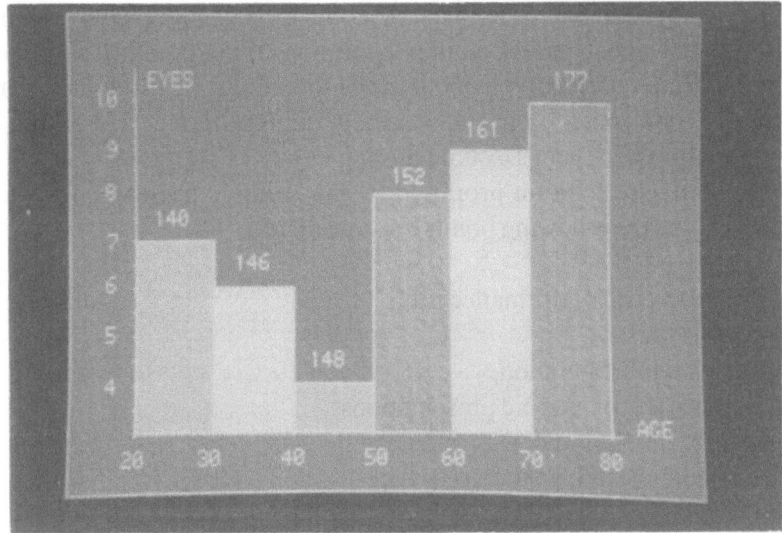

Fig. 5. Retinal thickness obtained for various age groups.

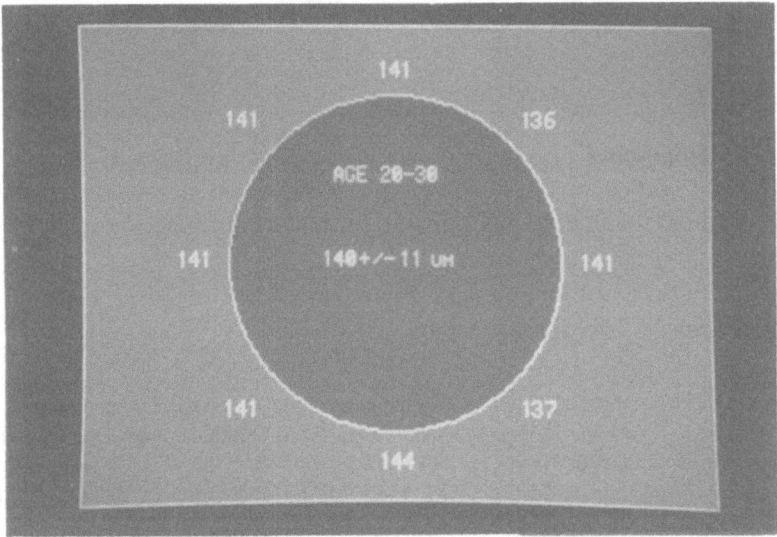

Fig. 6. Retinal thickness obtained at various meridians with the transducer applied on the equator of the globe for the age group 20—30 years.

Conclusion

The authors developed a system that permits accurate measurement of the posterior wall of living human eyes in vivo. The proposed system uses the DATA PRECISION 6000 for ultrasound signals acquisition, processing and storage. Since the rate of pulses send by the transmitter is about 1 KHz, some computations can be done in time interval between two pulses, while other, more complex operations must be done between two successive measurements. In both cases the medical operator obtains the necessary information on the selected output device during the time necessary for the patient's examination.

The hardware solution proposed by the Authors presents many advantages as far as the following points are considered:

(a) excellent cost/performance ratio,
(b) compactness,
(c) user-friendly operation,
(d) large variety of graphic presentations,
(e) storage on economic mass memories,
(f) easy and fast information retrieval.

By using the proposed system and the analysis of RF signals in time and/or frequency domain, it can be possible to measure thin layers with high accuracy. Further measurements in normal and pathologic subjects may help us to understand better the difference between the normal and morbid eyes.

Acknowledgement

The Authors thank Prof. F. Cennamo for his helpful suggestions.

References

Bayer AL, Thijssen JM. 1981. In vivo characterization of intraocular membranes. In: JM Thijssen and AM Verbeek (eds) Ultrasonography in Ophthalmology. Doc Ophthal Proc Ser, Vol. 29, Junk, The Hague, pp. 411–418.

Cennamo G, Daponte P, Savastano M. 1985. Misura dello spessore della retina in vivo. Riunione Annuale Societa Ecoftalmologica, Ferrara.

Cennamo F, Luciano AL, Savastano M. 1985. Real Time Analysis of Echographic Signal. IMACS Congress, Oslo.

Coleman DJ, Lizzi FL. 1979. In Vivo Choroidal Thickness Measurement. Amer J Ophthal 88: 369–375.

Daponte P, Landi C. 1986. The Universal Waveform Analyzer as Intelligent Measurement Apparatus. IMEKO Congress, Jena.

Daponte P, Savastano M. 1986. Noise Problems in Ophthalmic Echography. IMEKO Congress, Como.

Tane S, Kohno J, Horikoshi J, Kondo K, Ohasi K, Komatsu A, Kakehashi T. 1984. The study on the Microscopic Biometry of the Thickness of the Human Retina, Choroid and Sclera by Ultrasound. Acta Soc Ophthalmol, Jpn 88: 1412.

Trier HG, Decker D, Lepper RD, Irion KM, Reuter R, Kottow M, Muller R, Otto KJ. 1984. Ocular Tissue Characterization by RF-signal analysis: summary of the Bonn/Stuttgart in vivo-study. In: JS Hillmann and MM Lemay (eds) Ophthalmic Ultrasonography. Doc Ophthal Proc Ser, Vol. 38, Junk, The Hague, pp. 455—466.

Re-evaluation of scleral reflectivity in quantitative echography — where sclera is examined

A. YAMAMOTO, Y. BABA, T. HAYASHIDA AND A. SAWADA

Summary

Quantitative echography using A-scan equipment is one of the most effective procedures which have ultrasonic tissue differentiation more precise. In Ossoinig's method applicable to intraocular membranous structures, level of amplification of echoes from the target tissue is compared with those from the standard tissue, the sclera. The relation between histopathological findings and the value of dB has been investigated by many. However, the sclera as the standard tissue in quantitative echography has been scarcely studied. As the first step the scleral reflectivity was measured as the readings of the sensitivity control dial of the equipment, Kretztechnik 7200 MA, at the time when the peak of the spike reached to the marker line of 50% display height. The measurement was done in four direction of 3, 6, 9, and 12 o'clock meridians. The standard deviation was the smallest in the nasal meridian. No significant difference between the right and left eyes was found statistically in the superior and nasal meridians. From these results is was indicated that the scleral sensitivity in quantitative echography might be measured along with the nasal and superior meridians. To confirm these results the pattern of processed RF signals is to be studied.

Introduction

Quantitative echography using A-scan equipment, which has developed and been standardized by Ossoinig (1984) and others, is one of the most useful procedures for ultrasonic tissue differentiation. Quantitative echography is divided into two procedures according to the type of the lesion. To evaluate point-like and membrane-like lesions, it is necessary to know the difference between the two sensitivity settings for displaying the lesion spikes and the standard tissue spike to the definite level. As the standard

Department of Ophthalmology, Miyazaki Medical College, 5200 Kihara, Kiyotake, Miyazaki 889-16, Japan.

J. M. Thijssen (ed.) Ultrasonography in ophthalmology.
© 1988, *Kluwer Academic Publishers, Dordrecht. ISBN 978-94-010-7083-6*

tissue the sclera of the eye has been used. Up to date the relation between histological findings and the value of delta dB in quantitative echography has been investigated by many. However, the sclera as the standard tissue has been scarcely studied (cf. Purnell, 1980). As the first step of elucidation of reflectivity of the ocular coats including sclera, we studied the direction, in which the scleral reflectivity should be measured.

Methods and results

Study of scleral reflectivity with Kretztechnik 7200 MA

On 50 eyes of 25 individuals, 18—30 years old, without remarkable diseases except refractive errors, scleral reflectivity was studied. After local superficial anesthesia the probe was held on the bulbar conjunctiva 5—6 mm apart from the limbus in 6, 9, 12 and 3 o'clock meridian, successively. Such consecutive measurements around the cornea, clockwise in the right eye and counterclockwise in the left eye were repeated 10 times in each eye. The ultrasonic wave was aligned to hit the ocular coats perpendicularly through the center of the eyeball. When the probe was held in 6 o'clock meridian, the sclera in 12 o'clock meridian was checked. The results are shown in Table 1. The mean value in the inferior meridian was the smallest and the order was as follows:

inferior < superior < temporal < nasal

The standard deviation in the nasal meridian was the smallest and the order was as follows:

nasal < superior < inferior < temporal

The difference between two eyes in the same individual was not significant ($p < 0.05$) in the superior and nasal meridian, while it was significant ($p < 0.05$) in the inferior and temporal meridian (Table 2). The value of skewness was less than 1.00 in all four meridians. That meaned the measured values were symmetrical to the mode. The value of kurtosis was very close to 3.00 in four meridians, which meaned normal distribution. These statistical analysis showed that the measurement had high quality of confidence.

The ideal measurement should be done in those meridians, in which the measured values were stable and of the same in both eyes. On the point of view of standard deviation, reflectivity in the nasal meridian was the best and that in the superior meridian was the next. On bilaterality, the measured value in the nasal and superior meridian were equal.

Table 1. Results of measured scleral reflectivity in 4 directions.

	Mean + S.D. (dB)	Skewness	Kurtosis
Superior	36.43 ± 3.45	0.17	2.67
Nasal	38.12 ± 3.34	−0.02	2.85
Inferior	35.55 ± 3.64	0.59	3.24
Temporal	38.02 ± 3.65	0.17	3.05

Table 2. Difference in two eyes.

Superior	Not significant	($p < 0.05$)
Nasal	Not significant	($p < 0.05$)
Inferior	Significant	($p < 0.05$)
Temporal	Significant	($p < 0.01$)

Study of scleral reflectivity by deconvolution

While the values of scleral reflectivity in the preceding study were statistically stable, each value of those was not the same. For further investigation we transformed the echo signals of the ocular coats including sclera into RF signals and studied the direction, in which the pattern could be acquired best. RF signals from Kretztechnik 7200 MA were digitized and analyzed by the method of deconvolution with microcomputer.

To confirm the reliability of the analyzing system, investigation on the phantom was done. The phantom consisted of three plastic plates of 0.3 mm of thickness, arranged parallel in the water. Deconvoluted pattern from the phantom was regular. The system used in the experiment could meet the purpose.

Deconvoluted patterns of the posterior ocular coats in four meridians as mentioned before, were recorded. Those from the superior meridian were most regular and best separated into three layers (Fig. 1). These results indicated that echo patterns from the superior meridian were most stable.

Conclusion

From the results both on the direct readings of the sensitivity control dial of Kretztechnik 7200 MA and on the patterns of processed RF signals, the posterior ocular coats in the superior meridian should be used as the standard tissue in quantitative echography.

108

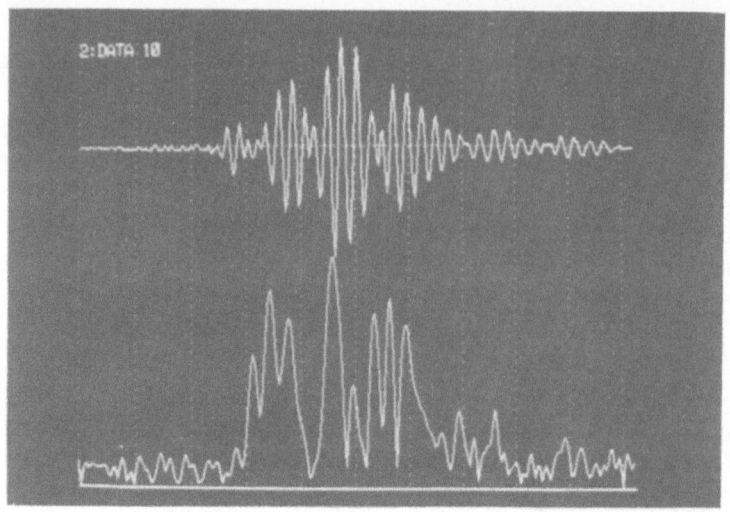

Fig. 1. Top, digitized RF signals. Bottom, signals processed by computer.

References

Ossoinig KC. 1984. Echographic detection and classification of posterior hyphemas. Ophthalmologica 189: 2—11.

Purnell EW. 1980. Ultrasonic biometry of the posterior ocular coats. Trans Am Ophthalmol Soc 38: 1027—1078.

Vitreoretinal and choroidal diseases

Ultrasonography as an aid in setting up an adequate therapy plan in the treatment of retinal detachment due to macular hole

S. CLEMENS, P. KROLL AND P. BERG

Summary

30 patients were treated at the University Eye Clinic in Münster because of retinal detachment due to a macular hole. Partial fluid gas exchange (SF_6), vitrectomy and SF_6 or vitrectomy and silicone oil instillation were used. 11 patients were examined pre- and postoperatively by ultrasonography with particular attention to the situation at the posterior pole. 18 eyes of 22 patients who were treated with SF_6 without vitrectomy were checked sonographically for staphyloma posticum. These echographical examinations enabled us to evaluate the following 3 criteria: 1. staphyloma posticum, 2. stiffness of the retina, and 3. vitreous adhesions. The presence of these conditions would mean that the prognosis could be worse if the SF_6 gas instillation was used alone. In these cases a vitrectomy should also be performed or a Klöti-Klemme procedure is useful when stiffness of the retina and staphyloma posticum is present. Preoperative ultrasonography is useful when setting up an adequate therapy plan.

Introduction

In surgery of retinal detachments due to macular holes the intraocular tamponade with SF_6 is the simplest and most atraumatic procedure besides other more invasive treatments. No disadvantage from coagulation at the macula or episcleral buckling procedure of the posterior pole in high myopic eyes has to be accepted.

Gonvers and Machemer (1982) and Tavakolian and Heimann (1985) observed vitreous adhesions at the posterior pole in retinal detachments due to macular holes which gave rise to the idea that the posterior situation of the retina and vitreous should be assessed both pre- and postoperatively. The vitreous adhesions described by these authors are usually not

Eye Hospital of the Westphalian Wilhelm's University, Münster, FRG.

J. M. Thijssen (ed.) Ultrasonography in ophthalmology.
© 1988, *Kluwer Academic Publishers, Dordrecht, ISBN 978-94-010-7083-6*

detectable by preoperative ophthalmoscopy but they are visible during vitrectomy or can be proved by synchronous swinging of the posterior detached retina when aspiration is applied. Oksala (1982) verified this phenomenon and found that early vitreous degenerations are more easily detected by ultrasonography than by ophthalmoscopy. He noted a direct correlation between vitreous degeneration and echo amplitude and quantity in A-mode (Oksala, 1978). McLeod (1979) reported on multiple vitreoretinal adhesions that are demonstrable by consecutive serial scanning of various levels within the eye. Mobile vitreous body gel that is settled against the retina should be excluded by movements of the eye so that the points of true vitreoretinal adhesions which might be tenuous could be identified (McLeod, 1977). Vitreoretinal adhesions are taken into account in surgery (Laqua, 1985). Clarkson (1984) performed a complete vitrectomy of the posterior pole to eliminate possible tractions, although vitreous adhesions could not be seen at the posterior pole pre- and intra-operatively. Lincoff (1984) reports on 7 out of 14 patients with vitreous adhesions at the posterior pole that were eliminated by vitrectomy. But vitrectomy is not a prerequisite for the gas injection. Adequate space for the injection is obtained by draining subretinal fluid (Lincoff, 1982).

The aim of these examinations was to find out

(1) how frequently a staphyloma posticum is found in a myopic eye with a macular hole and to which degree this staphyloma may hinder the reattachment of the retina;
(2) whether the detached retina is stiff or floating over the staphyloma;
(3) how much influence a vitreous adhesion can have on the reattachment of the retina.

Methods

From 1978 to 1985 30 patients were treated because of retinal detachment due to macular holes with no hole in the periphery. This rate amounts to about 1% of all our treated. retinal detachment cases, a rate that is in agreement with the literature (Smolin, 1965). Of 22 patients treated with SF_6, 11 underwent pre- and postoperative ultrasonography. 18 eyes of 22 patients who were treated with SF_6 without vitrectomy were checked sonographically for staphyloma posticum. The echographic examinations were performed with Triscan A- and B-scan (Biophysique Medical) and with Bronson Turner B-scan (High Stoy) and a Kretz 7200 MA A-scan device with contact scan. The high sensitivity of the receiver during echographic examinations permitted as many details of the vitreous to be detected as possible. Artefacts were excluded by moving the probe in axial and transverse directions. The display was free of distortion, as determined by a cylindric test reflector (Clemens, 1986). The operative treatment consisted primarily of partial fluid gas exchange (SF_6) and placing the patient in a prone position for a few days (Kroll et al., 1984). 3 cases undergoing SF_6 were primarily combined with vitrectomy. In two cases of redetachment SF_6 was combined with vitrectomy. In 10 cases a vitrectomy with silicone oil instillation was necessary; 5 of these cases were reoperations (Table 1).

The follow-up time in this study was 3 months on an average. In 11 out of 22 preoperatively examined cases, treated only with SF_6, a staphyloma posticum was detected (Fig. 1; Table 2). In all 11 cases the retinal detachment was found to be floating ultrasonographically. Of 11 patients

Table 1. Operative procedures used.

SF_6-gas tamponade without vitrectomy			Vitrectomy and SF_6-gas tamponade			Vitrectomy and intraocular silicone instillation		
Patient	Success		Patient	Success		Patient	Success	
1. W.A.	+							
2. E.D.	+							
3. W.H.	+							
4. H.E.	+							
5. B.M.	+							
6. W.W.	+							
7. T.H.	+					*Primarily*		
8. B.H.	+					26. L.F.	cataract	
9. T.H.	+					27. P.M.	+	
10. F.A.	+					28. S.A.	+	
11. W.A.	+		*Primarily*			29. L.A.	cataract; +	
12. S.H.	+		23. P.E.	+		30. R.L.	+	
13. K.M.	+		24. M.M.	+		*Secondarily*		
14. M.G.	+		25. S.M.	−	↔	25. S.M.	−	
15. S.K.	−			↔		15. S.K.	+	
16. F.E.	−			↔		16. F.E.	+	
17. W.M.	−			↔		17. W.M.	+	
18. M.G.	−			↔		18. M.G.	−	
			Secondarily					
19. G.R.	−	↔	19. G.R.	+				
20. M.G.	−	↔	20. M.G.	+				
21. W.J.	Reoperation							
22. V.G.	refused							

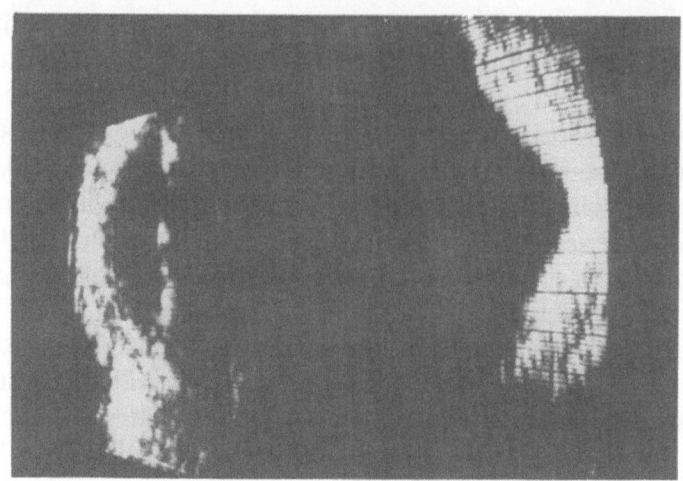

Fig. 1. B-scan of a myopic eye with staphyloma posticum 75 DB Triscan.

Table 2. Intraocular SF$_6$ gas tamponade without vitrectomy.

Patient	Preoperative visual acuity	Postoperative visual acuity	Myopia	Echographical staphyloma	Success
1. W.A.	FC	1/50	−11.0	+	+
2. E.D.	1/35	1/35	−18.0	+	+
3. W.H.	1/20	0.05	−11.5		+
4. H.E.	1/15	0.1	−14.0	−	+
5. B.M.	LP	0.1	−14.5	+	+
6. W.W.	1/35	1/20	−11.0	−	+
7. T.H.	0.05; a	0.15	−10.0	−	+
8. B.H.	MH	1/35	−8.0	−	+
9. T.H.	MH	1/15	−10.0	−	+
10. F.A.	MH	1/35	±0	−	+
11. W.A.	1/15	0.1	−20.0	+	+
12. S.H.	1/50	1/20	−2.0	−	+
13. K.M.	1/20	1/20	−5.0	+	+
14. M.G.	MH	0.1	−14.0	+	+
15. S.K.	MH; b	FC	−11.0	+	−
16. F.E.	1/25	LP	−12.0		−
17. W.M.	0.1; b	0.05	−16.0	+	−
18. M.G.	MH	0.1	−18.0	+	−
19. G.R.	LP; a	MH	−22.0	+	−
20. M.G.	First operation elsewhere; a		−12.0		−
21. W.J.	0.1; a	1/50	−8.5	+	Reoperation refused
22. V.G.	MH	MH	−15.0		

LP = light projection; MH = movements of hands; FC = finger counting; a = amblyopia; b = oculus ultimus.

examined by echography before and after instillation of SF_6 without vitrectomy in only 5 cases a connexion of the vitreous with the macular tissue was proved preoperatively. Postoperatively premacular condensation in the vitreous was found in 10 of 11 cases (Figs. 2—4; Table 3). After SF_6 and vitrectomy no echos from the premacular vitreous could be seen in any of these cases. 2 of 5 cases with preoperatively detected vitreoretinal adhesions could not be successfully operated on by SF_6 instillation alone (Fig. 4). In both cases there was also a staphyloma posticum. In 6 of the 11 echographically examined cases it was possible to achieve a reattachment of the retina only with SF_6 instillation. In 11 cases with preoperatively detected staphyloma posticum by ultrasound, 6 could be operated successfully by SF_6 gas alone (Table 4). In 7 cases without staphyloma all operative results were successful. The success rate of cases with preoperative vitreoretinal adhesions is equal to the rate of cases without adhesions (Table 5). In 3 cases of both preoperative vitreous adhesions at the macula and staphyloma posticum, only 1 case was successfully operated on (Table 6). In the 2 cases of no success, a condensated or adherent vitreous is seen in contact with the detached retina (Fig. 5). In one case of no success, there is no vitreoretinal adhesion (Fig. 6).

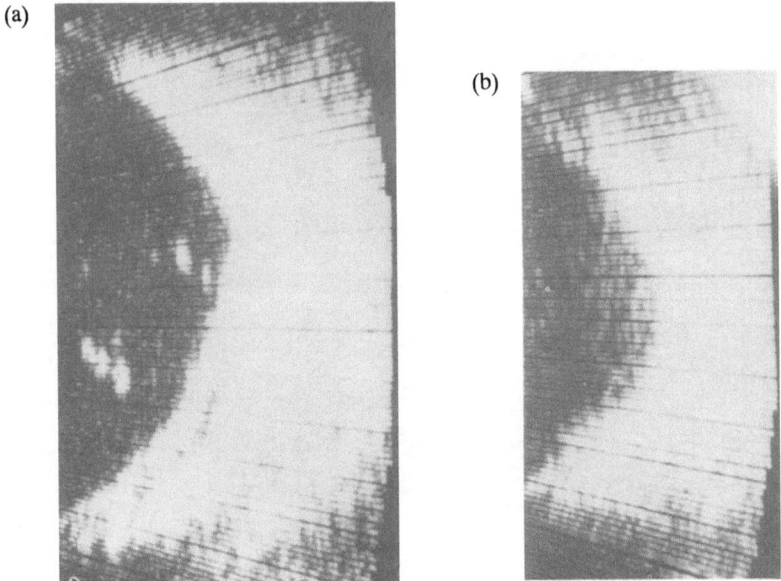

Fig. 2. (a) B-scan retinal detachment, vitreoretinal adhesions, staphyloma posticum before SF_6 gas instillation. (b) Situation after reattachment with SF_6 gas instillation. Augmented echoes in the vitreous cavity of the staphyloma. 85 DB Triscan.

116

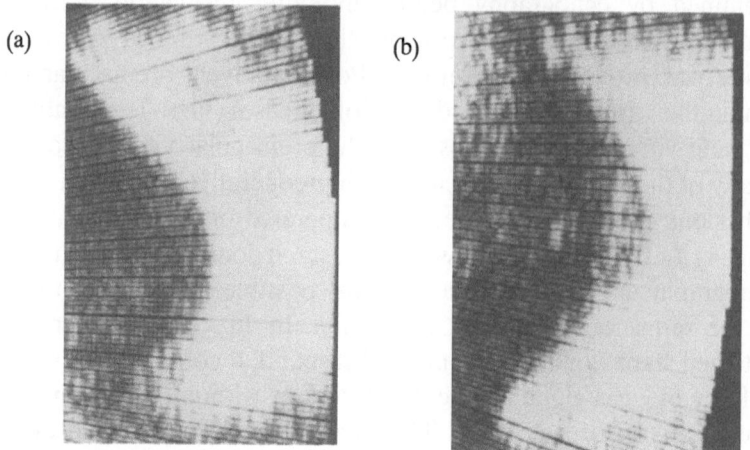

Fig. 3. (a) B-scan staphyloma posticum, retinal detachment (not visible because of high reflectivity in order to exclude vitreoretinal adhesions). (b) Same eye postoperatively after SF_6 gas instillation. Condensation of vitreous in the staphyloma. 85 DB Triscan.

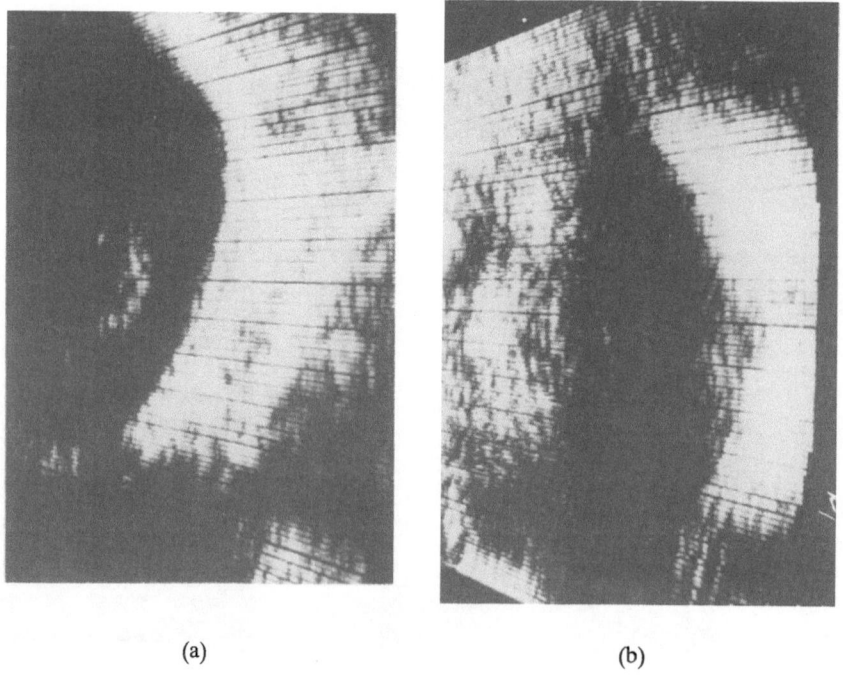

Fig. 4. (a) Retinal detachment, staphyloma posticum, echoes in the vitreous without connexion to the retina before SF_6 gas instillation. Right side: Same eye, staphyloma posticum with reattached retina and condensation of vitreous. 85 DB Triscan.

Table 3. Echographic detection of vitreous adhesions. Situation of posterior vitreous before and after operation, echographic detection of staphyloma, success.

Patient	Preoperative vitreous adhesions at the macula	Postoperative premacular vitreous condensation	Staphyloma	Success
1. W.A.	−	+	+	+
2. E.D.	−	+	+	+
5. B.M.	+	+	+	+
7. T.H.	+	+	−	+
11. W.A.	−	+	+	+
12. S.H.	+	+	−	+
15. S.K.	−	+	+	−
17. W.M.	+	+	+	−
18. M.G.	−	−	+	−
19. G.R.	−	+	+	−
21. W.J.	+	+	+	−

Table 4. SF$_6$ without vitrectomy staphyloma and success.

	Success	No success	Σ
Echographically no staphyloma	7	0	7
Echographically staphyloma	6	5	11
Total	13	5	18

Table 5. SF$_6$ without vitrectomy vitreoretinal adhesions and success.

	Success	No success	Σ
No vitreoretinal adhesions preoperatively	3	3	6
Vitreoretinal adhesions preoperatively proved	3	2	5
Total	6	5	11

Table 6. SF$_6$ without vitrectomy staphyloma and vitreoretinal adhesions and success.

No vitreoretinal adhesion, no staphyloma	0	0
Both vitreoretinal adhesion and staphyloma	1	2

118

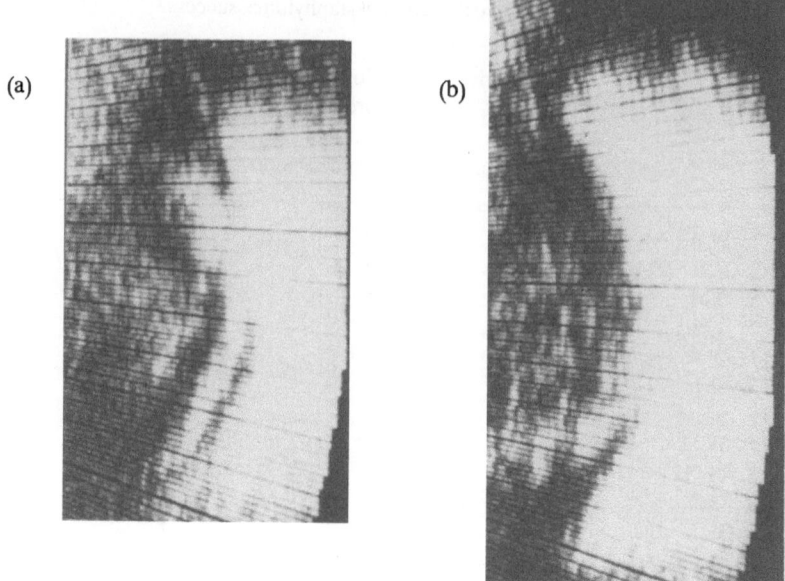

(a)

(b)

Fig. 5. (a) B-scan staphyloma posticum, retinal detachment, vitreoretinal adhesion after SF_6 gas instillation, no operative success. (b) Same situation in another eye, condensation of vitreous in both cases. 85 DB Triscan.

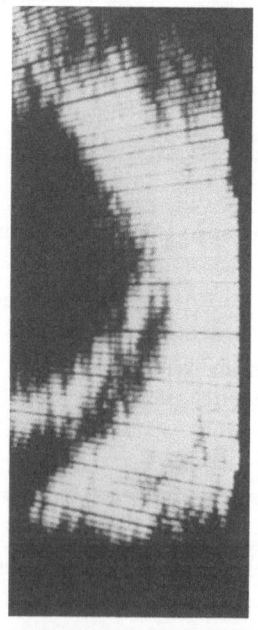

Fig. 6. B-scan retinal detachment, staphyloma posticum, no vitreoretinal adhesions, situation after SF_6 gas instillation, no operative success.

Discussion

According to these results in cases of staphyloma with floating retina a reattachment can be achieved by SF_6 gas instillation and prone positioning of the patient postoperatively. If the SF_6 gas instillation is not successful, combining SF_6 with vitrectomy or vitrectomy together with silicone oil instillation may result in reattachment (Kroll, 1984, 1985). Reattachment is possible with SF_6 gas instillation and prone positioning even in cases with preoperatively detected vitreous adhesions at the macula. Vitreous adhesion to the macular tissues may hinder reattachment in cases undergoing SF_6 gas instillation, as in some of these cases vitrectomy may be necessary in addition. No secondary vitreous adhesion at the posterior pole after vitrectomy was detected in our examinations. The augmentation of vitreous echos, particularly at the macula, after SF_6 gas instillation was surprising. This phenomenon confirms the theory of Lincoff and Machemer that SF_6 gas alone and prone positioning result in a compression of the vitreous against the macula (Lincoff, 1984; Machemer, 1983). In a primate model the alteration of vitreous after compression by a perfluorocarbon gas could be proven by electron microscopy. The hyaloronic acid content was diminished (Lincoff, 1984). These histological changes are suitable for augmentation of the sonographic vitreous signals. Zakov et al. (1983) found that vitreous adhesions are difficult to find ultrasonographically and during surgery. In our results vitreoretinal adhesions are detectable preoperatively by ultrasound and intraoperatively.

The success of the operation can be influenced particularly by a combination of staphyloma and preoperative vitreous adhesions. These conditions mean that the prognosis is worse if SF_6 gas instillation is used alone. When additionally vitrectomy or vitrectomy and silicone oil instillation were used, reattachment could be achieved in these cases.

References

Clarkson JG. 1984. Treatment of retinal detachment with macular holes. 14th Meeting Club Jules Gonin. Lausanne.

Clemens S, Kroll P, Busse H, Berg P (in press). Ultrasonography as a routine examination before treatment of retinal detachment due to macular hole. Graefe's Arch Clin Exp Ophthalmol.

Gonvers M, Machemer R. 1982. A new approach to treating retinal detachments with macular holes. Am J Ophthalmol 94: 468—472.

Kroll P, Clemens S, Busse H. 1984. Ultrasonic findings and treatment of retinal detachments due to macular holes. 14th Meeting Club Jules Gonin. Lausanne.

Kroll P, Busse H, Berg P. 1985. Intraokulare Therapie makulalochbedingter Netzhautablösungen. Klin Mbl Augenheilk 187: 499—502.

120

Laqua H. 1985. Die Behandlung der Ablatio mit Makulaforamen nach der Methode von Gonvers und Machemer. Klin Mbl Augenheilk 186: 13—17.

McLeod D et al. 1977. Rapid B-scanning of the vitreous. Brit J Ophthalmol 61: 437—445.

McLeod D, Restori M. 1979. Ultrasonic examination in severe diabetic eye disease. Brit J Ophthalmol 63: 533—538.

Lincoff H, Kreissig I, Brodie S, Wilcox L. 1982. Expanding gas bubbles for the repair of tears in the posterior pole. 13th Meeting Club Jules Gonin. Cordoba.

Lincoff H, Kreissig I. 1984. The nature of a "gas vitrectomy". 14th Meeting Club Jules Gonin. Lausanne.

Lincoff H, Kreissig I et al. 1984. Gas vitrectomy in a primate model. 14th Meeting Club Jules Gonin. Lausanne.

Machemer R. 1983. Vitreous compression instead of vitrectomy. Vail Vitreous Surgery Seminar. Vail, Colorado.

Oksala A. 1978. Ultrasonic findings in the vitreous body at various ages. Graefe's Arch Clin Exp Ophthalmol 207: 275—280.

Oksala A. 1982. Ultrasonic observation of the vitreous body immediately following cataract extraction. Graefe's Arch Clin Exp Ophthalmol 219: 292—294.

Smolin G. 1965. Statistical analysis of retinal holes and tears. Am J Ophthalmol 60: 1055.

Tavakolian U, Heimann K. 1985. Zur chirurgischen Behandlung von Amotiones mit zentralen Foramina bei hoher Myopie. Fortschr. Ophthalmol 82: 553—555.

Zakov ZN et al. 1983. Ultrasonographic mapping of vitreoretinal abnormalities. Am J Ophthalmol 96: 622—631.

Uveal effusion syndrome — idiophathic serous detachment of the choroid, ciliary body and retina

Clinical and Echographic features of a case examined with standardized echography

J. SCHUTTERMAN

Summary

A 72 year old woman who presented with what was clinically first thought to be an intraocular neoplasm in her left eye was examined clinically and with standardized echography. She was found to have a superior choroidal detachment combined with an inferior retinal detachment and dilated episcleral vessels. Her right eye showed only subtle changes. Following steroid treatment there was a regression after a few months. Less than a year later she presented with symptoms mainly from her right eye which was found to have a high bullous nonrhegmatogenous retinal detachment and a visual acuity which was highly dependent on her position. The echographic findings will be discussed.

Case report

A year ago a 72 year old Swedish lady was referred by a practising ophthalmologist to our Clinic in Södersjukhuset with a suspicion of a malignant melanoma behind a retinal detachment of her left eye. The lady had complained of curtainlike visual disturbances of her left eye for two or three weeks and the referring ophthalmologist had found corrected visual acuity in the right eye 20/30, left eye 20/35, slight conjunctival injection, slight lens opacities in both eyes and a superonasal retinal detachment of the left eye having been interpreted as harbouring a tumour.

IOP on admission was 14 right eye, 20 left eye and between 7 and 3 o'clock meridians were bullous choroidal elevations all the way to the ciliary body. At 3 o'clock posterior to the equator a horse shoe retinal tear was seen and below it a low retinal detachment. *Transillumination* failed to show any shadow either with diascleral or transpupillary approach.

Standardized echography of the left eye showed a kissing choroidal like

Dept. Of Ophthalmology, Südersjukhuset, Stockholm, Sweden.

J. M. Thijssen (ed.) Ultrasonography in ophthalmology.
© 1988, *Kluwer Academic Publishers, Dordrecht, ISBN 978-94-010-7083-6*

picture nasally and superiorly respectively. Centrally and inferiorly was a low somewhat stiff retinal detachment. The right *asymptomatic* eye showed pronounced choroidal thickening rendering the retinochoroidal layer 3 mm and the increased thickness was due to a thickened choroidal spike on standardized A-scan with lowered system sensitivity. Both *orbits* were echographically within normal limits.

The lady was sent home to await elective retinal surgery but on readmission the bilateral episcleral congestion was more pronounced and it was decided to regard the case as an inflammatory disorder and to treat it accordingly. Left eye had by now visual acuity of 20/60 and both topical and systemic highdose steroid treatment (60 mg Prednisolon daily) was installed.

A *medical screening* program was also effected before treatment. Physical examination disclosed a systolic cardiac murmur and chest X-rays showed cardiac enlargement (910/570 cc) but no pulmonary congestion. ECG showed coronary disease. There was also an arterial hypertension with blood pressure 170/90 with medication. Laboratory findings were slightly elevated polyclonal increase of IgM in serum and in CSF especially antibodies towards smooth muscles and glomeruli. Also LD 1/LD 2 isoenzyme ratio was increased and there was also a slightly increased level of LD 5 isoenzyme. However blood counts, ESR, ANF, reumatoid factor, complement C3, C4, CSF-IgG, serum-IgG and spinal protein ratio were all within normal limits.

The diagnosis of uveal effusion syndrome (idiopathic serous detachment of the choroid ciliary body and the retina) was now considered. On steroid treatment visual acuity left eye rose to 20/50 after 2.5 week and when it reached 20/35 treatment was tapered. On vacation in the Mediterranean however she was caught with a fever episode without headache or malaise and she had a relapse of visual complaints now also effecting her right eye soon thereafter. Visual acuity was right eye 20/25, Left eye 20/50. In the right fundus pigmentations were seen but no significant retinal or choroidal elevation. In the left eye there was a ciliary body detachment and bullous superior retinal detachment and choroidal detachment. A second steroid treatment period was installed, acuity rising to 20/25 right eye and 20/40 left eye and steroids were tapered again. A new visual deterioration followed. Visual acuity right eye came down to counting fingers 0.5 m despite 60 mg of Prednisolon and there was an anterior chamber flare.

Fluorescein angiography showed leopard spot pigment epithelial changes.

Echography of the right eye (Fig. 1) showed combined retinal and choroidal detachments with pronounced subretinal fluid shift. In supine position both A- and B-scan showed a high detachment over the entire posterior pole but in an upright position the detachment was located

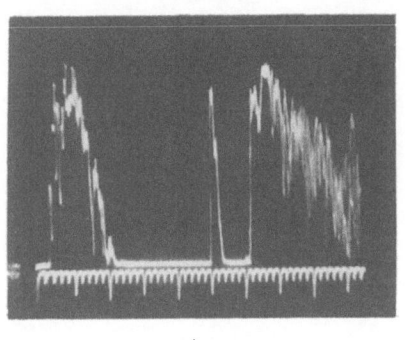 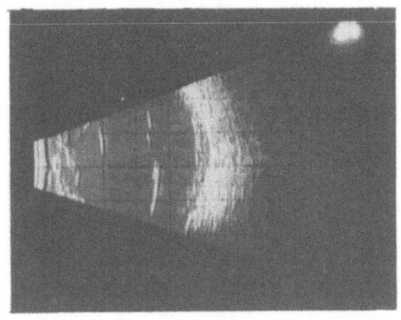

A   B

Fig. 1. A. A-mode of eye showing high retinal peak. B. B-mode of eye showing retinal detachment and choroidal thickening.

inferiorly. The pars plana was elevated 3—4 mm and there was also a significant choroidal thickening with retinochoroidal layer in 2.3—2.5 mm range in the posterior pole.

Systemic steroids now with Betametazon resulted in rising visual acuity and at latest examination April 14 visual acuity right eye was 20/90, left cye 20/40 and thc detachment right eye was now, in an upright position, not reaching the inferior arcade. Both eyes, especially left, showed increasing cataract changes.

Conclusion

A case of spontaneous idiopathic serous detachment of the choroid, ciliary body and retina examined with standardized echography and showing similar clinical and echographic changes as described by Gass and Jallow 1982 was described. The nature of this disease entity remains unclear, Gass and Jallow suggested "one or more congenital structural abnormality, including abnormal thickness of the sclera, aplasia, hypoplasia, and aberrant course of the vortex veins, that predispose the eye to develop obstruction to venous outflow".

References

Gass JDM, Jallow S. 1982. Idiopathic Serous Detachment of the Choroid, Ciliary body and Retina (Uveal Effusion Syndrome). Ophthalmology 89: 1018—1032.

Michaelson IC, Benezra D. 1980. Textbook of the Fundus of the Eye. Churchill-Livingstone, 3rd Ed, pp. 750—751.

Ossoinig KC. 1979. Standardized echography: Basic principles, clinical applications, and results. In: RC Dallow (ed) International Ophthalmology Clinics: Ophthalmic Ultrasonograpy: Comparative techniques 19/4: 127—210.

Fig. ... Appearance of ... growing bulk ... retinal ... B, B ... nerve of eye, showing retinal detachment and degenerative areas.

initiation. The pars plana was elevated 3–11 mm and there was also a significant choroidal thickening with peritumorical layer in 2.5–3.5 mm range in the posterior pole.

Systemic therapy now with Betamethasone resulted in tissue intact early and at tumor circumscribe ArcC 14 (L7.0) active figure was 20.0 at that level 20.0 and then clearing of right eye was seen, in tumoral peak re-appearing, the intraocular areas. Both eyes of each the left showed increasing tumoral change.

Conclusion

A case of spontaneous regression across detachment of retina detected under and retina examined with simultaneous ultrasonography and showing similar clinical and histogenetic changes as described by Reese and Jahnke 1962 was described. The nature of this disease entity carries unclear. Cross-challenge suggested one or more genetically structural abnormality in finding anomalous thickness of the sclera, splasm, hyperplasia, and abnormal control of the vortex veins that predispose the eye to developing changes to the vascular outflow.

References

Reese AB, Jahnke S (1962) Magnetic resonance examination of the retinal. Collect. Collect. Trans. Ophthalmology conference ASCo Ophthalmology 88: 601–607.

Michaelson R, Hanover I (1960) Textbook of the biology of the eye. Churchill, Edinburgh, pp 67–74.

Osterlin K (1978) Scandinavian ophthalmology. Basic physiological clinical applications and aspects. In: Proc international Ophthalmology Congr. Ophthalmol. Conf. clinical ophthalmology symposium 1978, pp 91–102.

Echographic follow-up of Coats's disease

V. MAZZEO, L. RAVALLI[1], G. GALLI AND P. PERRI

Summary

Coats' disease is the more common differential diagnosis with retino-blastoma. While many cases were examined only once, 5 cases were followed up with echography for different periods (from 6 months up to 5 years). Depending on the stage of the disease different echopatterns were found. They went from an increased retino- choroidal layer thickness to a total retinal detachment in which the retina was no more recognizable. The subretinal fluid changed its acoustic characteristics from case to case and in the long run. It was rather echogenic in the majority of cases. Some cases seem to have a slower tendency to reach the total detachment stage, while others seem to belong to a "rush type".

Introduction

Coats's disease is a unilateral vascular disorder of the retina. Its cause is unknown, but electron microscopy studies in the early stages seemed to have shown a break-down of the blood-retinal barrier at the endothelial layer of retinal vessels, followed by aneurysmal dilatations and teleangiec-tasis (Tripathi and Ashton, 1971).

The purpose of this paper is to describe in detail the pathological changes in the retina, occurring with time, together with the echographic patterns. The echopatterns of Coats's disease have been almost invariably considered as differential diagnosis with retinoblastoma. This diagnosis is not always easy especially in the advanced stages where a complete retinal detachment has already occurred. At the last SIDUO meeting, Haik et al. (1984) stressed the importance of other ancillary tests, such as Compu-terized Tomography and Nuclear Magnetic Resonance, in order to achieve a correct diagnosis.

[1] University Eye Clinic, Ophthalmic Department U.S.L., Ferrara, Italy.

J. M. Thijssen (ed.) Ultrasonography in ophthalmology.
© 1988, *Kluwer Academic Publishers, Dordrecht, ISBN 978-94-010-7083-6*

Materials and methods

This paper is mostly based on 5 cases of Coats's disease. The average follow-up was 38 months (from 7 to 64 months), the mean age of the subjects (4 males and 1 female) was 73 months when examined for the first time, the youngest being 10 months, the oldest 18 years. Each subject had a unilateral form of the disease and was examined with the A-scan technique (Kretztechnik 7200 MA) and since 1981 also with contact B-scan technique (Ophthalmoscan 200, Cilco Inc.). Because of the age of the subjects, only two of them underwent an immersion technique examination for the latter method.

No patient was submitted to any kind of treatment.

Results

After the aneurysmal dilatations an teleangiectasis have occurred in the retinal vessels, the plasma leakage gives origin to the intraretinal and sub-retinal exudates. Thus in this stage a marked thickening of the attached retina occurs and later the thickened or normal retina can detach (Fig. 1). It must not be forgotten that all the pathological lesions of this disease occur in and under the retina.

As clearly shown in the micrograph reported in Spencer's Ophthalmic Pathology (1985) large areas of retinoschisis can occur because of the marked intraretinal fluid accumulation, thus forming a kind of retinal cyst. Intra- and/or subretinal haemorrhages are frequent while blood is mixed to the lipid-rich exudate. If organization of this detachment occurs fibrous tissue can develop, with a lipid-rich exudate presenting some cholesterol slits. When this occurs in the macular area this organization gives origin to a disciform sar. A hyperplastic retinal pigmented epithelium and some calcification can easily be found into this scar (Fig. 1, 4th row).

The evolution of the disease may differ from case to case. Sometimes the retina appears to reattach spontaneously, when the fluid of the exudate is absorbed and subsequent organization takes place (Fig. 1, 2nd and 3rd rows). A complete retinal detachment can be expected, but the time-lag between the discovery of the illness and its occurrence is unknown. Among our cases, apart from the oldest patient who had already had a total retinal detachment, a rather rush-type of the disease was seen in the only girl (Fig. 2, 1st and 2nd rows). In one of the boys on the other hand, it took five years to progress from retinal thickening to a complete retinal detachment, in which the retina was no longer recognizable (Fig. 2, 3rd row). In other cases the completely detached retina assumed a convoluted appearance

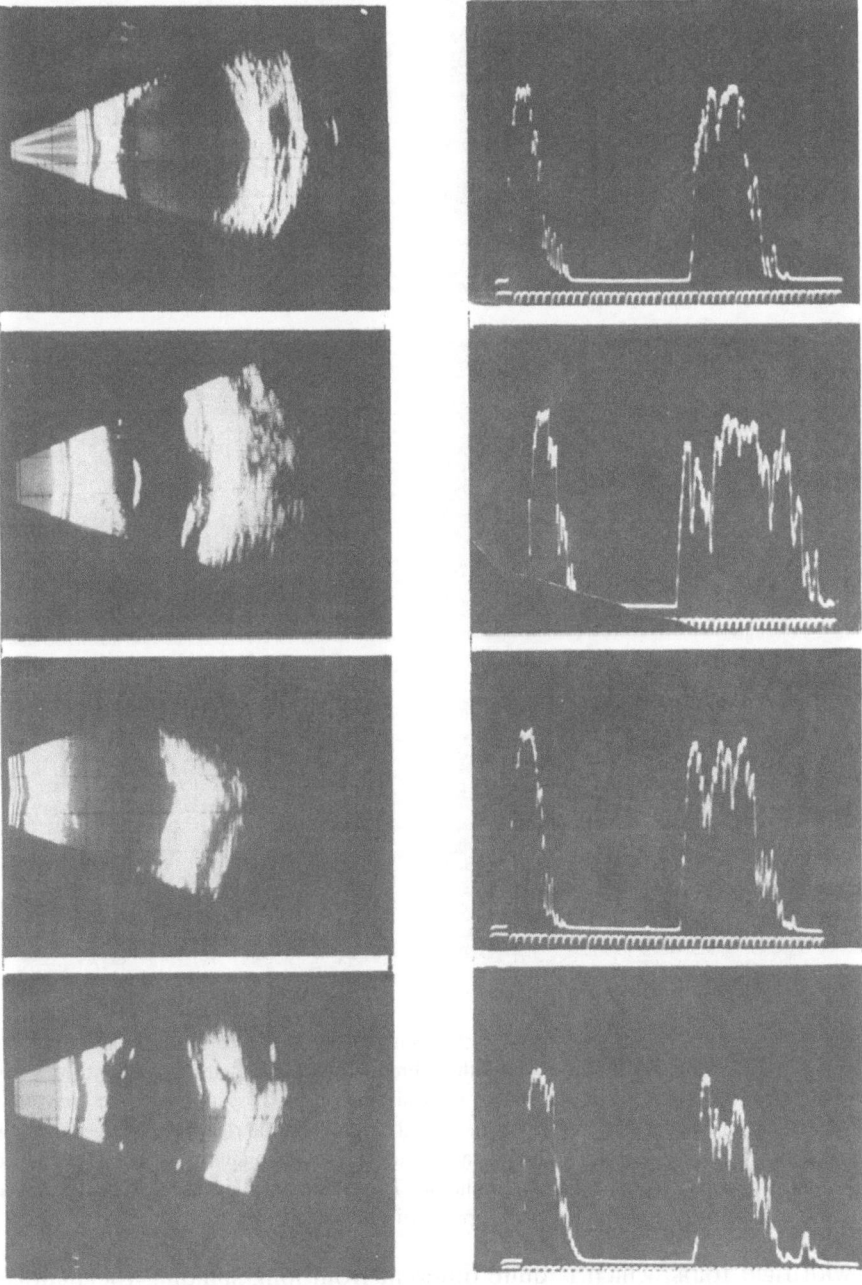

Fig. 1. Coat's disease at different clinical stages. 1st row (from above): irregularities of the retina are clearly visible on both B- and A-scans. 2nd row: the detached retina is thickened, a subretinal fluid exists. 3rd row: same case of row 2. The thickened retina spontaneously reattached. 4th row: organized subretinal exudate containing calcification creates acoustic shadowing.

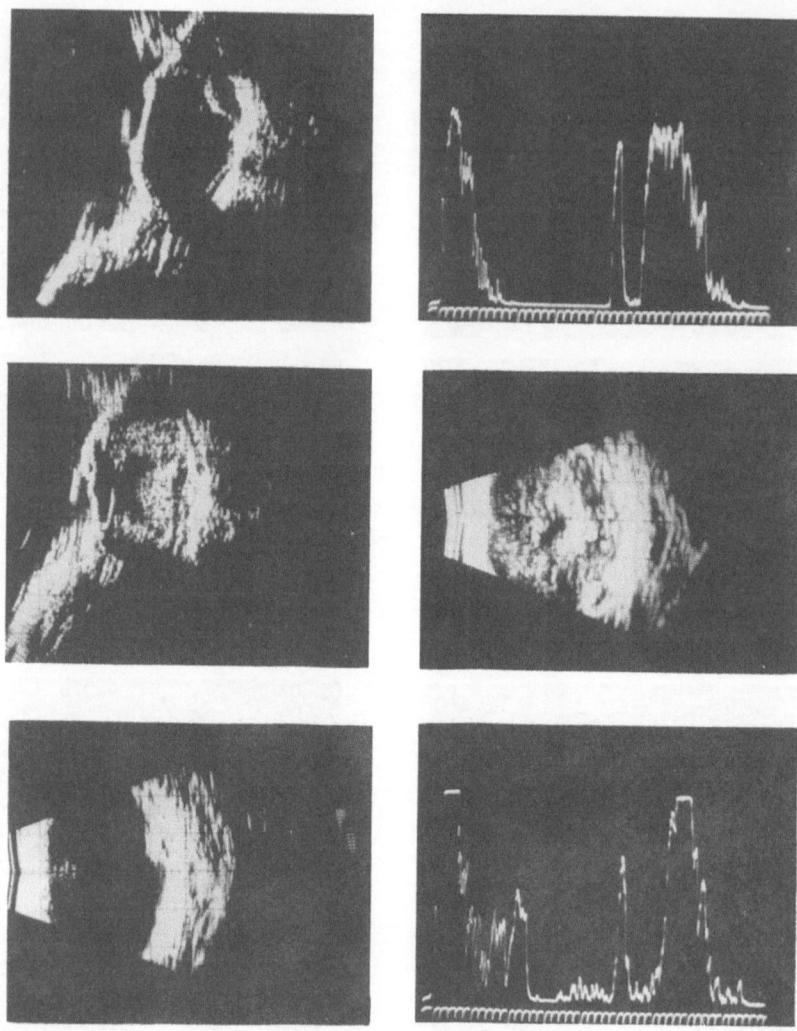

Fig. 2. Coat's disease progression. 1st row from above: total retinal detachment. The retina clearly shows leaflets with different width. Subretinal fluid is not clear. 2nd row: same case after 7 months. The retina is no longer recognizable on the B-scan, notice the convoluted appearance of what is supposed to be the retinal surface. On the right side the A-scan shows the typical pattern of a total retinal detachment. The retinal leaflet near to the transducer produces a large echo of medium amplitude. The subretinal fluid near to the transducer shows fast movements produced by the lipid particles.

with rigid folds, which is quite different from long standing rhegmatogen retinal detachment.

Comments

In our experience the echopattern of Coats's disease seems to adhere very well to the pathological findings. The irregularly distributed retinal thickening, which invariably occurs both in early and late stages is, in our opinion, the real pathognomonic echopattern of this disease. The characteristics of the subretinal fluid change widely, by going from proteinaceous material to lipid-rich fluid or blood. When organized this simulates a solid retinal detachment. These characteristics had already been mentioned by Diamond et al. (1981), Mazzeo (1985), Mazzeo et al. (1985). The typical fast movements of free cholesterol particles (Till and Hauff, 1981) do not seem to belong to all cases of Coats's disease or to the early stages of the retinal detachment, especially in the juvenile form of the disease.

A very difficult echographic diagnosis concerns the retinal angiomatosis of von Hippel, if single or multiple hamartomatous masses are not clearly visible. When these angiomatous tumours are present they create one or more dome-shaped masses whose echographic characteristics have not yet been well established owing to the rarity of this disease. In the long run, von Hippel's disease also gives origin to a diffuse, quite regular retinal thickening, except for the vascular hamartomas and to a total retinal detachment.

The presence of calcification in the organized subretinal tissue can simulate retinoblastoma. A few cases of pseudogliomas containing calcification and false positive echographic diagnosis of retinoblastomas have been reported in the literature (Ossoinig, 1982). One case of Coats's disease containing calcification was reported by Goes (1984) and two cases by Varene and Poujol (1984). On the other hand one must always remember the existence of retinoblastomas without calcifications (Galli et al., 1984; Ossoinig and Reshef, 1984), even if very rare, because their misdiagnoses is life threatening.

When a total retinal detachment has already occurred, thus creating a leukocoria and problems of differential diagnosis at clinical inspection, one must look for the retinal thickening and its convoluted appearance.

As suggested by Haik et al. (1984) when the echographic diagnosis is controversial all clinical methods must be used in order to avoid a false negative diagnosis of retinoblastoma.

References

Diamond DJ, Ossoinig KC, Fischer JL. 1984. Ecografia. In: GA Peyman, DR Sanderson and MF Goldberg (eds) Oftalmologia. Principi e pratica Verduci — Roma, pp. 1384—1469.

Galli G, Perri P, Mazzeo V. 1984. Retinoblastoma of the diffuse type on the A- and B-scan. S.I.D.U.O. X, abstract book, St Petersburg Beach, Fl, p. 54.

Goes F. 1984. Ultrasonographic aid in the diagnosis of retinoblastoma cases. Docum Opthtalmol Proc Series 38: 81—92.

Haik BC, Ellsworth RM, Smith ME, Saint Louis L. 1984. Ancillary diagnostic testing in the differentiation of Retinoblastoma and advanced Coats' disease. S.I.D.U.O. X Abstract book. St Petersburg Beach Fl, p. 53.

Mazzeo V. 1985. Ultrasonography in early diagnosis of pathologic conditions which produce a visual handicap in infancy. Acta Med Romana 23: 323—332.

Mazzeo V, Rossi A, Galli G, Perri P. 1985. Pediatric eye diseases: a challenge for ultra-sound. In: RW Gill and M Dadd (eds) "WFUMB 85". Pergamon Press, Sidney, p. 427.

Ossoinig KC. 1982. Advances in diagnostic ultrasound. Acta XXIV International Congress of Ophthalmology, I, pp. 89—114.

Ossoinig KC, Reshef DS. 1984. The echographic diagnosis of non-calcified retinoblastoma. S.I.D.U.O. X Abstract book, St Petersburg Beach, Fl, p. 54.

Spencer WH. 1985. Ophthalmic pathology. An atlas and Textbook. Vol. 2, Saunders, Philadelphia.

Till P, Hauff W. 1981. Differential diagnostic results of clinical echography in intraocular tumours. Doc Ophtalmol Proc Series 29: 91—95.

Tripathi R, Ashton N. 1971. Electron microscopical study of Coat's disease. Brit J Ophtal 55: 289—301.

Varene B, Poujol J. 1984. Apport de l'echographie au diagnostic des retinoblastomas J Fr Ophtal 7: 51—56.

Intraocular foreign body localization by A- and B-scan echography

S. RIZZO, M. P. BARTOLOMEI, M. PUCCIONI AND A. ROMANI[1]

Summary

Six patients with intraocular foreign bodies of various nature have been examined by A- and B-scan echography; the value of A- and B-scan echography in order to assess the location of the foreign bodies and the vitreo-retinal situation is discussed.

Introduction

Echography is an important examination technique for the localization of intraocular foreign bodies (I.O.F.B.) and for evaluating damage to the eye caused by trauma.

The value of echography in the diagnosis of intraocular foreign bodies (I.O.F.B.) was emphasized in 1959 by Oksala, successively by Bronson (1965), Penner and Passmore (1966), Ossoinig (1969) and Bellone and Gallenga (1969a, b), Coleman (1971).

Ultrasonographic examination has proved to be an essential compliment to radiography in the diagnosis of I.O.F.B.: with this technique it is also possible to detect nonradiopaque foreign bodies (Bronson, 1964; Coleman et al., 1977; Penner and Passmore, 1966; Poujol, 1981).

Subjects and methods

Six patients with an I.O.F.B. were examined. In all these patients a X-ray examination of the orbit and echography of the eyeball were performed: the echographic examination was performed with a ES-100 (Topcon), Scanner 10 MHz. (cases III and IV) and a Xenotec (Cooper Vision), Scanner 8 MHz. (cases I, II, V, VI).

[1] Viale Petrarca, 2, 50124 — Firenze, Italy.

J. M. Thijssen (ed.) Ultrasonography in ophthalmology.
© 1988, Kluwer Academic Publishers, Dordrecht, ISBN 978-94-010-7083-6

132

Case reports

Case I

36-year-old man with I.O.F.B. in the left eye. Retinography confirmed the presence of an epiretinal foreign body along the supero-temporal vessels together with a preretinal haemorrhage. The B-scan ultrasonogram demonstrated an I.O.F.B. at the back of the eye and at a lower sensitivity shows the I.O.F.B. to lie anterior to the retina above the macula.

Case II

56-year-old man with I.O.F.B. in the left eye. X-ray showed a small foreign body with metallic density localized in the posterior part of the eyeball. The B-scan ultrasonogram showed a high-amplitude echo persisting at a lower sensitivity.

Case III

32-year-old man with I.O.F.B. in the left eye. X-ray showed a metallic foreign body localized anteriorly in the eyeball. The B-scan ultrasonogram demonstrated, peripherally in the vitreous a characteristic high-amplitude echo returned from I.O.F.B.

Case IV

56-year-old woman with I.O.F.B. in the right eye. X-ray displayed a radiopaque foreign body localized in the median part of the eyeball. The B- and A-scans demonstrated a foreign body in the inferonasal side of the eye. A-scan pattern shows the characteristic high-amplitude echoes returned from metallic foreign body which approach and exceed the echo amplitude of the vitreoretinal interface.

Case V

24-year-old man with I.O.F.B. in the right eye. X-ray showed a radiopaque foreign body localized in the lower posterior part of the eyeball. The B-scan ultrasonogram revealed a foreign body, indicated by a bright, high-amplitude echo seen in the premacular area.

Case VI

42-year-old woman with I.O.F.B. in the right eye. The B-scan ultrasono-gram demonstrated a traumatic cataract, vitreous haemorrhages and posterior vitreous detachment. In the vitreous cavity a high-amplitude echo caused by an I.O.F.B. is seen.

Conclusions

A major use of ultrasound in ophthalmology has been the localization of intraocular foreign bodies, the determination of their magnetic properties and the evaluation of ocular damage caused by trauma (Bronson, 1964, 1965, 1968; Clay et al., 1970).

The combined use of radiographic and ultrasonographic examinations overcomes many limitations present in either method when used alone (Coleman and Trokel, 1971). In the presence of a nonradiopaque foreign body the ultrasonic examination may be the only method by which the foreign body can be detected and localized.

The echographic method provides the most accurate information of I.O.F.B.'s position with relation to the ocular structures and the demonstration of simultaneous intraocular pathologies such as dislocation of the lens, vitreous haemorrhage and retinal detachment.

The ultrasound scan is useful in determining the I.O.F.B.'s magnetic properties using a pulsed magnet (Coleman et al., 1977; Penner and Passmore, 1966; Poujol, 1981). A significant advantage is that ultrasono-graphy is a simple, non traumatic examination which can be performed at the patient's bedside.

Ultrasound is useful in the following cases:

— to distinguish an I.O.F.B. that is nonradiopaque and therefore not visible by radiological investigation;
— to locate I.O.F.B. with a diameter larger than or equal to 0.5 mm; often it can be used to detect I.O.F.B. with smaller diameters;
— to identify the position: intraocular, intramural, or orbital;
— in the demonstration of other simultaneous intraocular pathologies such as dislocation of the lens, vitreous haemorrhage and retinal detachment;
— in the demonstration of other simultaneous intraocular pathologies such as dislocation of the lens, vitreous haemorrhage and retinal detachment;
— in the determination of magnetic properties using pulsed magnet.
— in axial length measurements to augment X-ray localization.

134

References

Bellone G, Gallenga PE. 1969. Diagnostic echography of Ophthalmic foreign bodies. Part I. Foreign bodies located in the anterior segment. Arch Rass Ital Oftal 37: 296.

Bellone G, Gallenga PE. 1969. Diagnostic ultrasonography for ophthalmic foreign bodies. Part II. Foreign bodies located in the posterior segment. Arch Rass Ital Oftal 37: 317.

Bronson NR, II. 1964. Nonmagnetic foreign body localization and extraction. Am J Ophthalmol 58: 133.

Bronson NR. 1965. Techniques of ultrasonic localization and extraction of intraocular and extraocular foreign bodies. Am J Ophthalmol 60: 596.

Bronson NR. 1968. Management of intraocular foreign bodies. Am J Ophthalmol 66: 279.

Clay C, Rousselie F, Offret G. 1970. Ultrasonographie dans le diagnostic des corps étrangers intra-oculaires. Arch Ophthalmol, Paris 30: 619.

Coleman DJ, Trokel SL. 1971. A protocol for B-scan and radiographic foreign body localization. Am J Ophthalmol 70: 84.

Coleman DJ, Lizzi FL, Jack RL: Ultrasonography of the eye and orbit. Lea & Febiger, Philadelphia, pp. 255—264.

Oksala A, Lehtinen A. 1959. Use of the echogram in the location and diagnosis of intra-ocular foreign bodies. Brit J Ophthalmol 43: 744.

Ossoinig K, Seher K. 1969. Ultrasonic diagnosis of intraocular foreign bodies. In: CV Mosby, K. Gitter et al. (eds) Ophthalmic Ultrasound, St Louis, pp. 311—320.

Penner R, Passmore JW. 1966. Magnetic vs nonmagnetic intraocular foreign bodies. An ultrasonic determination. Arch Ophthalmol 76: 676.

Poujol J. 1981. Echographie en ophthalmologie. Masson, Paris, pp. 53—55.

Echographic evaluation of bulbar phthisis

A. MELE[1], G. CENNAMO[1], N. ROSA[2] AND R. BENEDETTO[3]

Summary

"Phthisical" is useful and acceptable for a clinical designation that connotes an end-stage eye. Congenital microphthalmia should be distinguished from phthisis bulbi, which usually represents an acquired shrinkage of the eye following trauma, inflammation, and so forth rather than a primary development defect. The term of phthisis bulbi should be reserved for cases in which specific histopathologic criteria as described below are met. The Standardized A-Scan and B-Scan echography help us to distinguish the phthisis bulbi from atrophy of the eyeball without shrinkage and atrophy of the eyeball with shrinkage.

Introduction

"Phthisical" is a useful and acceptable clinical designation that denotes an end-stage eye. Congenital microphthalmia should be distinguished from phthisis bulbi, which usually represents an acquired shrinkage of the eye consecutive to trauma, inflammation, and so forth rather than a primary developmental defect. The term of "phthisis bulbi" should be reserved for cases which meet specific histopathological criteria as described below (D. J. Apple et al., 1978). Standardized A-Scan and B-Scan echography can help us to distinguish phthisis bulbi from other ocular pathologies. We have carried out a retrospective study of echographic features observed in 35 cases of phthisis bulbi from 1976 to date. Standardized A-Scan echography with Kretz 7200 MA apparatus was used. In B-Scan echography both the immersion technique with Sonometric Ophthalmoscan 200 and the contact technique with Topcon echographic apparatus were utilized. In addition, echobiometry of the ocular globe was carried out in all cases, with standardized A-Scan echography using Ossoinig immersion shells (Gallenga et al., 1984; Guthoff et al., 1984; Ossoinig, 1979).

[1] Cardarelli Hospital, Naples, [2] University Eye Clinic, Naples, [3] University Eye Clinic, Modena, Italy.

J. M. Thijssen (ed.) Ultrasonography in ophthalmology.
© 1988, *Kluwer Academic Publishers, Dordrecht, ISBN 978-94-010-7083-6*

Results

This study has identified 4 characteristic features of bulbar phthisis:

(1) Shorter axial length.
(2) Total "disorganization" of intraocular structures, especially vitreous and retina.
(3) Thickened retina — choroid layer with retinal folds.
(4) Bone formation in the choroidal layer.

The decrease of ocular dimensions is most evident along the antero-posterior axis, which is at least 25% shorter than mormal values (Fig. 1).

This decrease is principally due to the compressive action of the muscles: rectus muscles having an antero-posterior action, and oblique muscles acting in the opposite direction. Intraocular structures, especially the vitreous, are completely altered with an irregular, medium-high or low reflectivity. Often there are high reflectivity interfaces due to vitreous membranes, or retinal and/or choroidal detachment. In these cases, with quantitative echography of type II, it is not possible to differentiate vitreal from retinal pathology, due to the complete alteration and disorganization of these structures and also due to tissue wrinkling. Sometimes, it is possible to discern a structure with a very high reflectivity within the vitreous body, similar to a "foreign body", this is due to a calcified lens (Fig. 2a, 2b).

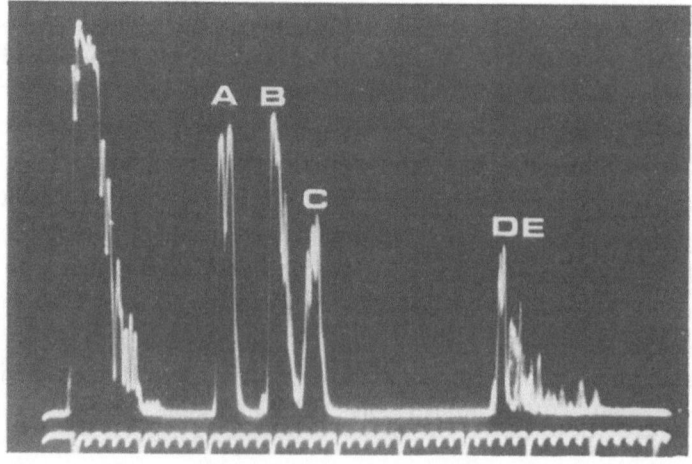

Fig. 1. The globe is small, measures less than 20 mm in diameter A. Cornea. B. Anterior surface of the lens. C. Posterior surface of the lens. DE. Thickness of retino-choroid.

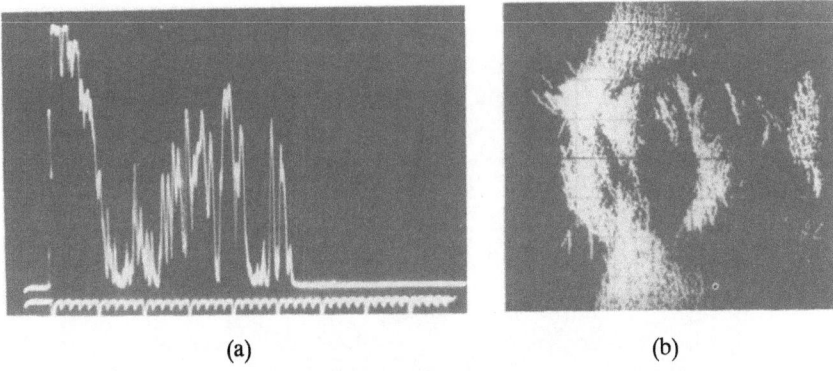

(a)   (b)

Fig. 2a, b. Total disorganization of intraocular structures.

The marked thickening of retino-choroidal layers, is always 100% greater than normal values. The reflectivity of these structures is medium low and irregular (Fig. 3a, 3b, 3c). Moreover it is very difficult to point out a single, steeply rising peak (Fig. 4); this is due to the retino-choroidal folds that are always present in this disease. For this reason, the first peak of the retino-choroidal complex will not be steeply rising because of the oblique incidence of the ultrasonic beam on the retinal surface.

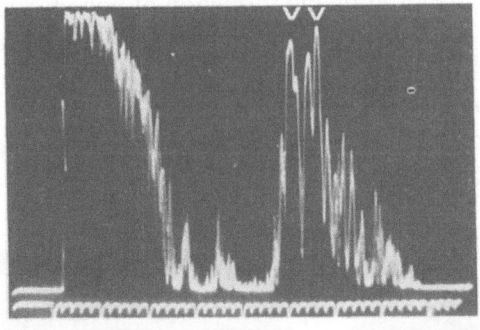

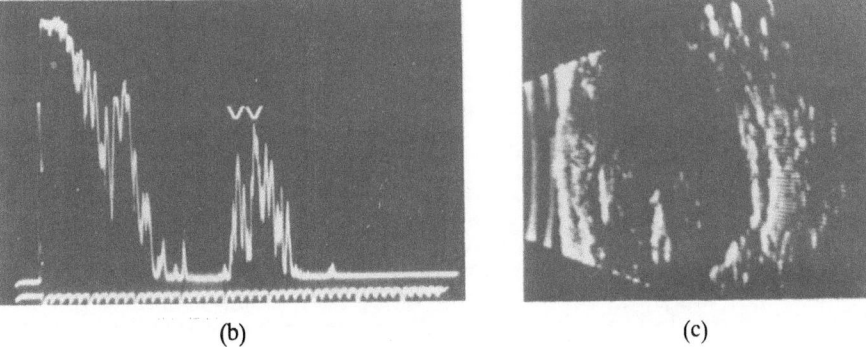

(b)   (c)

Fig. 3. Retina, choroid and sclera show marked thickening and are wrinkled or indented, with medium-low and irregular reflectivity. (a) A-Scan tissue sensitivity. (b) A-Scan low level of amplification. (c) B-Scan.

138

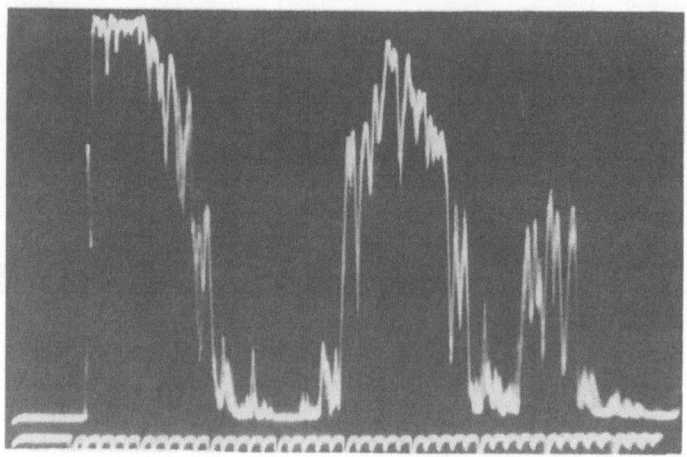

Fig. 4. Impossibility of obtaining a steeply rising retinal peak.

The presence of these three conditions signifies the presence of a bulbar phthisis in an irreversible phase. The fourth characteristic, the acoustic shadowing of retrobulbar tissues, is present only in a very advanced stage of this disease. It is caused by the formation of bone tissue in the choroidal layer. In this case, the presence of tissue with a high reflectivity is the direct cause of the acoustic shadowing (Fig. 5). However, shadowing can be present in the absence of choroidal calcification, when it could be caused by a very irregular reflectivity, due to the more or less marked changes of the internal surfaces of the ocular globe.

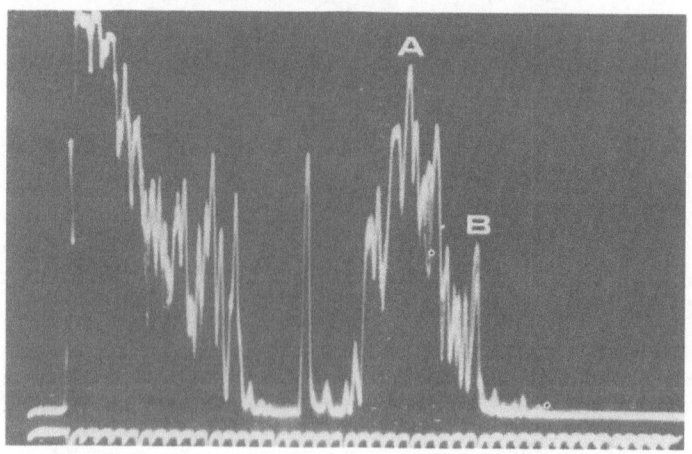

Fig. 5. Intraocular bone formation (shadowing in the orbital fat tissue).

We wish to point out a possible characteristic of a pre-phthisical eye in a reversible phase: a thickening of the retino-choroidal layers, even when more than 100%, but with a medium high and regular reflectivity, with the absence of a complete vitreous body disorganization. In these cases steroid therapy brought about a regression of this initial pre-phthisis (Fig. 6). The differential diagnosis must in particular be made between phthisis bulbi and non-colobomatous microphthalmos (Cennamo, 1985; Osborn, 1984). In the latter case, the absence of vitreous changes, the decrease in ocular volume (not only of antero-posterior axis, but also of transverse axis) but most particularly the presence of a markedly thickened retino-choroid with a high and regular reflectivity (Figs. 7, 8) will permit an exact diagnosis to be made.

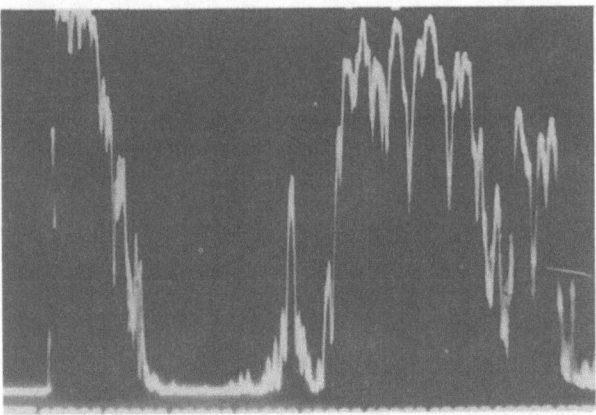

Fig. 6. Thickening of retino-choroid with medium high and regular reflectivity.

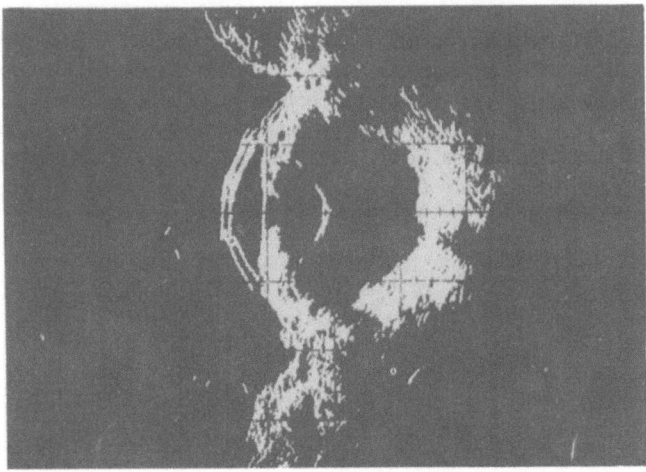

Fig. 7. Short axial length in hypermetropic eye.

140

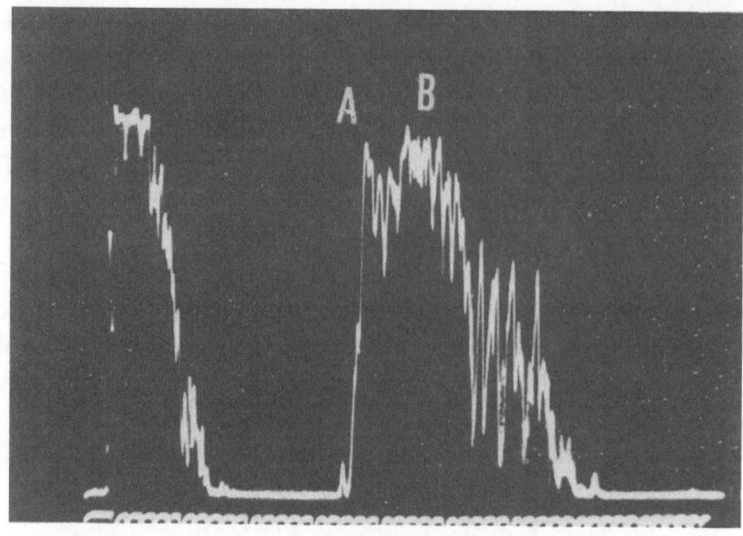

Fig. 8. Hypermetropia-microphthalmos. Decrease of antero-posterior and transverse length of the eye globe. A, B. Thickening of the retino-choroid with medium high and regular reflectivity.

References

Apple DJ, Rabb MF. 1978. Clinicopathologic Correlation of Ocular disease. Mosby, Saint Louis, pp. 196—200.

Cennamo G, Magli A, Corvino C. 1985. Genetic and Ultrasound Study of Ereditary Microphthalmos. Proc II Joint Meeting of International Society for Paediatric Ophthalmology, Ghent, Belgio 1984, Ophth Paed 2 Gen 6, pp. 1—2.

Gallenga PE, Cennamo G, Rosa N. 1982. Echographic Study of Microphthalmos Proc VII Congress S.O.E. Helsinki, Finland.

Guthoff R, Berger RW, Draeger J. 1984. Measurements of Ocular Coat Dimensions by Means of Combined A- and B-Scan Ultrasonography. Ophthalmic Res 16: 289—291.

Osborn DR, Foulks GN. 1984. Computed Tomographic Analysis of Deformity and Dimensional Changes in the Eyeball. Radiology 153: 669—674.

Ossoinig KC. 1979. Standardized Echography: Basic, Principles, Clincal Applications and Results. Int Ophthalmol Clin 19 (4): 127—210.

B-scan echography in 40 eyes treated by trabeculectomy

A. FEDE, S. PALAZZO AND G. GORGONE

Summary

The authors studied the echographic patterns of 40 eyes which underwent trabeculectomy in the attempt to extrapolate characteristic morphological aspects. An immersion B-scan method, using a 15 MHz probe, was carried out to perform preoperative and postoperative echography. The authors point out that, due to the higher resolution power of the 15 MHz probes, it is possible to analyze the morphological features of the examined structures.

Materials and method

A Sonometrics Ophthalmoscan 200 A with 15 MHz immersion probe was used. 39 patients (24 female, 15 male) affected by glaucoma (36 eyes open-angle and 4 closed-angle glaucoma) and undergoing trabeculectomy, according to Cairns technique, have been considered.

Each patient was investigated with ultrasounds on 4 occasions — 1 preoperative and 3 postoperative. Standardization criteria concerning the distance probe-eye and the amplification have been applied. The scanning was performed in the sagittal plane (axis 12—6 o'clock) with the eye rotated downwards.

Discussion

B-scan echography with high resolution probe is considered useful in the study of the region of anterior chamber angle. The echograms of patients operated by Cairns trabeculectomy show a significant change in the morphology of the region examined: the picture demonstrates anatomical

Clinica Oculistica, Università degli Studi, Catania, Italy.

J. M. Thijssen (ed.) Ultrasonography in ophthalmology.
© 1988, Kluwer Academic Publishers, Dordrecht, ISBN 978-94-010-7083-6

modification following surgery. It can be appreciated that beside the filtering bleb there is a lack of tissue due to the excision of the corneo-scleral flap.

Conclusions

From our observations, we stress that echography is a convenient up to date method of investigation in the postop follow up of patients operated for glaucoma. With the increase of cases considered it is possible to start drawing important morphological-functional correlations.

Recurrent spontaneous choroidal detachment: echographic follow-up

L. FALCO, A. DENAPOLI AND A. CAPACCINI

Summary

A case of choroidal effusion has been described and followed echographically. Alternate phases of choroidal swelling associated with a detached retina considered secondary, have been echographically demonstrated.

Introduction

Choroidal effusion is a type of pathology which has been known for some time. In 1834 Wardrop noted that it had been first mentioned in Zinn's works in 1755. Von Graefe (1858), Verhoeff (1931), and Stallard (1954) have also contributed some observations on this condition. It is, however thanks to Schepens and Brockhurst (1973) that a closer study has been made.

Clinically speaking, choroidal effusion is a collection of fluid in the potential suprachoroidal space which is external to the main structural and functional layers of the choroid and ciliary body. Choroidal effusion can be distinguished: the lobar, the flat, and the annular forms (depending on the different ways in which the liquid collects in the space above the choroid).

As the choroid remains immersed in the liquid "at length", pigment accumulates in the folds of the retinal layers. The moment these folds are distended, the pigment remains, following the course of the preexisting retinal folds (Verhoeff's sign).

Etiologically, four types of choroidal effusion can be distinguished:

1. after surgery or trauma;
2. that which is associated with the Vogt-Kojanagi-Harada Syndrome;
3. idiopathic;
4. that known as the Schepens and Brockhurst Syndrome or the choroidal effusion syndrome.

U.S.L. 18, H.S. Giuseppe. Div. Oculistica, Empoli, Firenze, Italy.

J. M. Thijssen (ed.) Ultrasonography in ophthalmology.
© 1988, Kluwer Academic Publishers, Dordrecht, ISBN 978-94-010-7083-6

The pathogenesis in surgical choroidal effusion or the post traumatic form seems to be either hypotension or trauma to the blood vessels caused by surgery or vitreal traction. The so called idiopathic form and the Schepens and Brockhurst form have not been clearly defined pathogenetically. The type associated with the Voght-Koyanagi-Harada Syndrome seems to be related to a viral etiology.

Most of the authors believe that over a period of time, both retinal detachment (R.D.) and cases of detached choroid resolve spontaneously.

This paper presents a case of choroidal effusion associated with R.D. in which onset, evolution and resolution have been echographically documented. As is often the case in this type of pathology, the clinical pre-echographic diagnosis was compatible with a choroid melanoma.

Clinical case

P.D. 72 years old, operated three months previously for bilateral cataracts, complained of decreasing vision, particularly in the nasal sector of the right eye.

The objective examination demonstrated the bilateral presence of gerontoxon, the anterior chamber of normal depth and optically empty, the pupils round and reacting, and surgical aphakia.

Visual acuity was "Hand movements" in the right eye and in the left eye +9 sph +1.50 cyl (175) = 8/10.

The eye pressure was the same in both eyes and equal to 14 mmHg (Goldmann).

The ophthalmoscopic examination performed with maximum mydriasis, and the biomicroscopic examination using three mirror lenses showed a serous type of retinal detachment in the nasal sector of the right eye and a solid type in the temporal zone. On the temporal side of the macula there was a rounded area with clearly defined margins and dark in color. This aspect seemed to indicate a detachment secondary to a choroidal melanoblastoma.

Figure 1 presents immersion echography performed with CGE equipment for internal medicine with a 5 MHz linear probe, since nothing else was available. Although the echographic examination was not very specific because of the type of apparatus used, the probe established the complete detachment of the retina but no indication of a melanoma type neoplasm in the choroid.

As we were aware of the limitations of the apparatus used, the next day the patient was re-examined echographically (Ocuscan 400, Sonometrics, Fig. 2) and the diagnosis of total detachment of the retina was confirmed.

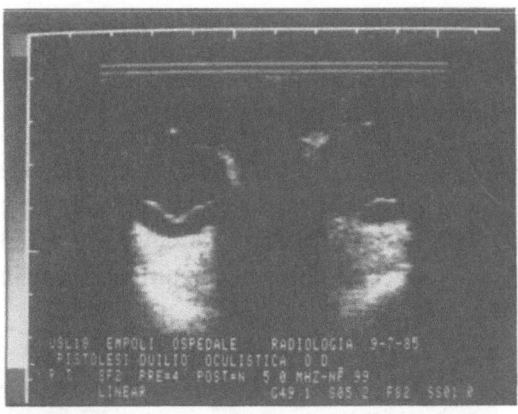

Fig. 1. B-mode echogram obtained with 5 MHz probe (CGE equipment). Eye with complete retinal detachment.

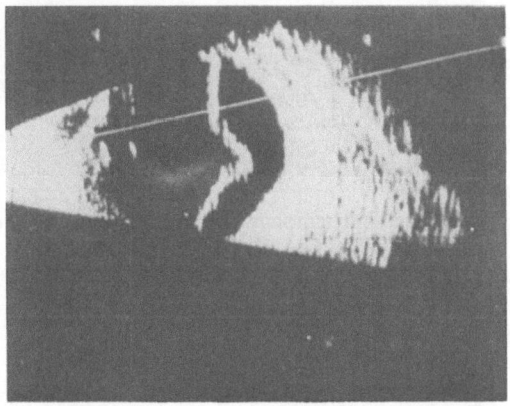

Fig. 2. Same case as in Fig. 1, examined with 10 MHz probe (Ocuscan 400, Sonometrics).

The diagnosis was as follows: total R.D. associated with previous annular choroidal effusion which was responsible for residual pigmentation in the temporal para-macular site.

As the R.D. persisted in the right eye, and since it was total, surgery was planned but not carried out because on the day of the operation the patient had developed acute uveitis in the right eye (Corneal edema with large folds in Descemet's membrane, heavy flare both in the anterior chamber and the vitreous, pupils miotic with some synechiae and intraocular pressure normal on digital assessment).

The same day, the echographic examination was reported (Sonometrics Ocuscan 400, Fig. 3) revealing, apart from R.D., the presence of a detached choroid in the posterior pole and temporally. This evidence confirmed the previous diagnosis of choroidal effusion. The echographic examination performed in the following days with different equipment (Biophysic Medical, Ophthascan, Figs. 4, 5 and CGE Fig. 6) did not show significant change in the right eye.

Only five days after the last examination a further control (Biophysic Medical, Ophthalscan, Fig. 7) established the permanence of R.D. and a thickening of the choroid in the posterior pole and temporally but no longer showed choroidal detachment. A later echographic examination confirmed that the retinal and choroidal picture had remained unchanged.

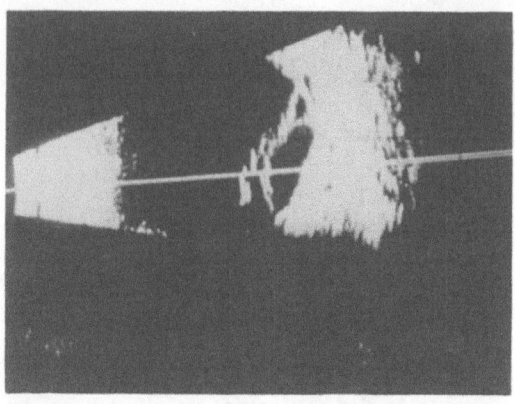

Fig. 3. Preoperative B-mode echogram showing choroidal detachment (posterior, temporal).

Fig. 4.

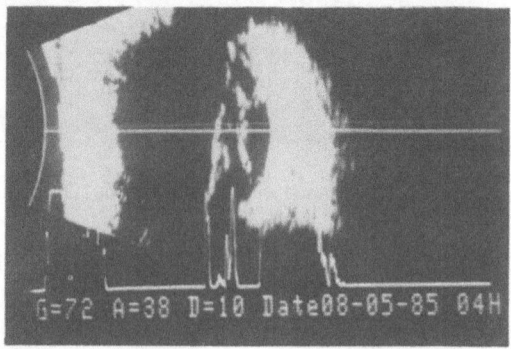

Fig. 5.

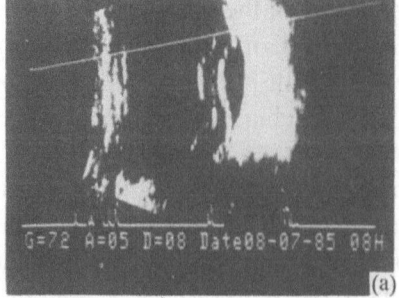

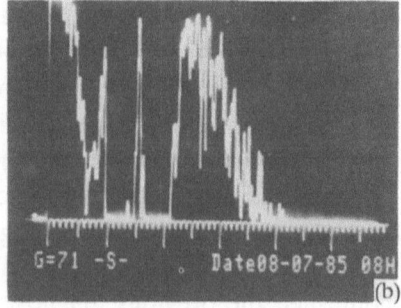

Fig. 6.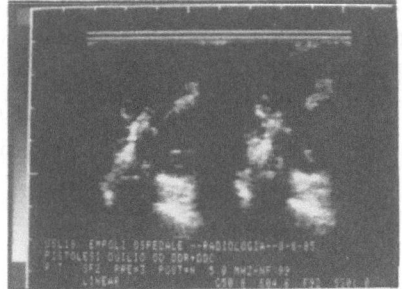

Fig. 4 to 6. Serial B-mode echograms on subsequent days. Figs. 4 and 5 with Ophthascan B, Biophysic Medical, Fig. 6 with CGE equipment.

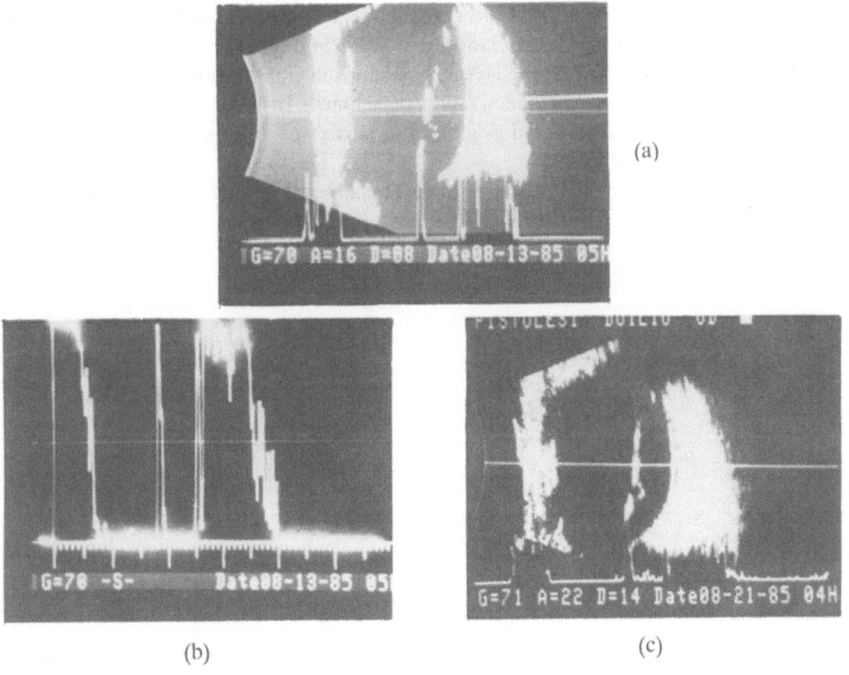

(a)

(b)   (c)

Fig. 7. Echogram obtained five days after last examination (Fig. 6). Persistence of retinal detachment, no choroidal detachment, thickened choroid.

Discussion

The case presented here manifests a clinical peculiarity. In fact, as the problem arose some time after the cataract removal, we can speak of a picture of post-operative choroidal effusion, but we are uncertain as to the origin of the uveitis, which would lead us to suspect an idiopathic form.

148

However, aside from pathogenetic clinical observations, we were interested in demonstrating the reality of the case echographically. The fact that we were able to follow (with different types of equipment) the evolution of this pathology seems worthy of note. It confirms the spontaneous capacity of the eye to reabsorb the fluid underneath the choroid during a case of choroidal effusion.

References

Brockhurst RJ, Lam KW. 1973. Uveal effusion: II. Report of a case with analysis of subretinal fluid. Arch Ophthalmol 90: 399.

Duke-Elder S, Perkins ES. 1966. Cilio-choroidal detachments. In: S Duke-Elder, System of Ophthalmology, Vol. 9, Disease of the Uveal Tract. St Louis.

Schepens CL, Brockhurst RJ. 1963. Uveal effusion. Arch Ophthalmol 70: 189.

Stallard HB. 1954. Annular peripheral retinal detachment. Brit J Ophthalmol 38: 115.

Verhoeff F. 1931. The nature and origin of the pigmented streaks caused by separation of the choroid. JAMA 92: 1873.

Warddrop J. 1934. The morbid anatomy of the human eye. London: Churchill, Vol. 2, p. 72.

Intraocular tumours and leukokoria

Ophthalmic ultrasonography of pathologically proven ocular melanomas with a high resolution real-time small parts scanner

D. T. C. LIN[1], P. L. MUNK[2], A. L. MABERLEY[3],
P. L. COOPERBERG[2], AND J. ROOTMAN[1]

Summary

The authors present a series of 13 patients with intraocular melanomas imaged using high resolution Small Parts Ultrasonography. All patients underwent enucleation and subsequent histopathologic examination. On ultrasonography, patients were assessed for the presence of retinal detachment, choroidal excavation, rupture through Bruch's membrane, retroorbital fat shadowing, and acoustic texture. Correlation with histopathology demonstrated that using traditional criteria, the majority of rupture through Bruch's membrane was missed due to the limits of instrument resolution. No patients with a homogeneous acoustic texture showed evidence of tumour necrosis or haemorrhage, while the vast majority of those with an inhomogeneous texture did. The authors suggest that high resolution small parts scanning may result in an alteration in the traditionally accepted criteria for the B-Scan diagnosis of choroidal melanoma.

Introduction

Ocular B-Scan echography is a diagnostic method that was popularized in the early 1970's by D. J. Coleman and his associates (1973). N. R. Bronson (1973) introduced the use of contact real time echography. There are now many commercially available B-Scan units including the Ocuscan 400 (Sonometrics), Ultrascan 2 (Cooper) and the Renaissance (Storz). B-Scan echography of choroidal melanomas has been extensively investigated (Char, 1980; Coleman et al., 1977; Fuller et al., 1979; Hodes, 1977; Shammas, 1984; Shields and Tasman, 1977). However, due to the limited image resolution properties of the previously available real time scanners, many investigators resorted to the use of standardized A-Scan echography

Department of [1] Ophthalmology and [2] Radiology University of British Columbia and Vancouvar General Hospital, 855 West 12th Avenue, Vancouver, B.C., Canada, V5Z 3N9; [3] 2550 Willow Street, Vancouver, B.C., Canada, V5Z 3N9.

J. M. Thijssen (ed.) Ultrasonography in ophthalmology.
© 1988. *Kluwer Academic Publishers, Dordrecht, ISBN 978-94-010-7083-6*

as popularized by K. C. Ossoinig (1983) for the evaluation of intraocular tumours including choroidal melanomas (Coleman et al., 1977, Shammas 1984; Ossoinig, 1983; Farah et al., 1984). Recent advances in ultrasonography have overcome some of the image resolution difficulties of the earlier real time scanners and images with excellent resolution are currently available.

Real Time Small Parts Unit has been used extensively in radiology primarily for the evaluation of superficial structures and the peripheral vasculature. This imaging system has been extensively discussed in a recent review (Walter, 1985). The advantages of this unit include improved image resolution with 64 shades of gray, larger field of view with magnification, and depth gain control settings. There have been no previous publications concerning the use of this high resolution real time scanner in the evaluation of intraocular melanomas. The purpose of this paper is to correlate the ultrasonographic features of 13 choroidal melanomas with their histopathology using the Real Time Small Parts Scanner.

Materials and methods

Since March 1983, the Department of Radiology and Ophthalmology of the University of British Columbia at the Vancouver General Hospital have been using the Real Time Small Parts Scanner manufactured by Diasonics (DS-10) routinely in the evaluation of intraocular and intraorbital lesions. During a 2 year period (March 1983—March 1985), 13 patients had both ocular ultrasonography and enucleation for choroidal melanoma. Only one patient in this series received preoperative radiation therapy. All ultrasounds on these eyes were reviewed by the authors. The ultrasonographic features that were analyzed included the presence or absence of choroidal excavation, retro-orbital fat shadowing, scleral and extrascleral extension, tumour homogeneity (homogeneous defined as no echo poor areas within the tumour, and inhomogeneous defined as large echo poor areas within the tumour). Ultrasonographic evidence for rupture through Bruch's membrane (mushroom stalk configuration), and presence or absence of retinal detachment were noted. All enucleations were performed within two weeks of the analyzed ultrasound. The pathology was read by one ocular pathologist. The pathologic features that were analyzed included histologic cell type, scleral or extrascleral extension, presence or absence of retinal detachment. Tumour homogeneity was defined according to the presence of necrosis, haemorrhage and sinusoidal spaces within the tumour. Tumour shape including microscopic evidence for rupture of Bruch's membrane was evaluated. The ultrasonographic features were compared to the histopathologic features.

Results

Using convertional B-scan criteria for the evaluation of choroidal melanomas (Table 1), only 6/13 showed evidence of choroidal excavation 0/13 showed evidence of retro-orbital fat shadowing. The acoustic structure was homogeneous in 4/13, and inhomogeneous in 9/13. Tumours with homogeneous acoustic structures by ultrasonography showed no evidence of necrosis or haemorrhage by pathology. Likewise the majority of tumours with inhomogeneous acoustic structures showed evidence of haemorrhage or necrosis by histology (Table 2). Typical mushroom stalk appearance of choroidal melanomas occurred in only 2/13. It was observed that the sclera immediately posterior to the tumour often showed an apparent decreased thickness. This is a subjective finding noted in 8/13 patients, and was difficult to measure in an accurately reproducible manner. On the other hand choroidal excavation could be identified with confidence in only 6/13 cases. In comparing choroidal melanoma ultrasonographic features to histopathological features, it was noted that of 13 histologically proven retinal detachments, 3/13 were missed by ultrasound. Of the 10 tumours proven to have broken through Bruch's membrane by histopathology, only 2 were noted to have the traditional criteria of a mush-

Table 1. Ultrasound of choroidal melanomas using a real time parts scanner.

Characteristics	Frequency
Lesions seen	13/13
Retinal detachment	10/13
Choroidal excavation	6/13
Rupture through Bruch's (mushroom)	2/13
Retro-orbital fat shadowing	0/13
Acoustic structure — homogeneous	4/13
— inhomogeneous	9/13

Table 2. Tumour acoustic structure versus tissue architecture.

Ultrasound	Histopathology
4/13 homogeneous	0/4 haemorrhage
	0/4 necrosis
9/13 inhomogeneous	7/9 haemorrhage
	3/9 necrosis
	3/9 both

room stalk shaped tumour configuration on ultrasound. Of the remaining 8, 3 displayed a globular shape with short, broad necks. 2/13 eyes showed evidence of extrascleral extension by histopathology that were not picked up by ultrasound. These extrascleral extensions were very small. In one case the patient had a small epibulbar nodule less than 2 mm in diameter. In the other case, the patient had one emisserial vein filled with tumour cells.

Discussion

Traditional B-Scan criteria of choroidal melanomas as described by H. J. Shammas (1984) and others have included choroidal excavation, retro-orbital fat shadowing, and acoustic homogeneity were found in a minority of cases in our series. The classic mushroom stalk appearance of choroidal melanomas has been considered pathognomonic for rupture of Bruch's membrane. This was found in a minority of cases analyzed in spite of the presence of rupture on histopathology (Fig. 1). Several cases of rupture of Bruch's membrane demonstrated by pathology did not demonstrate the classic mushroom shaped configuration. Instead microscopic breaks through Bruch's membrane could be demonstrated (Fig. 2). Large extra-scleral extensions of choroidal melanomas have previously been diagnosed by ultrasound by J. A. Martin (1983). In our series, a small epibulbar nodule (less than 2 mm in diameter) and an emisserial vein extension of tumour cells could not be picked up by a high resolution Small Parts Scanner. This is most likely secondary to the small size of the extraocular masses, which approached the limits of instrument resolution. Acoustic inhomogeneity was found to correlate well with areas of haemorrhage and necrosis within the tumour (Fig. 3). The 3 missed retinal detachments may well have been too shallow for detection, although this could not be confirmed in in the histology specimens since fixation procedures preclude accurate measurement of detachment depth. The most widely accepted subjective criteria in the diagnosis of melanoma has been the presence of choroidal excavation (Coleman et al., 1974), a finding seen in less than half of our subjects. However, another subjective finding, that of apparent scleral thinning posterior to the tumour, was identified in a majority of cases. In no instance was a histopathological correlate present for either subjective sign.

Small parts B-Scanning offers unprecedented excellent gray scale and high resolution images of intraocular melanomas. Although this is a pre-liminary study, small parts B-Scanning may lead to a reassessment of traditionally accepted criteria for their diagnosis in particular tumour homogeneity, retro-orbital fat shadowing and tumour shape.

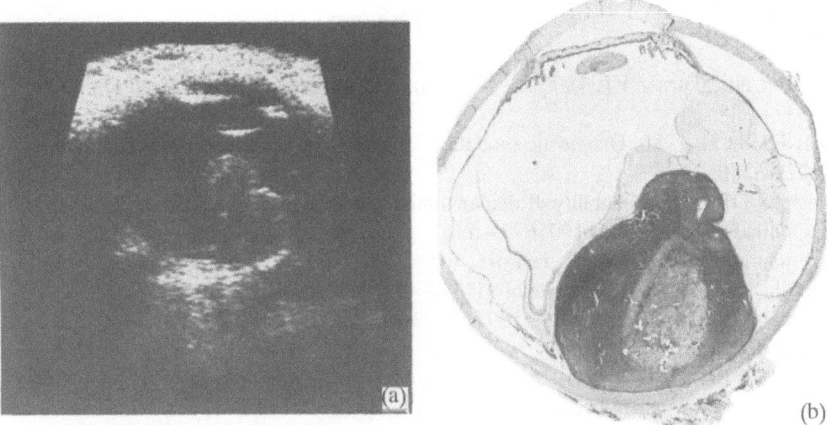

Fig. 1. (a) High resolution ultrasound and (b) histopathology of a choroidal melanoma on which the "mushroom" cap and stalk of a rupture through Bruch's membrane is clearly seen.

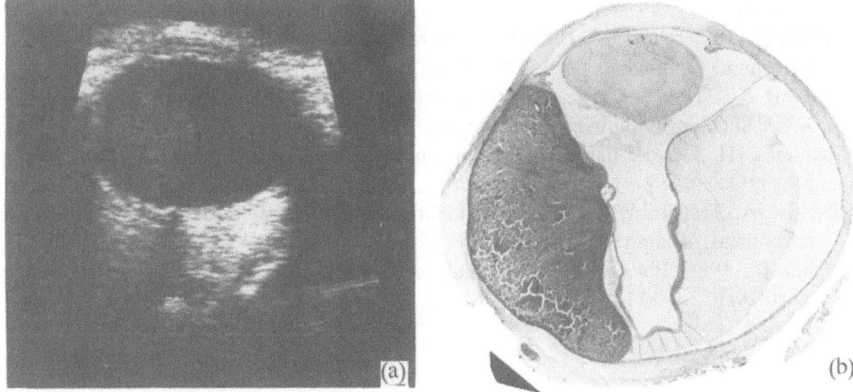

Fig. 2. (a) Ultrasound of a globular-shaped melanoma with a homogeneous acoustic texture. No evidence of a "mushroom" indicating rupture through Bruch's membrane. (b) On histopathology, a small break is demonstrated.

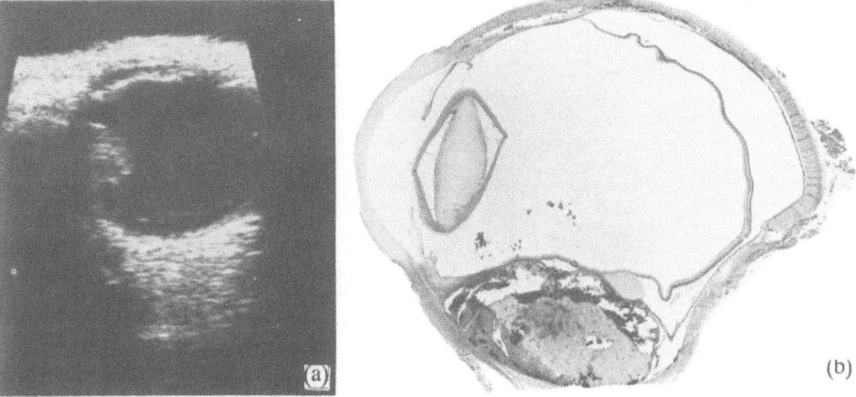

Fig. 3. (a) Ultrasound of a melanoma which demonstrates acoustic non-homogeneity with numerous echo-poor areas. A retinal detachment is present. (b) Histopathology shows numerous areas of haemorrhage and necrosis.

References

Bronson NR, Turner FT. 1973. A simple B-scan ultrasound scope. Arch Ophthalmol 90: 237—238.

Char DH et al. 1980. Diagnostic modalities in choroidal melanoma. Am J Ophthalmol 89: 223—230.

Coleman DJ. 1973. Reliability of ocular tumour diagnosis with ultrasound. Trans Am Acad Ophthal and Otolaryngol 77: 677—686.

Coleman DJ, Albramson DH, Jack RL, Franzen LA. 1974. Ultrasonic diagnosis of tumours of the choroid. Arch Ophthalmol 91: 344—354.

Coleman DJ, Lizzi FL, Jack RL. 1977. Ultrasonography of the eye and orbit. Philadelphia: Lea & Febiger.

Farah ME, Bryne SF, Hughes JR. 1984. Standardized echography in uveal melanomas with scleral or extraocular extension. Arch Ophthalmol 102: 1482—1485.

Fuller DG, Snyder WB, Sutton WL, Vaiser A. 1979. Ultrasonographic feature of choroidal malignant melanomas. Arch Ophthalmol 97: 1465—1472.

Hodes BL. 1977. Ultrasonographic diagnosis of choroidal malignant melanoma. Surv Ophthalmol 22: 29—40.

Martin JA, Robertson DM. 1983. Extrascleral extension choroidal melanoma diagnosed by ultrasound. Ophthalmol 90: 1554—1559.

Ossoinig KC. 1983. Advances in diagnostic ultrasound. In: P Henkind et al. (eds) Acta XXIV: Int Cong Ophthalmol. Philadelphia: J.B. Lippincott, pp. 93—98.

Shammas HJ. 1984. Atlas of ophthalmic ultrasonography and biometry. St Louis: C.V. Mosby Co.

Shields JA, Tasman WS. 1977. B-Scan ultrasonography of lesions simulating choroidal melanomas. Mod probl Ophthalmol 18: 57—63.

Walter JP. 1985. Physics of high-resolution ultrasound — practical aspects. Radiol Clin North Am 23: 3—11.

Analysis of a recent series (254 cases) of choroidal tumours

J. POUJOL AND M.-C. CHAINTRON

Summary

We thought it could be useful to bring up to date the present-day possibilities and reliability of modern echography in the field of choroidal tumours with specially designed equipment for this purpose. Our aim was to study a homogeneous sample. With this object, though we use ultrasound since 1964, we only reviewed our echographic examinations performed from September 1980 to December 1985. Both equipment and the operators were the same, so as to enable comparisons and conclusions to be drawn. On the whole 527 patients suspected to present a choroidal tumour were examined during this period, of which 254 actually had a tumour. The B-mode data of these tumours are analysed and discussed as well as the diagnostic accuracy and the causes of error.

Introduction

We thought it would be useful to update the present-day possibilities and reliability of modern echography in the field of choroidal tumours with equipment specially designed for this purpose.

Material and method

Selection of patients

Our aim was to study a homogeneous sample. With this objective, although we have been using ultrasound since 1964 (32538 examinations), we only reviewed our examinations performed from September 1980 to December 1985 (Table 1), that is to say 14213 patients. Among them 527 were suspected of a choroidal tumour and 254 actually had one.

Laboratoire d'Echographie du Centre National d'Ophtalmologie des Quinze-Vingts, 28, rue de Charenton, 75012 — Paris, France.

J. M. Thijssen (ed.) Ultrasonography in ophthalmology.
© 1988, *Kluwer Academic Publishers, Dordrecht, ISBN 978-94-010-7083-6*

158

Table 1. Number of Examinations.

Total: March 1964—December 1985: 32558 ex.	
— Patients suspected to have a choroidal tumour:	1204 (4%)
— Patients actually having a choroidal tumour:	745 (2%)
Present series: September 1980—December 1985: 14213 ex.	
— Patients suspected to have a choroidal tumour:	527 (4%)
— Patients actually having a choroidal tumour:	254 (2%)

Both the equipment and the operators were the same, so as to enable comparisons to be done and conclusions to be drawn.

Examination techniques

We used the TRISCAN instrument (Biophysic Médical), a contact sector B-scanner. It incorporated a digital memory with storage capacity of 256 × 256 × 4 bits (16 levels of grey) with a rate of presentation of 50—60 Hz (Fig. 1). Since January 1986 we have been using the OPHTHASCAN B

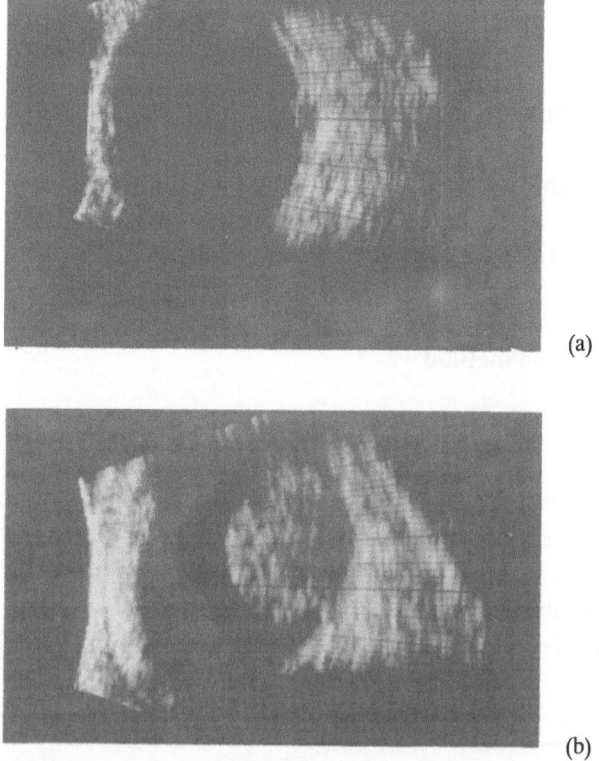

(a)

(b)

Fig. 1. Choroidal melanomas. (a) Small melanoma (less than 1 mm high). It is nevertheless well visible thanks to the choroidal excavation. (b) Very large melanoma (20 mm high). Choroidal excavation is visible at the lowest part of the tumour.

(Biophysic Médical) with 64 levels of grey. The measurements of the tumours were performed with a caliper so that not only the height of the tumour could be measured but its lateral diameter too, which is possible only with B-scan.

A-scan was used for the measurement of reflectivity as previously described (Massin and Poujol, 1977; Poujol, 1984; Poujol, 1986) and occasionally for the evaluation of the Kappa-angle i.e. attenuation (Fig. 2). With our new instrument all these data can be extracted directly from the B-scan picture.

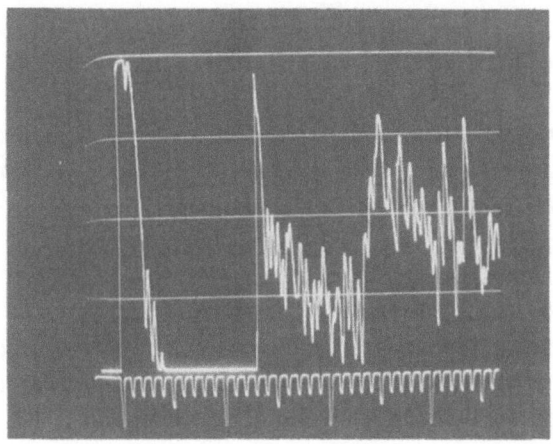

Fig. 2. Choroidal melanoma (10 mm high). The reflectivity (measured on the first echo) is 20 dB and the kappa-angle 30°. Direct measurement with logarithmic amplification, 40 dB dynamic range.

Verification of echographic diagnosis

A histological diagnosis was performed in about half of the cases of melanoma. Otherwise we considered the cases as true melanomas or other choroidal tumours when the echographic diagnosis was consistent with other methods, mainly fluorescein angiography and clinical findings (metastases for instance).

Results

Size of tumours (Table 2)

— The *height* of melanomas went up to 22 mm with the most frequent around 5 mm. The average height of metastases was the same with the

Table 2. Size of 254 choroidal tumours.

	Height	Diameter
Melanomas:	0.5 mm—22.0 mm	4.2 mm—20 mm
Most freq.:	5 mm	
Metastases:	1.0 mm—6.5 mm	5.5 mm—15 mm
Most freq.:	5 mm	
Angiomas:	1.0 mm—10.0 mm	8.0 mm—10 mm
Most freq.:	2 mm	

highest no more than 6.5 mm. The average elevation of angiomas was 2 mm with a unique maximum of 10 mm.

— The *diameter* of melanomas went up to 20 mm, but compared with their height, the metastases were usually wider. Angiomas were fairly wide too as compared to their elevation.

Reflectivity (Table 3)

The less reflective tumours were choroidal melanomas whereas melanomas of the ciliary body were a little more reflective than choroidal metastases. Angiomas were the most reflective tumours on average.

Choroidal excavation (Table 4)

We noted the presence or absence of choroidal excavation in 124 histologically verified melanomas. It was absent in 3 cases and uncertain in 3 cases only. Coleman found a choroidal excavation in 42% of the melanomas he examined (Coleman, 1977).

It was observed in about half of the metastases and in no case of angioma.

Table 3. Reflectivity of 254 choroidal tumours.

	Range (dB)	Average (dB)
Melanomas		
— Choroid	8—25	15.55
— Ciliary body	15—24	19.00
Metastases	12—22	18.20
Angiomas	16—25	21.60

Table 4. Choroidal excavation in 124 histologically verified melanomas and other choroidal tumours.

	Excav. +	Excav. ±	Excav. −
Melanomas			
— of the choroid (106)	104	0	2
— of the ciliary body (18)	14	3	1
Metastases (19)	8	3	8
Angiomas (16)	0	0	16

Choroidal excavation was present in 95% of melanomas and absent in only 3 cases of very large melanomas (15 mm, 16 mm and 20 mm)

Melanomas in eyes with opaque media (Table 5)

In eyes with opaque media we found 21 choroidal melanomas. Among them 2 were false-positive due to very large hemorhagic retinal detachments.

Diagnostic errors in melanomas (Table 6)

We were able to verify positive echographic diagnosis in 221 cases. Among them were 7 erroneous diagnoses (3%).

Correlation between reflectivity, kappa-angle and histology in choroidal melanomas (Table 7)

We tried to establish a correlation between the reflectivity, kappa-angle and histological findings in 20 cases of choroidal melanomas (ruling out ciliary body melanomas). No reliable correlation was found.

Table 5. Melanomas in eyes with opaque media.

Cataracts:	5 melanomas
Vitreous hemorhage:	8 melanomas
Absolute glaucoma:	6 melanomas
	19 cases

False positive: 2 cases

Table 6. Diagnostic errors in melanomas.

Echographic diagnosis	Height	Chor. excav.	Final diagnosis
Melanoma ++/Metast ±	7 mm	+	Metastasis
Melanoma ++	23 mm	±	Hemor. ret. det.
Melanoma ++	2 mm	±	Retinal hematoma
Melanoma +	9 mm	±	Hemor. ret. det.
Melanoma +	5 mm	±	Inflam. ret. det.
Melanoma −	−	−	Large hemor. mel.
Metastase +	−	+	Infl. ch. ret. atrophy

Total: 5 false positive (2 eyes with opaque media)
 1 incomplete positive
 1 false negative

Table 7. Correlation between reflectivity, kappa-angle and histology in 20 cases of choroidal melanoma.

	Nr.	Reflect.		K-angle	
Epithelioid	(1)	16 dB	(16)	22°	(22)
Spindle cell	(9)	10−25 dB	(18)	17°−40°	(33)
Mixed	(7)	8−18 dB	(15)	16°−45°	(32)
Indifferentiated	(3)	8−18 dB	(14)	23°−33°	(27)

Treated tumours

These were mainly melanomas (Stallard disks, conventional radiotherapy and proton irradiation). The dimensions did not change very quickly: the height usually decreased slightly only one year after the treatment. In some cases the tumour increased and enucleation was performed.

Discussion

Melanomas

Most errors did occur with very large tumours and, choroidal excavation, although not pathognomonic of a choroidal tumour (Poujol and Le Roy, 1983) was dubious in 5 cases out of 7 erroneously diagnosed cases.

In the 5 false-positive melanomas, 2 were diagnosed in eyes with opaque media and both of them were large retinal detachments with dubious choroidal excavation.

Metastases

In these cases choroidal excavation was present in 42% and dubious in 16% of these metastatic tumours.

Angiomas

Choroidal excavation was absent in all cases of angiomas which concords with the opinion of Coleman (1977) and disagrees with the findings of Fuller et al. (1979). In fact, the disagreement appears to be due to the difference in instruments since modern ones show the acoustic characteristics much better thanks to their grey scale.

Melanomas in eyes with opaque media (Table 5)

Among these 21 cases there were 2 diagnostic errors and both of them were cases of large melanomas where choroidal excavation was dubious.

Conclusion

The diagnostic accuracy of choroidal tumours has improved over the past five years due to the development of new instruments with grey scale. Ultrasound appears at the moment to be the most reliable technique for the diagnosis of these tumours. It will become even more reliable with new equipment (Fig. 3).

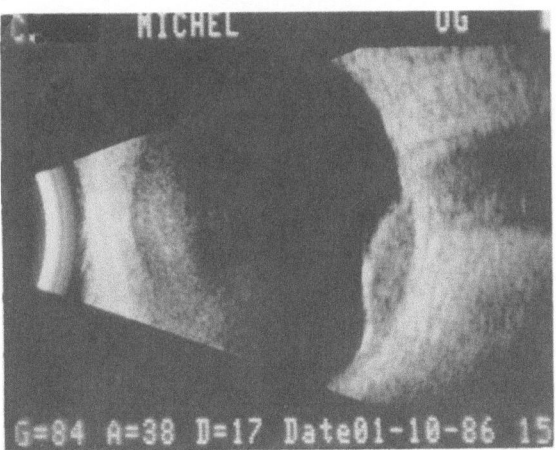

Fig. 3. Recent choroidal melanoma. Ophthascan B (Biophysic Medical). 64 levels of grey. New probe.

References

Coleman DJ, Lizzi FL, Jack RL. 1977. Ultrasonography of the Eye and Orbit. Lea & Febiger, Philadelphia.

Fuller DG, Snyder WB, Hutton WL, Vaiser A. 1979. Ultrasonographic Features of Choroidal Malignant Melanomas. Arch Ophthalmol 97: 1465–1472.

Massin M, Poujol J. 1977. Direct quantitative echography using logarithmic amplification. In: DN White and RE Brown (eds) Ultrasound in Medicine, Vol. 3B, Plenum, New York.

Poujol J. 1984. Echographie en Ophtalmologie. Masson, Paris.

Poujol J, Le Roy M. 1983. Echographic modifications of the choroid in its tumours and pseudotumours. In: JS Hillman and MM LeMay (eds) Ophthalmic Ultrasonography. Junk, The Hague, pp. 57–62.

Poujol J. 1986. Echography in Ophthalmology. Masson, New York.

Echographical follow-up of choroidal melanoma after irradiation with Iodine 125

A. STANOWSKY[1,2] AND I. KREISSIG[1]

Summary

Nine patients with malignant choroidal melanomas treated with radioactive Iodine 125 have been followed up since 1984 with the B-scan and the standardized A-scan procedures. Within the first month after beginning of treatment the echograms showed differences among the tumours in prominence, structure and inner reflectivity.

In contrast to this all tumours showed an increase in vascularisation. This became particularly clear with video-echography.

Later on an increase of reflectivity and an inhomogeneity of the inner structure were predominant, as is the case with other radiation procedures. Tumour prominence decreased in all patients.

Our impression is that the echographically determined degree to which vascularisation increases after irradiation is an indicator of the therapy's effectiveness.

Introduction

Because of its high accuracy echography has decisive importance for the diagnosis of malignant choroidal melanoma (Ossoinig, 1979; Coleman et al., 1977). Since the introduction of localized irradiation therapy with episcleral applicators (Stallard, 1960) it has become surgically indispensable as well.

Preoperatively it is used to determine the exact size of the tumour — a conditio sine qua non for preparing the radioactive applicator. Postoperatively it ensures the reliability of follow-ups. These are important because during the operation the sclera is exposed to a high dose of radiation and may perforate if tumours recur.

In addition one hopes that such echographical parameters as inner

[1] University Eye Clinic Tübingen, Ophthalmology III: Diseases of the Posterior Eye, 7400 Tübingen, FRG; [2] Zentralklinikum Augsburg, Stenglinstrasse 2, 8900 Augsburg, FRG.

J. M. Thijssen (ed.) Ultrasonography in ophthalmology.
© 1988, *Kluwer Academic Publishers, Dordrecht, ISBN 978-94-010-7083-6*

structure and the degree of reflectivity give early indication of the therapy's effectiveness.

Reports have already appeared on follow-ups after irradiation with Ruthenium 106 (Lüllwitz et al., 1979; Hasenfratz, 1985). With this therapy malignant melanomas with a prominence of up to 5 mm can be treated (Lommatzsch, 1979).

Packer and Rotman were the first to treat malignant melanomas with Iodine 125 (Packer et al., 1984). In this treatment tumours may have a prominence of up to 10 mm and a base diameter of up to 15 mm. Following is a report on the echographical characteristics of these tumours after irradiation with Iodine 125.

Material and methods

Since 1984 we have used Iodine 125 to treat 9 patients with choroidal melanomas. These were 5 women and 4 men between 26 and 72 years of age (average age: 57 years). The tumour prominence ranged from 6.3 µs to 10.9 µs (average: 8.5 µs) and the base diameter from 9.4 µs to 18.5 µs (average: 13.7 µs). The tumours were less than 2 mm from the disc in 1 patient and extended to the macula in 2 others. The ciliary body was not involved in any of the patients.

The examinations were performed with the Kretz 7200 MA standardized A-scan unit (determination of prominence) and the Ocuscan 400 B-scan unit (determination of base diameter). The eye and the probe were kept as stationary as possible (a fixation light was used), and the A-scan was recorded with a video system. The video camera was positioned in front of the screen, and the images recorded with a VHS recorder. When the tape was played back and stop-action used, vascularized portions of the tumour continued to be highly indistinct and showed spontaneous movements, since the video system's resolution speed was too slow for exact registration of the high-frequency vertical oscillations within vascularized areas of the tumours. These areas near the lower reversal points of the amplitudes were measured in µsec and the results added up. The sum was then divided by the total tumour prominence and this result designated as the "per cent degree of vascularisation" within the tumour. Individual pictures with remnants of movement, even within the orbit or the upper amplitude reversal points, were not evaluated. They were caused by movements of the eye and/or the probe.

The examinations were done the day before surgery, weekly for 4 weeks after applicator removal, monthly for the next 3 months, and finally once every half year. The radiation dose measured between 28,000 and 42,700 rads at the tumour base and between 5,700 and 8,140 rads at the tumour apex. The follow-up period ranged from 8 to 18 months, with an average of 12 months.

Results

Prominence

Within the first month after radiation therapy this increased by up to 0.6 μsec in 2 patients and decreased in another 7 patients by up to 3.8 μsec. Thereafter it decreased in all patients (Table 1).

Structure

Preoperatively it was regular in all patients. It became temporarily irregular in 3 patients between the 2nd and 10th weeks, but was again regular in all tumours from the 10th week on.

Reflectivity

Its preoperative height was 10% to 50%. It diminished by up to 10% in 3 patients and increased by up to 10% or stayed the same in the others within the first month after irradiation. Thereafter it uniformly exceeded the initial height more and more (Table 2). Only photographs showing maximal tumour prominence were evaluated.

Table 1. Tumour prominence in μsec preoperatively and after irradiation (* designates patients in whom it increased after 1 month).

	Before irradiation	After irradiation	
Pat.		1 Month	6 Months
M.P.*	10.9 μsec	11.5 μsec	6.0 μsec
W.U.	6.8 μsec	5.3 μsec	4.4 μsec
S.K.	10.6 μsec	7.0 μsec	1.5 μsec
H.H.	9.0 μsec	6.0 μsec	5.0 μsec
B.K.	8.4 μsec	7.3 μsec	5.6 μsec
A.G.	8.8 μsec	5.0 μsec	4.0 μsec
F.R.	8.0 μsec	7.5 μsec	6.8 μsec
R.A.	6.3 μsec	5.4 μsec	3.0 μsec
D.W.*	8.0 μsec	8.5 μsec	6.0 μsec

Table 2. Degree of reflectivity in per cent preoperatively and after irradiation. Approximate results (≈) are due to irregularity of the inner tumour structure.

Pat.	Before irradiation	After irradiation	
		1 Month	6 Months
M.P.	30%	≈ 20%	40%
W.U.	30%	≈ 40%	60%
S.K.	20%	30%	50%
H.H.	10%	20%	60%
B.K.	50%	≈ 40%	70%
A.G.	20%	20%	50%
F.R.	30%	40%	50%
R.A.	10%	20%	70%
D.W.	30%	20%	50%

The per cent degree of vascularization

Preoperatively it was between 10% and 30% and rose by a minimum of 10% and a maximum of 30% in all patients within the first month after irradiation. Thereafter it remained at a constant high level for at least 6 months (Table 3).

Table 3. Per cent degree of vascularisation before and after irradiation. Note the uniform increase after only 1 month and the constant high level after 6 months.

Pat.	Before irradiation	After irradiation	
		1 Month	6 Months
M.P.	30%	40%	40%
W.U.	20%	30%	40%
S.K.	20%	30%	40%
H.H.	30%	40%	50%
B.K.	10%	40%	40%
A.G.	30%	40%	50%
F.R.	20%	40%	50%
R.A.	30%	40%	40%
D.W.	20%	30%	40%

Discussion

The results to date show tumour prominence, inner structure and reflectivity to be highly variable within the first weeks after irradiation. They therefore hardly constitute a reliable yardstick for measuring the subsequent results of therapy.

The per cent degree of vascularisation, on the other hand, increased uniformly in all patients during the first treatment period. Thereafter the tumours grew steadily smaller and more highly reflective, the inner structure again regularized. The degree of vascularisation in per cent remained at a constant high level during this period.

It therefore seems possible to obtain early and reliable information about the subsequent effectiveness of irradiation with Iodine 125 from the degree of vascularisation. This may be helpful in deciding on the length of the application period or radiation dose.

The group of patients treated by us is however still too small and the follow-up time too short to state this firmly. Due to the disease's comparatively rare incidence, a final clarification of the issue may be achieved only when several clinics join together in a multi-institutional study.

References

Coleman DJ, Lizzi FL, Jack RL. 1977. Ultrasonography of the eye and orbit. Philadelphia: Lea & Febiger.

Hasenfratz, G. 1985. Echographische Befunde bei Aderhaut-Melanoblastomen nach Ruthenium-Therapie. Fortschr Ophthalmol 82: 453—456.

Lommatzsch PK. 1979. Radiotherapie der intraocularen Tumoren, insbesondere bei Aderhautmelanomen. Klin Mbl Augenheilk 174: 948—958.

Lüllwitz W, Hallermann D, Schröder W. 1979. Zum klinischen Verlauf des malignen Melanoms der Aderhaut nach Strahlentherapie mit Ru^{106}/Rh^{106} — Applikator. Ber Dtsch Ophthalmol Ges 76: 181—183.

Ossoinig C. 1979. Standardized echography: basic principles, clinical applications and results. In: RL Dallow (ed) Ophthalmic ultrasonography: comparative techniques. (Int Ophthalmol Clin 19/4), Little, Brown & Co., Boston.

Packer S, Rotman M, Salanitro P. 1984. Iodine-125 irradiation of choroidal melanoma. Ophthalmology 91: 1700—1708.

Stallard HB. 1960. Malignant melanoma of the choroid treated with radioactive applicators. Trans Ophthalmol Soc U.K. 79: 373—392.

Ultrasonically diagnosed cystic ciliary body melanomas

R. D. STONE[1] AND D. R. SHAPIRO

Summary

We present five cases of malignant melanoma of the ciliary body which appear cystic on ultrasound, including a histopathological correlation in one case. Such a histopathologic correlation has, to our knowledge, never been documented in the literature before. Histopathology of this case showed numerous small cystic spaces whose interiors were Alcian Blue and PAS negative. Regions of individual cells showing balloon degeneration were also seen.

Introduction

It is well known that malignant melanomas are the most common primary intraocular tumours. While they can occur anywhere in the uveal tract, 9% have been previously reported to occur in the ciliary body (Scheie and Albert, 1977). The A-mode and B-mode ultrasound characteristics of intraocular melanomas have been extensively described elsewhere (Baum, 1967; Coleman, 1974; Oksala, 1963; Ossoinig, 1969; Poujol, 1971). Skalka has already pointed out the importance of ultrasonography as a tool for detecting these malignancies in eyes with media opacity (Skalka, 1978). In one series, 21% of eyes with malignant melanomas had opaque media rendering visualization impossible (Mackley and Teed, 1958). Even when the media are clear, ultrasound has a vital role. In a study of eyes with clear media and lesions which were ophthalmoscopically visible and which had been diagnosed as melanomas without the aid of ultrasound, the diagnosis was incorrect in 19% of cases (Ferry, 1964). Furthermore, as Coleman points out, ultrasound is of even greater importance in the particular case of ciliary body melanomas as the ciliary body is an area not routinely examined and these tumours often precipitate cataracts which make visuali-

[1] The Department of Ophthalmology, University of California, 400 Parnassus Avenue, Room A-775, San Francisco, CA 94143, USA.

J. M. Thijssen (ed.) Ultrasonography in ophthalmology.
© 1988, *Kluwer Academic Publishers, Dordrecht, ISBN 978-94-010-7083-6*

zation difficult (Coleman, 1977). Coleman mentions the existence of acoustic quiet zones in sonograms of ciliary body melanomas, but no such cases have been histopathologically correlated in the literature (Coleman, 1977). We would like to describe five cases of ultrasonically cystic (by quantitative A-mode and B-mode) ciliary body melanomas, including one case with histopathologic correlation. These five cases were found from our review of our cross referenced ultrasound files on 534 ocular melanomas, 62 (12%) of which involved the ciliary body and/or iris and which were examined in our laboratory over the 10 year period 1974—1984.

Materials and methods

All patients were examined in the Ophthalmic Ultrasound Laboratory at the University of California Medical Center in San Francisco upon referral from our Ocular Oncology Unit over the 10 year period 1974—1984. Cross referenced diagnostic ultrasound files on 534 ocular melanoma patients seen in this laboratory over this period were reviewed to identify these cases. Three males and two females are described with ages ranging from 18 to 76. All patients ultimately exhibited an ultrasonically "cystic" tumour of the ciliary body during our ongoing long-term study protocol at this institution. B-mode examinations were performed with the Sonometrics 150 instrument using immersion techniques and a 10 MHz transducer. A-mode examinations were performed with the Kretz 7200 MA instrument using contact techniques and the 8 MHz transducer. One eye was eventually enucleated. Pathologic specimens were treated with H and E, PAS, and Alcian Blue stains and examined in the University of California Eye Pathology Laboratory.

Case reports

Case One

A 23 year old white male with a vague history of remote trauma to his right eye was referred to the Ocular Oncology Unit because of an unusual appearing darkly pigmented mass of the ciliary body and anterior choroid of the right eye. He was aware of decreased vision in the right eye of recent onset. Examination revealed a best corrected visual acuity of 20/70 in the right eye and 20/20 in the left eye. Behind the right lens, a cystic appearing, but highly vascularized lesion, was seen between the 1:00 and 5:00 o'clock meridians. It appeared slightly translucent on transillumination. The intraocular pressures were 15 mmHg by applanation. Indirect ophthalmoscopy and contact lens examination revealed a localized ciliary body-choroidal mass lesion which involved the nasal periphery and obscured visualization of the right disc. The most unusual clinical feature of the lesion was its intense vascularity. This vascularity appeared deep in the mass and appeared to be of choroidal origin. Examination of the left fundus was normal. Fluorescein angiography was most consistent with a ciliary body melanoma.

B-mode ultrasonography of the right eye (Fig. 1) revealed a nasally situated "cystic" mass of the anterior globe which appeared to be based at the iris root anteriorly and to elevate the ciliary body, pars plana, and anterior retina. It appeared to displace the lens temporally. Its posterior configuration was similar to a haemorrhagic choroidal detachment (its posterior acute angled insertion was at approximately the equator). The mass was distinctly cystic ultrasonically in B-mode and had thick anterior and posterior walls which were connected at the crest of the mass, where the thinnest wall was noted. There was a complex membrane pattern corresponding to the posterior wall of the mass which was suggestive of multiple "cystic" changes in this "cystic" lesion's wall. This feature, however, was not able to be confirmed ophthalmoscopically at the time of examination due to the lesion's large size.

Quantitative A-mode ultrasonography (Fig. 2) confirmed the cystic

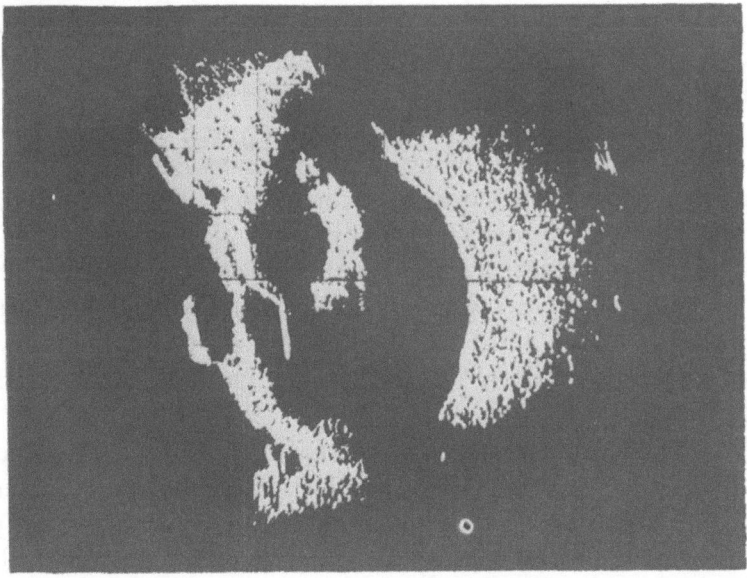

Fig. 1. B-mode sonogram, Case One. Note the small, multiple "cysts" in the posterior wall of this cystic appearing melanoma.

174

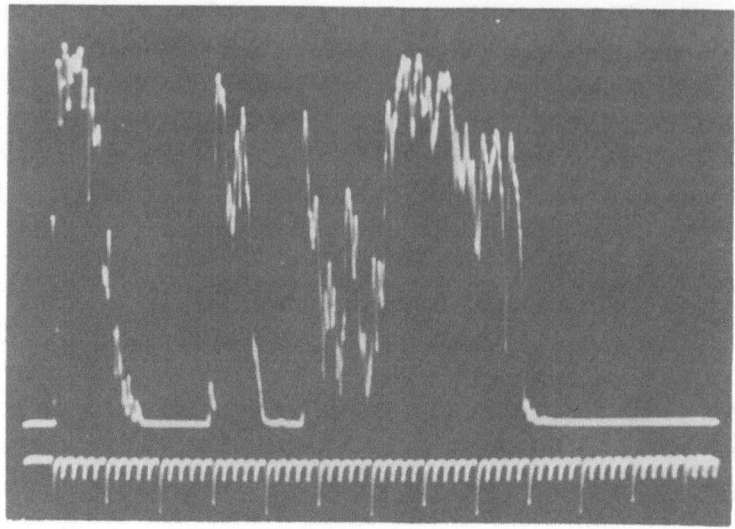

Fig. 2. A-mode sonogram, Case One. Note that the tracing falls to baseline, indicating an acoustically homogeneous interior.

nature of the mass. The fact that the A-mode trace fell to baseline was quite striking. The tracing also revealed true heterogeneity and high amplitude spikes associated with the walls of the mass. A-mode examination also showed the tumour thickness to be 10.55 mm.

The ultrasonic differential diagnosis of the lesion included: an unresolved, possibly organized, choroidal detachment (there was a vague history of trauma), a ciliary body cyst, and an extremely atypical cystic ciliary body malignant melanoma.

Because the lesion was large and very atypical and the diagnosis was unresolved, a fine needle biopsy was performed. Because of its equivocal results, an iridocyclectomy was performed one week later. Initially, the tumour appeared to have been removed with clear margins at the time of surgery. The presence of an opaque media caused by vitreous haemorrhage postoperatively, created problems in the clinical management of this case. However, serial follow-up ultrasound examinations revealed a residual mass posteriorly with documented growth. Therefore, the right eye was enucleated.

The fine needle aspirate showed a few clusters of tightly packed small round to spindle shaped cells with a high N/C ratio. Nucleoli were small but conspicuous and the chromatin pattern finely granular. No pigment was seen. The diagnosis was considered equivocal, but felt to be most consistent with melanoma. Other types of neoplasms such as neurilemmoma were not able to be ruled out.

The iridocyclectomy specimen (Figs. 3, 4) also showed predominantly

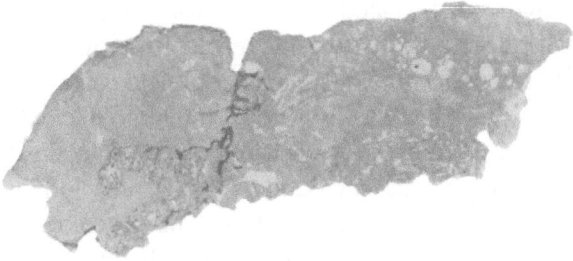

Fig. 3. Iridocyclectomy specimen, Case One, showing fluid filled pseudocysts, and larger cleft presumed to be collapsed larger pseudocyst.

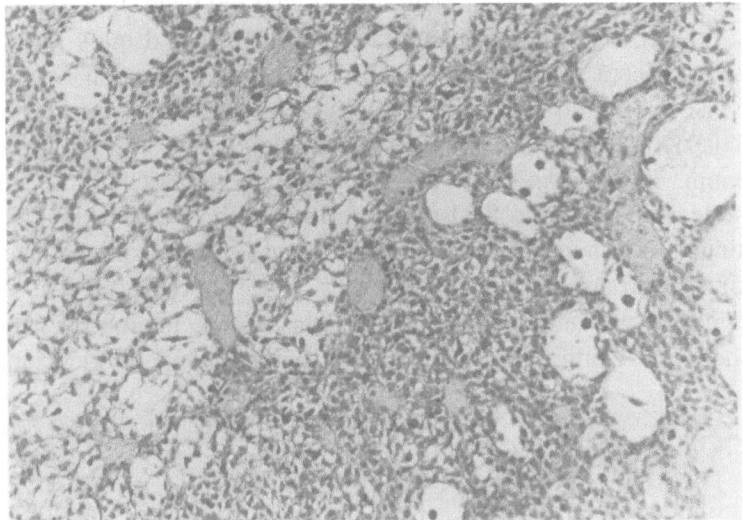

Fig. 4. Iridocyclectomy specimen, Case One, (10×), shows regions of balloon degeneration.

spindle cells with numerous cells showing small nucleoli. No epitheliod component was noted. Most important for our discussion here, unusually large fluid filled spaces without an endothelial lining were seen (Fig. 3). These pseudocysts measured approximately 0.05 to 0.50 mm and were separated by walls 3—4 cells thick or by homogeneous tumour stroma of thickness equivalent to these spaces. The interior of these pseudocysts were Alcian Blue negative (indicating there was no mucopolysaccharide present) and PAS negative. There were regions of widespread balloon degeneration of individual cells (Fig. 4) which could appear as sonolucent regions on ultrasound and therefore sonographically look like the pseudocysts. A large cleft was noted and interpreted to be consistent with the largest collapsed cyst, although this might also have been an artifact caused by folding of the specimen.

176

The enucleated eye revealed that the nasal ciliary body was absent (secondary to iridocyclomectomy) and residual tumour was found posterior to the border of the previously made surgical resection. The tumour consisted of spindle shaped cells with prominent nucleoli. No mitoses were seen. Melanin pigment was seen interspersed in the tumour mass. Posteriorly, the tumour was surrounded by chronic inflammatory cells, which were felt to be of surgical evocation. The pathologic diagnosis was ciliary body and choroidal melanoma of the spindle B type.

Case Two

On B-mode ultrasonic examination, a 75 year old male showed an acoustically (immersion B-mode, quantitative A-mode) solid mass located temporally adjacent to the lens equator occupying the region of the ciliary body. The solid ultrasonic interior was typical for malignant melanoma of the ciliary body (Fig. 5). A-mode examination showed a tumour height of 8.23 mm. 10 months later, the tumour had increased in thickness on A-mode examination to 8.81 mm. On B-mode, however, while the tumour continued to be acoustically solid in its anterior portion, it had developed a striking cystic appearance in its posterior portion (Fig. 6). The A-mode examination was noted to be difficult due to the tumour's location, but did not yield confirmation of cystic pattern seen on B-mode examination

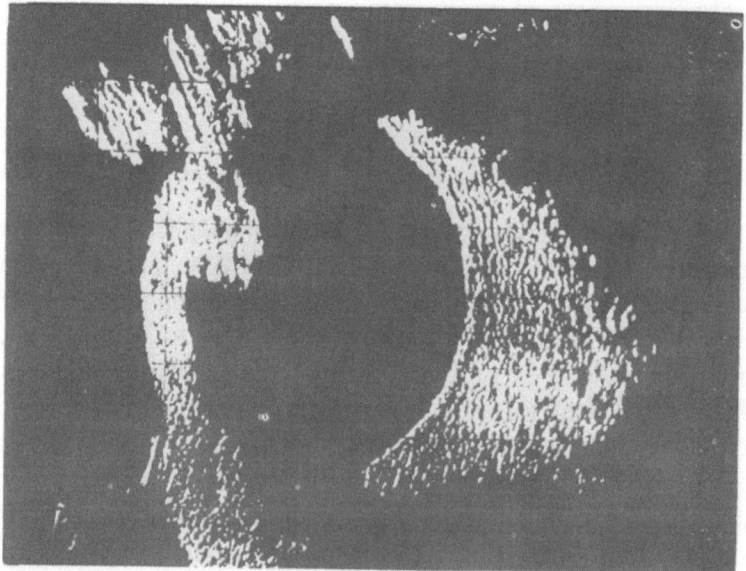

Fig. 5. Initial B-mode sonogram, Case Two. This solid pattern is typical for ciliary body melanomas.

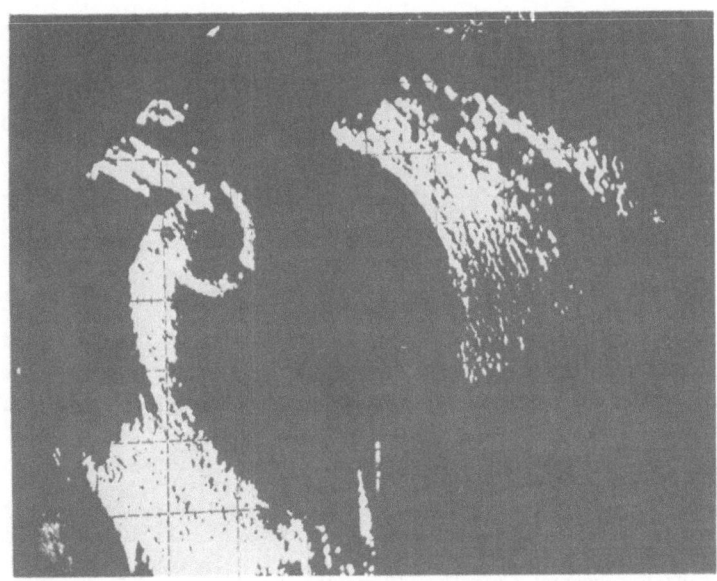

Fig. 6. B-mode sonogram, Case Two. 10 months after Fig. 5. Note the posterior cystic appearance of the lesion.

(Fig. 7). 13 months later, however, follow-up A-mode examination (Fig. 8) also revealed a cystic pattern for the posterior portion of the tumour consistent with the B-scan, which had continued to appear cystic posteriorly. The ultrasonic diagnosis was malignant melanoma of the ciliary body. The patient is still being followed.

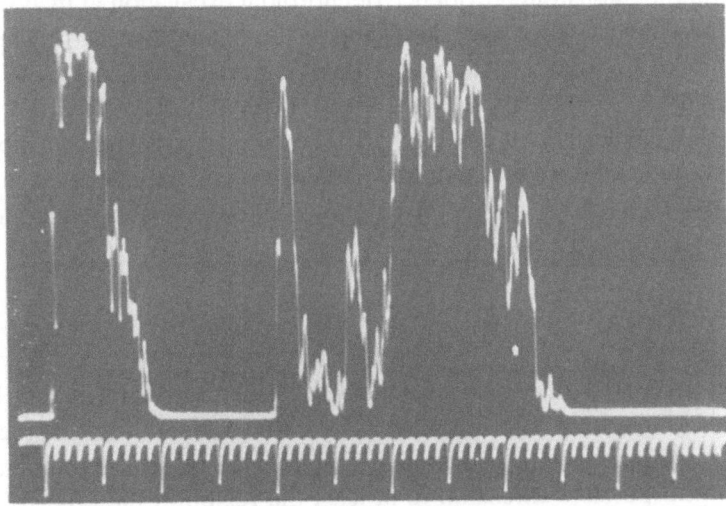

Fig. 7. A-mode sonogram, Case Two at the time of Fig. 6. The trace does not return to baseline and thus does not confirm the presence of internal acoustic homogeneity seen on the B-mode in Fig. 6.

178

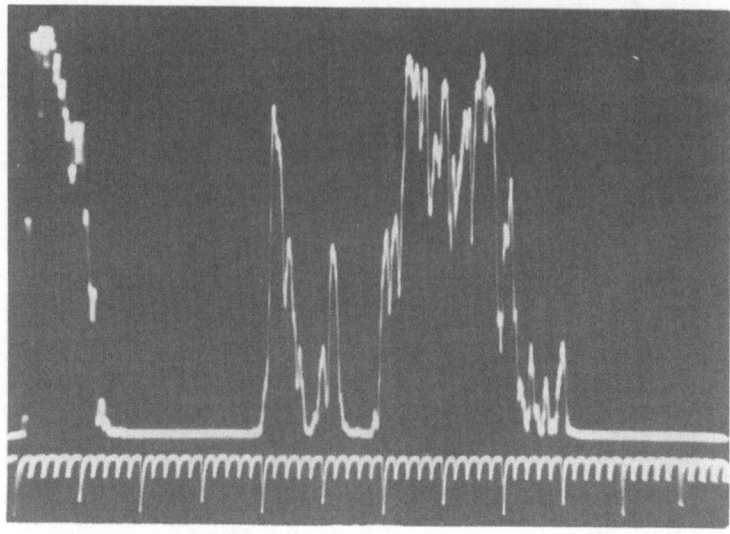

Fig. 8. A-mode sonogram, Case Two. 13 months after Figs. 6 and 7 were recorded. The trace now does return to baseline.

Case Three

B-mode examination of the right eye of this 70 year old male revealed a cystic appearing choroidal mass involving the ciliary body, pars plana and choroid of the superior quadrants to approximately the equator (Fig. 9). The retina was on its surface and it exhibited acoustic quiet zones internally and demonstrated evidence of choroidal excavation at its border with normal choroid. Acoustic shadowing in the orbital fat echo complex was also present. A-mode examination demonstrated a high degree of internal homogeneity consistent with the cystic B-mode appearance as well as a high degree of attenuation (Fig. 10). The A-mode tracing also showed the maximum height of the lesion to be 8.43 mm. The ultrasonic diagnosis was malignant melanoma of the ciliary body and the patient continues to be followed.

Case Four

A 76 year old female was evaluated for a mass in her left eye. B-mode examination of the eye suggested a shallowing of the anterior chamber nasally associated with a mass involving the area of the iris root and ciliary body with possible extension to at least the region of the ora serrata. The anterior portion of the mass appeared acoustically solid but the posterior portion appeared cystic (Fig. 11). The A-mode pattern suggested that the

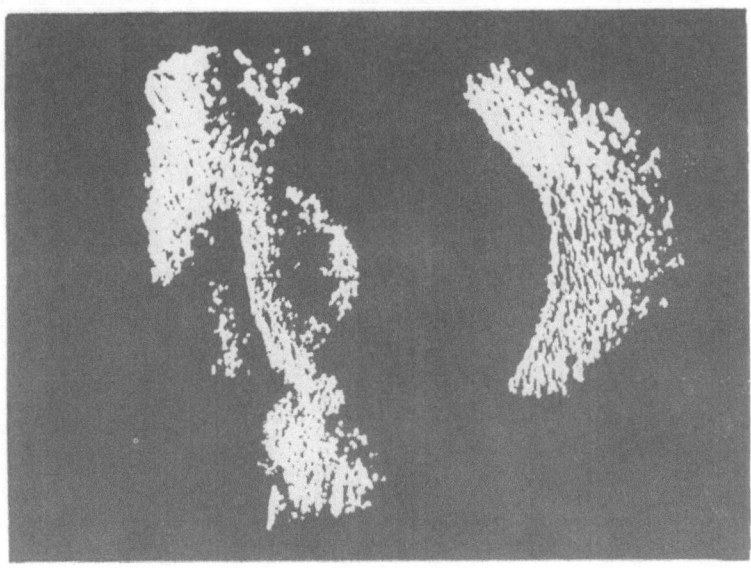

Fig. 9. B-mode sonogram, Case Three.

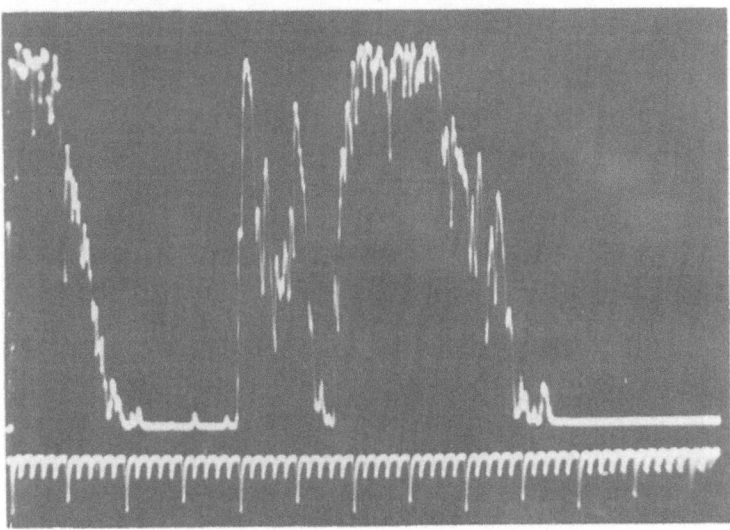

Fig. 10. A-mode sonogram, Case Three, confirms the cystic appearance seen in Fig. 9.

mass was solid throughout despite its cystic appearance on B-mode (Fig. 12). A-mode measurements showed a tumour thickness of 5.17 mm. Four months later, the A- and B-scan patterns had not changed but the tumour had increased in thickness to 6.70 mm. The patient is still being followed.

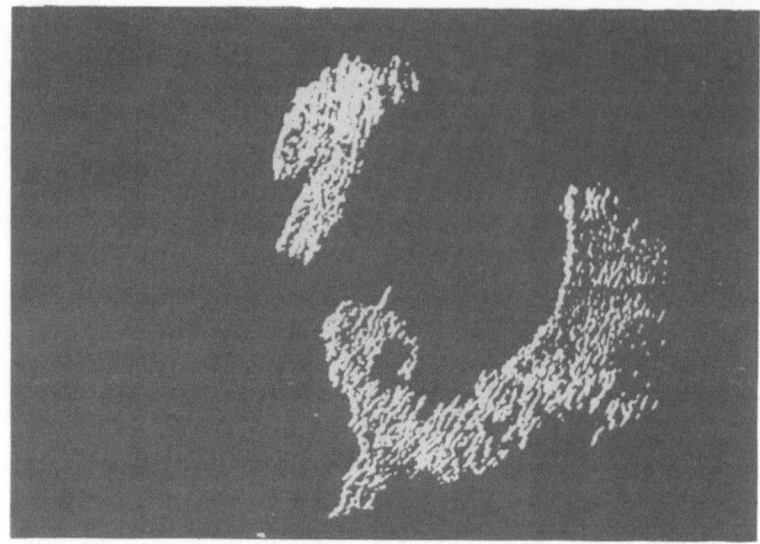

Fig. 11. B-mode sonogram, Case Four. Note the posterior cystic appearing space in the lesion.

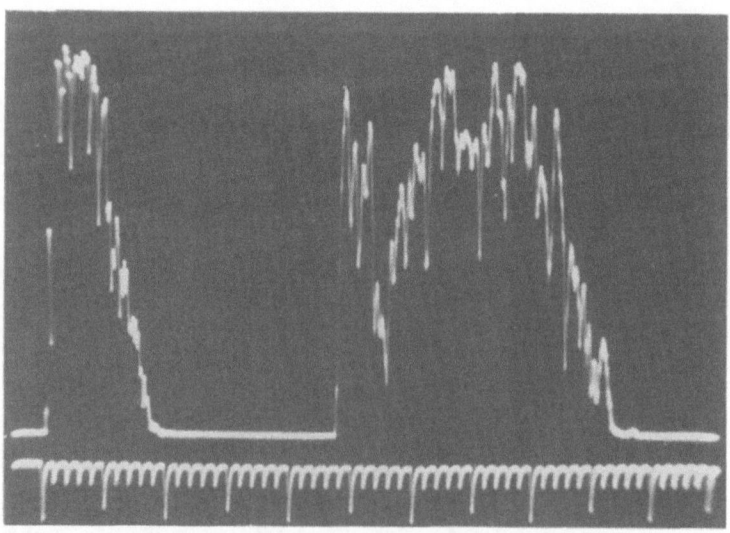

Fig. 12. A-mode sonogram, Case Four. The tracing suggests a solid pattern throughout, in contrast to the B-mode sonogram in Fig. 11.

Case Five

An 18 year old male was evaluated for a mass of the ciliary body of his right eye. It had a cystic appearance on B-scan without evidence of choroidal excavation or acoustic shadowing (Fig. 13), while the A-mode demonstrated a fairly high degree of internal homogeneity and attenuation of the ultrasound. No cystic A-mode features have been detected thus far however, and the patient continues to the followed.

Discussion

While the A-mode and B-mode ultrasound characteristics of intraocular melanomas is extensively described elsewhere, the ultrasound character of these five cases is quite unique due to the cystic qualities demonstrated. Usually, these are ultrasonically solid when in the ciliary body, in contrast to our cases being presented, although the existence of acoustic quiet zones in the sonograms of ciliary body melanomas has been described (Coleman, 1977).

Coleman points out that the B-mode displays can be viewed as the summation of the A-mode acoustic characteristics. Choroidal excavation, an indentation in the choroidal contour on B-scan, is a prominent feature of posterior choroidal melanomas but not of ciliary body melanomas and was not seen in the series we present here. Acoustic shadowing can occur with ocular melanomas but was not prominent in our cases. Coleman's final B-scan acoustic characteristic, acoustic quiet zones, is of the most

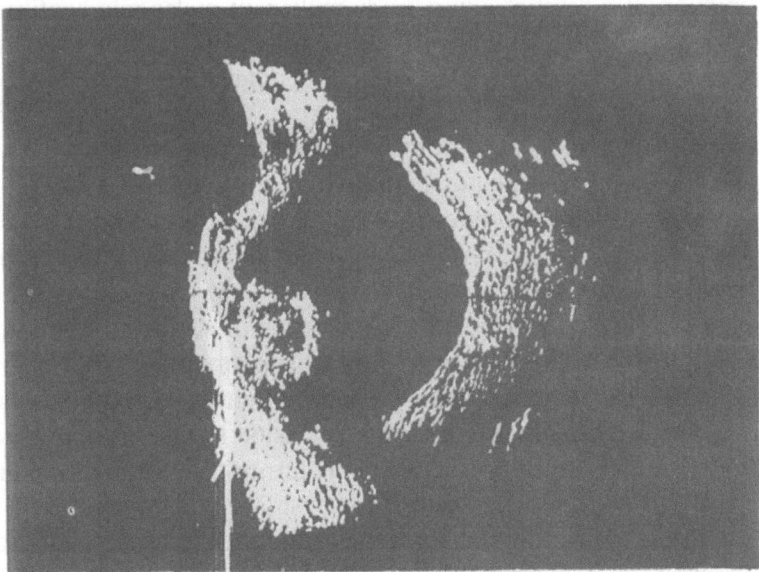

Fig. 13. B-mode sonogram, Case Five. Note the cystic appearance of the lesion. As in Case Four, the A-mode sonogram in this case did not confirm this cystic appearance.

interest to the discussion of the cases we are reporting since we have confirmation that the acoustically quiet or "cystic" zones in ciliary body melanomas can actually arise from histologically cystic spaces. Coleman points out that in relatively avascular melanomas elsewhere there is a lack of significant internal acoustic interfaces resulting in an acoustic "quiet zone". This quieting phenomenon is accentuated on B-mode while the A-mode tracing reveals echoes of moderate, but declining, amplitude throughout the solid tumour. Coleman also points out that if the lesion were actually hollow and filled with fluid, the A-mode would show absence of echoes after the initial leading echo. Finally, Coleman notes that acoustic quiet zones at the posterior part of a ciliary body melanoma can be seen, but comments that he has not had extensive experience with this phenomenon.

A-mode examination with the Kretz 7200 MA instrument was most helpful in predicting the histolopathologically cystic nature of the melanoma in Case One. Ossoinig (1969) summarizes the quantitative A-mode ultrasonic characteristics of melanoma of the choroid and ciliary body. He includes characteristics of: a three dimensional lesion with a chain of spikes in all sound beams passing through the lesion, low to medium reflectivity with spike height of 10—60%, hard consitency with no after-movements, strong sound attenuation with·a large "angle Kappa", and decreased reflectivity of sclera at the tumour base.

Our cases include an actual case report of the ultrasonically unusual presentation of a "cystic" ciliary body malignant melanoma confirmed by histopathology. The quantitative A-mode tracing in the lesion did, in fact, return to baseline as one would expect if it contained a cyst. On pathologic examination the lesion was found to be a spindle B type malignant melanoma. The homogeneity of this type of tumour alone however, cannot account for the acoustically cystic pattern seen so far in Cases One, Two and Three, but might account for the features of Cases Four and Five, in which the A-scan revealed a non-cystic interior despite a cystic appearance on B-scan. It is possible that the melanoma in Case One actually was filled by a large cyst which was collapsed at the time of needle aspiration biopsy or subsequently by the excision. This is supported by the cleft in the specimen which may represent the remnants of such a large central cyst.

Case Two adds another interesting dimension to the series. In this case, both the B-mode and the A-mode sonograms initially showed the tumour to be solid, then, 10 months later, B-mode showed the tumour to be cystic while the A-mode tracing remained solid, and then finally, an additional 8 months later, both the B-mode and the A-mode sonograms were cystic. The tumour had increased in size by 0.38 mm since the initial evaluation. The B-mode sonogram revealed sonolucencies earlier than a quantitative

A-mode tracing, as it uses a higher threshold level for recording echoes than the A-mode instrument. It seems that we caught a dynamic process at three separate windows in time as the tumour went from less to more homogeneity internally. As we have no pathological correlation we can only speculate on the changes involved. Perhaps small cysts were forming, each one too small to be resolved individually, but once they reached a threshold size, they resulted in a large ultrasonic quiet zone similar to the process in Case One. Alternatively, perhaps an actual cyst has developed which first appeared on B-mode examination and then, as the cyst became larger, also appeared on A-scan. Case Three, like Cases One and Two, is cystic on both B-mode and A-mode sonograms. Cases Four and Five, however, follow more the pattern Coleman mentions, having an acoustic quiet zone on B-scan but appearing solid on A-scan.

Acknowledgements

Marvin Zielinski, COT, Sharon Humphrey, RDMS, and Ann Welling, RDMS, were technicians in the Ultrasound Laboratory, University of California, San Francisco, during this study. Nancy King typed the manuscript, which was processed on an IBM PC-XT, with Wordstar software.

The authors have no financial, commercial, or proprietary interest in either the Sonometrics 150 A/B-mode instrument or the Kretztechnik 7200 MA A-mode instrument.

Pathological examinations were performed in the Eye Pathology Laboratory, Department of Ophthalmology, University of California School of Medicine, San Francisco, by J. Brooks Crawford, M.D., and Edward L. Howes, M.D.

This study was supported, in part, by an unrestricted grant from research to prevent blindness, Inc.

References

Baum G. 1967. Ultrasonic characteristics of malignant melanoma. Arch Ophthalmol 78: 12—15.

Coleman DJ, Abramson DH, Jack RL, Franzen LA. 1974. Ultrasonic diagnosis of tumours of the choroid. Arch Ophthalmol 91: 344—354.

Coleman DJ, Lizzi FL, Jack RL. 1977. Ultrasonography of the Eye and Orbit. Philadelphia, Lea and Febiger.

Ferry AP. 1964. Lesions mistaken for malignant melanomas of the posterior uvea: a clinico-pathologic analysis of 100 cases with ophthalmoscopically visible lesions. Arch Ophthalmol 72: 463—469.

184

Mackley TA, Teed RW. 1958. Unsuspected intraocular malignant melanomas. Arch Ophthalmol 60: 475—478.

Oksala A. 1963. Ultrasound diagnosis in intraocular melanoma. Ann NY Acad Sci 100: 18—27.

Ossoinig K, Till P. 1969. Methods and Results of Ultrasonography in Diagnosing Intraocular Tumours. In: K Gitter et al. (ed) Ophthalmic Ultrasound. The CV Mosby Company, St Louis.

Poujol J. 1971. Clinical Echography in Intraocular Tumours. In: J Boeck and K Ossoinig (eds) Ultrasonographia Medica (SIDUO III). Verlag der Wiener Med Akad, Vienna, pp. 275—290.

Scheie HG, Albert DM. 1977. Textbook of Ophthalmology. Philadelphia, WB Sanders Company.

Skalka HW. 1978. Unusual ophthalmic melanomas: the value of ultrasonography. Ann Ophthalmol 10: 42—46.

A mushroom-shaped pigmented pseudomelanoma
(case report)

J. SCHUTTERMAN AND U. AXELSSON

Summary

A 52 year old woman of Asian origin presented with a highly elevated pigmented mushroom-shaped fundus mass lesion which on transillumination showed a definite shadow. P^{32}-examination gave borderline results. In the contralateral eye a slightly elevated smaller mass lesion showed positive results on P^{32}-examination. Clinical, P^{32}, echographic and histopathological features will be described.

Report

A 52 year old lady of Asian origin was referred with a two week history of a shadow in the visual field of her left eye by a practising ophthalmologist to the Eye Clinic at Karolinska Hospital. He had found a highly protruding tumour between the 5.30 and 8 o'clock meridians in her left fundus. She had no history of any other disease and had no medical treatment prior to presentation.

On admission the right eye had 20/20 visual acuity, normal IOP by palpation and slight posterior pole lens opacities. In the fundus the optic disc and macula were within normal limits ophthalmoscopically. At 10 o'clock in the midperiphery there was a 7—8 disc areas blackish brown non elevated pigmented lesion that looked like a common naevus. The left eye had a 20/25 visual acuity, normal IOP by palpation and in the fundus a circumscribed pigmented area with some depigmented spots and slight elevation from which a dark pigmented mushroom-shaped tumour was seen protruding far into the vitreous cavity, from below the inferior arcade almost to the ora serrata. The basis of the mass was considerably more narrow than the top. The distance of the mass from the optic disc was 3 discdiameters. There was an exsudative retinal detachment on either side and peripherily.

Department of Ophthalmology, Södersjukhuset, Stockholm, Sweden.

J. M. Thijssen (ed.) Ultrasonography in ophthalmology.
© 1988, *Kluwer Academic Publishers, Dordrecht, ISBN 978-94-010-7083-6*

186

Both diascleral and transpupillar *transillumination* gave a definite shadow from the tumour area. *Fluorescein angiography* showed marked blocking of background fluorescense due to heavy pigmentation of the mass. P^{32}-*examination* at Södersjukhuset with a bare sclera approach gave a maximum 88% uptake over tumour area. Adjacent parts of the tumour area had 55% or less. (In the right eye at the pigmented non elevated fundus lesion 92% uptake was recorded with a trans-conjunctival approach.) The results were interpreted as borderline positive.

The fundus lesion of the left eye was also examined with *standardized echography* at Södersjukhuset with a Kretz Technik 7200 MA and the Sonometrics Ocuscan 400. Between 4 and 9 o'clock behind the equator a solid lesion with a mushroom- of collarbutton-shape was detected. (Fig. 1) The reflectivity was high, sometimes extremely high, but never below 75% and the internal structure was heterogeneous. There was no pronounced attenuation and the vascularity was slight. The maximum tumour height over scleral inner surface, examined with standardized A-scan and decreased system sensitivity, was found to be at least 10 mm; the width of the lesion was roughly estimated to be at least 16 mm by B-scan examination. (The fundus of the right eye was screened with B-scan and no elevated lesion was detected.) The mass lesion in the left eye was considered echographically not typical for a malignant melanoma of the choroid because of its high reflectivity and lack of signs of significantly increased vascularity, despite its mushroom-shape so common in large melanomas. From the echographic standpoint a metastatic lesion was considered the most likely diagnostic alternative although an "atypical melanoma could not completely be ruled out".

A *medical screening* for a primary neoplastic lesion was carried on: The physical examination, laboratory tests as blood counts, electrolytes, hepatic and thyroid tests, chest X-rays and mammograms were all within normal limits.

On follow up visual acuity left eye decreased during the next few

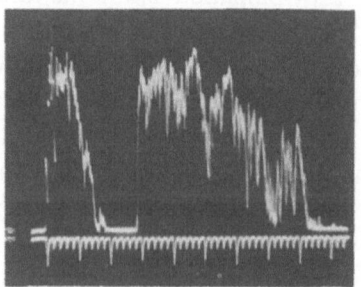 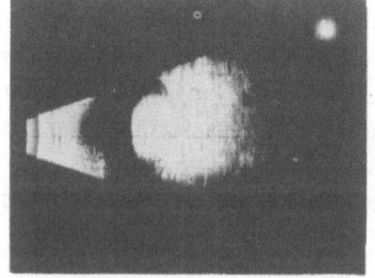

(a) (b)

Fig. 1. (a) A-scan picture (Kretztechnik 7200 MA) through lesion, note high lesion echoes. (b) B-scan showing regular, highly reflective tumour.

months to 20/50 and ophthalmoscopically both tumour size and extension of the retinal detachment were considered possibly slightly increased. The patient was now suggested an enucleation on clinical suspicion of a malignant melanoma but the patient did not accept and the decision was postponed for another 2.5 months. At that point visual acuity was down to counting fingers 3 m and there was a definite growth of the tumour and enlarged retinal detachment now including parts of the macula. There was another period of hesitation from the patient and finally she accepted enucleation and visual acuity was by then only counting fingers 20 cm. Enucleation was performed after linear accelerator preoperative radiation treatment 5 × 4 Gy which is our routine procedure for treatment of those uveal melanoma patients that are not treated in other ways.

Histopathology report was as follows: Under the retina there is pigmented tumour, originating from the pigment epithelium cell layer. The tumour is well vascularized and consists of the pigmented cells on a thin connective tissue stroma. Tumour cells show some polymorfism. The tumour is rich in vacuols containing a proteinous exsudate. The tumour is well outlined against Bruch's membrane but infiltrates the retina all the way to the internal limiting membrane. The tumour is diagnosed as a benign adenoma of the retinal pigment epithelial cells. It is considered benign because there is no infiltration into the choroid nor through the internal limiting membrane. Still it is obviously destructive to the eye. The borderline positive P^{32}-results seemed to be due to proliferation of cells.

Conclusion

In this case standardized echography turned out to be more correct than the total clinical impression. This kind of lesion is obviously extremely infrequent.

References

Duke JB, Maumenee AE. 1959. An unusual Tumour of the Retinal Pigment Epithelium. Br J Ophthalmology 47: 311.

Garner A. 1970. Tumours of the Retinal Pigment Epithelium. Br J Ophthalmology 54: 715.

Michaelson IC, Benezra D. 1980. Textbook of the Fundus of the Eye, Churchill-Livingstone, 3rd Ed, pp. 527—528.

Ossoinig KC. 1979. Standardized echography: Basic principles, clinical applications, and results. In: RL Dallow (ed) International Ophthalmology Clinics: Ophthalmic Ultrasonography: Comparative techniques 19(4): 127—210.

Shields JA. 1983. Diagnosis and Management of Intraocular Tumours. C.V. Mosby Comp, St Louis, pp. 144—170.

Errors in the diagnosis of retinoblastoma

R. SAMPAOLESI[1] AND J. ZARATE

Summary

We have studied 60 retinoblastomas over a period of 8 years in the Buenos Aires University Hospital. 40 cases were enucleated after diagnosis and pathology was performed on each eye.

The echographic diagnosis was performed with the 7200 Kretz unit echograph, and lately with the Ocuscan: Sonokretz 400 ST — Both with A-mode with S shaped amplification.

The diagnosis was correct in 36 cases and of the four remaining cases, two were false negative and two false positive.

Diagnosis of retinoblastoma

Figure 1 corresponds to the typical pattern of a retinoblastoma. In Fig. 1c (B-mode) the echogram shows a solid mass with a cyst anterior to it. In Fig. 1a, spike q corresponds to the anterior wall of the cyst, the many spikes at t belong to the echoes of the tumour; the spike ca has a very high reflectivity and corresponds to the presence of calcium in the tumour; e corresponds to the sclera. The most important element for the diagnosis, however, was the very low reflectivity of the orbital echoes o due to the acoustic shadow caused by the calcium. Figure 1b corresponds to the contralateral normal eye, e is the sclera wall, and the orbital echoes have a very high reflectivity. (o) The reflectivity of these normal echoes should be compared with the pathological ones with very low reflectivity.

The Fig. 1c lower right diagram illustrates the tumour, the cyst and the orbital tissue, the probe and its direction, the ultrasound beam and the corresponding echograms. This pattern was described in 1981 by Ossoinig.

Figure 2, with the B-mode, shows the mass of the tumour and the

---

[1] Dept. of Ophthalmology, School of Medicine, University of Buenos Aires, Parana 1239-1A, 1018 Buenos Aires, Argentina.

J. M. Thijssen (ed.) Ultrasonography in ophthalmology.
© 1988, *Kluwer Academic Publishers, Dordrecht, ISBN 978-94-010-7083-6*

190

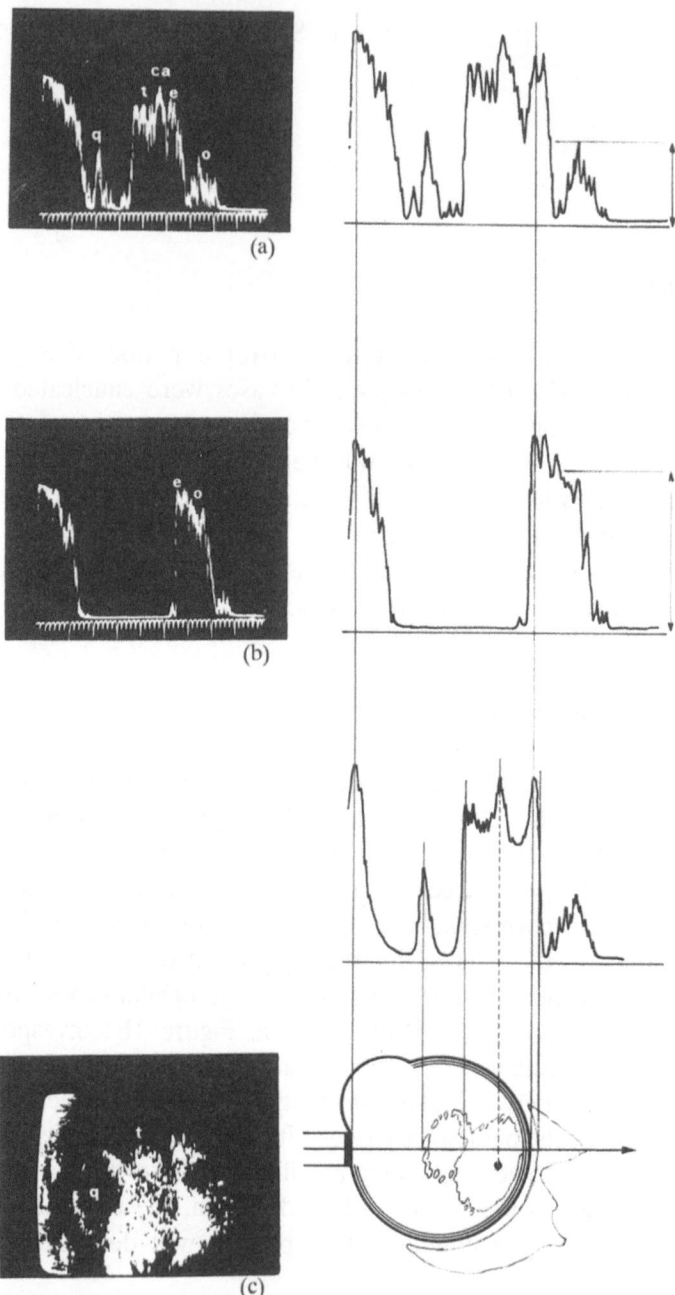

Fig. 1. Echogram typical of retinoblastoma (a) contralateral normal eye (b) B-mode echogram of retinoblastoma q = cyst (c).

acoustic shadow (s a.). On lowering the decibels from 80 to 40 the echoes which remain correspond to the calcium in the tumour (ca). With com-

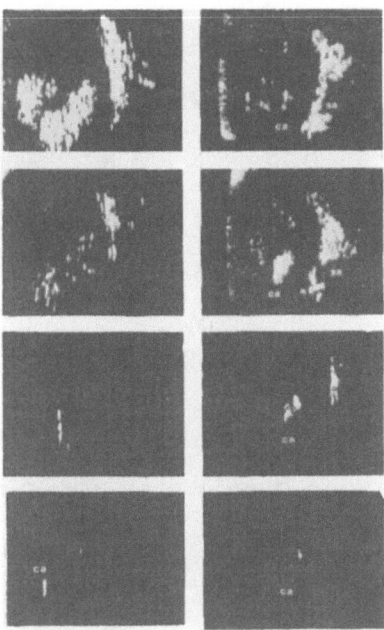

Fig. 2. B-mode echograms of retinoblastoma at four different sensitivity settings of equipment (rows from top to bottom at 80 dB through 40 dB, respectively).

puterised tomography, it is also possible to detect the calcium content in the tumour.

In each case we performed echobiometry. The axial length is usually normal for the age or perhaps larger when secondary glaucoma is present.

These findings contrast with the echobiometry in leucocoria, in which we generally find a decrease of the axial length as Bertenyi and co-workers have found.

Figure 3, on the left side, shows the pathology of different retinoblastomas with different calcium contents. In Fig. 3a, there is a well differentiated retinoblastoma with high calcium content which corresponds to echoes a a a. o are the orbital echoes with very low reflectivity. Figure 3b is a semi-differentiated retinoblastoma with rosettes and a small quantity of calcium and Fig. 3c is an undifferentiated retinoblastoma without calcium and in the echogram the orbital echoes are normal. In cases like this it is very difficult, even impossible, to make a diagnosis with echography.

In four cases we made a wrong diagnosis: two were false positive and two were false negative. In the first two cases, the echographic diagnosis was retinoblastoma and the histopathological diagnoses were in the first case choroidal haemangioma and in the second Coats' disease.

In the third case the echographic diagnosis was Panuveitis and in the

192

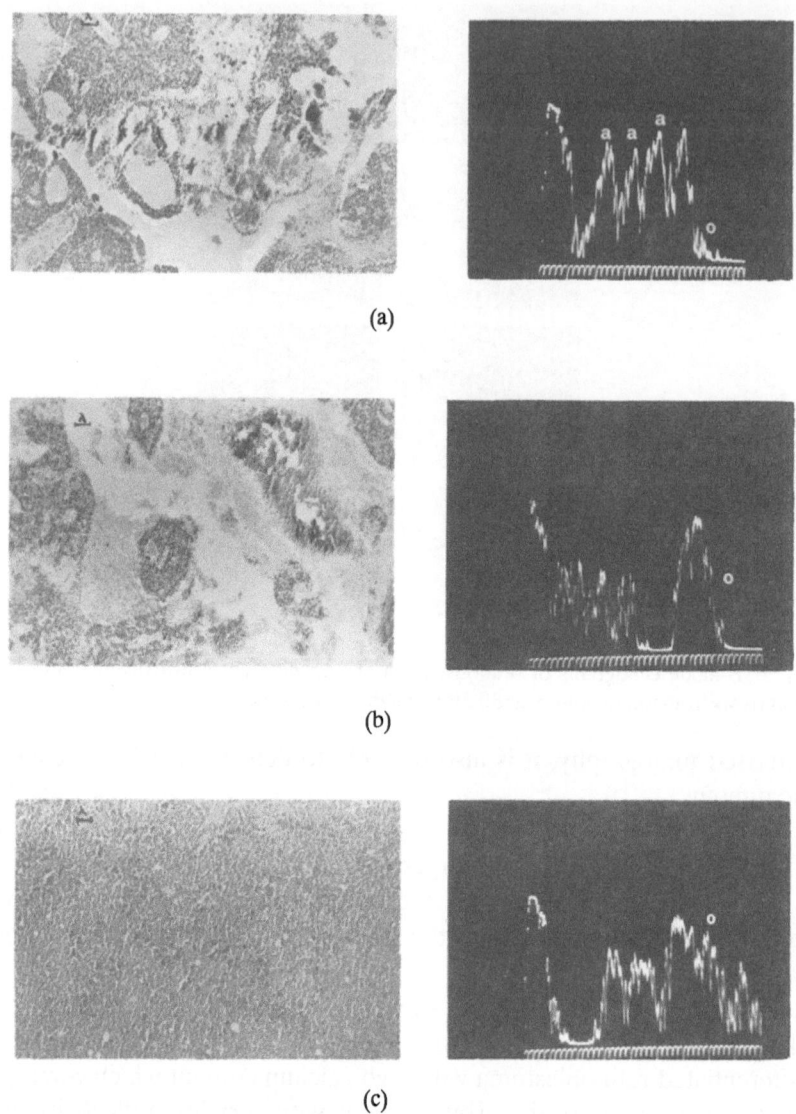

(a)

(b)

(c)

Fig. 3. Comparison of histology and A-mode echography of retinoblastoma, o = orbital echoes, a = calcium spikes.

fourth case it was vitreous haemorrhage. The histopathological diagnosis in these two last cases was in fact retinoblastoma.

Erronic cases

Case No. 1

6-year-old female presenting with a right eye retinal detachment with a solid appearance. In the echogram (Fig. 4a) the spike r corresponds to the detached retina followed by many echoes with high reflectivity produced by the tumour, and o corresponds to the orbital echoes with very low reflectivity. We performed an enucleation. In Fig. 4b, the histopathology shows an unusually thick haemangioma. Near the choroid we observed a proliferation of the vascular walls, melanocytes and melanophages. The lumen of the large vessels are full of red corpuscles.

In summary, the echographic diagnosis was retinoblastoma and the histopathology shows a choroidal haemangioma.

Case No. 2

16-month male presenting with leucocoria. During the examination under general anesthesia we observed a detached retina with two bags and a white mass behind the retina. Intraocular pressure was 28 mmHg. Figure 5a: the spikes S correspond to the detached retina, and ca, of high reflectivity, to the possible contents of calcium; o are the orbital echoes with very low reflectivity. Figure 5b shows the histopathology with many cholesterol crystals (negative areas).

In summary, the echographic diagnosis was retinoblastoma and the histopathology shows a Coats' disease.

Case No. 3

6-year-old male presenting with a uveitis with hypopyon, pain and an intraocular pressure of 66 mmHg in the right eye which did not respond to medical treatment. We carried out a trabeculectomy.

The excised trabeculectomy tissue showed a haemorrhagic inflammatory reaction at the trabeculum, a fibrino-leucocyte exudate, pigment and pigment thrombus in the Schlemm Canal and the ciliary muscle with

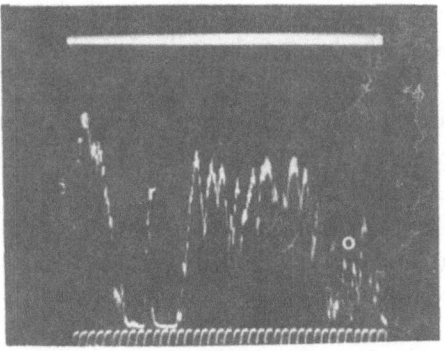

(a)

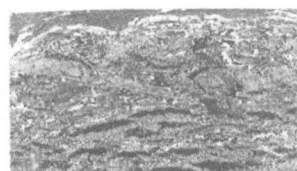

(b)

Fig. 4. A-mode echogram and histology of case 1, o = orbital echoes.

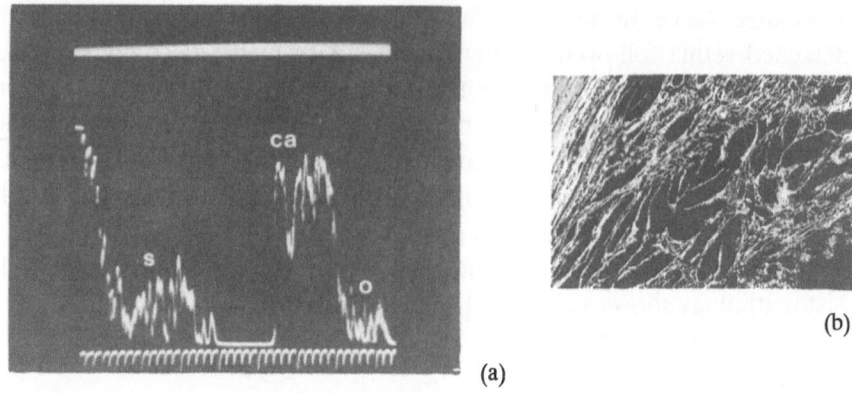

(b)

(a)

Fig. 5. A-mode echogram and histology of case 2, ca = calcium, s = retinal spikes.

oedema and inter-fibrillar haemorrhages. Figure 6 shows the echogram: d, corresponds to some celular débris in the vitreous body, r to the retina followed by many spikes corresponding to the tumour and the orbital echoes with normal reflectivity.

Because the eye continued to be painful with ocular hypertension and had no vision it was enucleated. The histopathology showed a diffuse infiltrating retinoblastoma instead of a panuveitis as the echographic diagnosis had indicated.

This kind of retinoblastoma produces a pseudo-hypopyon and infiltration of the vitreous body. It was described for the first time in 1887 by Grollman, in 1916 by Leber, in 1926 by Velhagen, in 1926 by Kuchle and in 1960 by Schofield. In the 4 cases of Schofield and diagnosis was performed by anterior chamber puncture which showed tumour cells and the tumours were of small size as in our case.

Case No. 4

4-year-old male presenting with vitreous haemorrhage with loss of vision, shallow anterior chamber, and ocular hypertension. Figure 7 shows the echogram. a are the spikes indicating the haemorrhage. b, the sclera and c, the orbital echoes.

Because the diagnosis was not clear, we performed computed tomography. The result confirmed the diagnosis of haemorrhage in the vitreous body. Two years later, because the eye was blind and painful it was enucleated. The diagnosis was undifferentiated retinoblastoma. Notice (Fig. 8a) tumour proliferation and large necrotic foci and haemorrhages. In Fig. 8b: homogeneous proliferation of tumour cells with even vascularization and homogeneous structure.

In summary, although the echographic diagnosis was vitreous haemor-

195

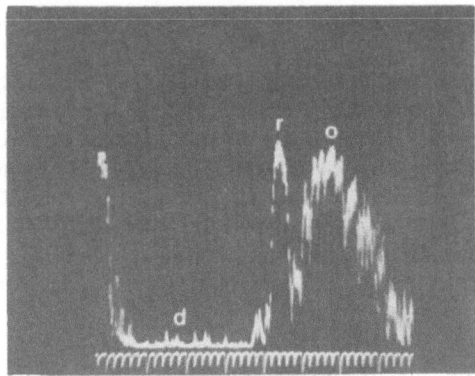

Fig. 6. A-mode echogram of case 3, d = debris, r = retina, o = orbital echo spikes.

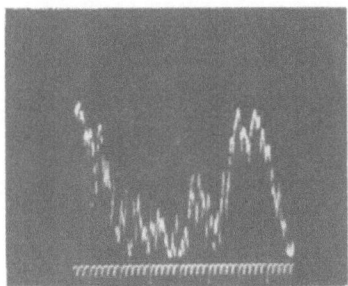

Fig. 7. Echogram of eye with vitreous haemorrhage of case 4, a = haemorrhage, b = sclera, o = orbit.

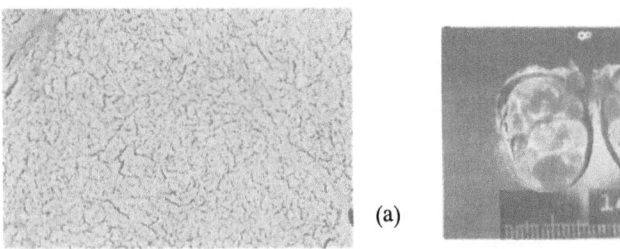

(a)

(b)

Fig. 8. (a) Enucleated eye of case 4, showing tumour. (b) Histological slice through tumour, diagnosis: retinoblastoma.

rhage, in fact the histopathology proved that it was an undifferentiated retinoblastoma.

References

Grolman W von. 1887. Beitrag zur Kenntnis der Netzhautgliome. Albrecht V. Graefes Arch Ophthalm 33/II: 47.

Kuchle HJ, Resky H, Sttler R. 1958. Diagnosis of gliomatous Pseudo-Uveitis. Amer J Ophthal 45: 439.

Leber Th. 1916. Die Krankheiten der Netzhaut II. (XV Die Geschwulstbildungen der Neutzhaut) In: Graefe-Saimisch-Hess: Handbuch der gesamten Aungenheilkunde. Leipzig.

Ossoinig KC, Cennamo G, Green RL, Weyer NL. 1981. Echograpic results in the diagnosis of retinoblastoma. In: JM Thijssen and AM Verbeek (eds) Ultrasonography in Ophalmology. Doc Ophthal Proc Series, Vol. 29, Junk, The Hague, pp. 103—108.

Schofield PB. 1960. Diffuse infiltrating retinoblastoma. Brit J Ophthal 44: 35.

Velhagen K. 1926. Gliom und Vorderkammer. Klin Augenheilk 77: 76.

Ultrasonographic correlations in retinoblastoma

R. D. STONE[1,2], D. R. SHAPIRO[1]

Introduction

Retinoblastoma is a childhood intraocular malignancy which, despite once being nearly always fatal, can now be recognized and treated early enough to preserve vision as well as life (Shields, 1983). Much of the most recent success in diagnosing retinoblastoma stems from ultrasonic and CT imaging systems. Even with these systems, however, there is still room for improvement. In a study of 618 histologically proven retinoblastomas, 92 cases (14.9%) were initially misdiagnosed as a non-retinoblastoma lesion (Howard et al., 1965). Conversely, Margo and Zimmerman found that, of all eyes enucleated for retinoblastoma in the United States and Canada between 1974 and 1980, 26.8% did not contain a malignant tumour (Margo et al., 1983).

The ultrasonic A-mode characteristics of retinoblastomas have been described elsewhere (Koch et al., 1983; Ossoinig et al., 1974; Ossoinig et al., 1969). Sterns, Coleman, and Ellsworth have described two retinoblastoma appearances on B-mode ultrasound: "cystic" and "solid". They pointed out that they were uncertain of a histologic basis for this division, but postulated that the cystic pattern relates to larger, older, more necrotic tumours (Sterns et al., 1974). Rather than the terms "cystic" and "solid", we describe these two sonographic appearances either as the presence or absence of internal acoustic quieting.

The CT characteristics of retinoblastoma have also been described (Danziger et al., 1979; Katz et al., 1984; Arrigg et al., 1983; Char et al., 1984). In addition, Char, Hedges, and Norman have described two modes of appearance of retinoblastomas on CT: tumours with "nonhomogeneous" and with "homogeneous" calcification patterns (Char et al., 1984).

In view of the continuing error rates in diagnosing retinoblastoma, the subtlest and most exacting knowledge of the ultrasonic and CT presentation of retinoblastoma becomes important. In this retrospective study, we

[1] The Department of Ophthalmology, University of California School of Medicine, San Francisco, USA; [2] The Ophthalmic Ultrasound Laboratory, University of California, 400 Parnassus Avenue, Room A-775, San Francisco, CA 94143, USA.

J. M. Thijssen (ed.) Ultrasonography in ophthalmology.
© 1988, *Kluwer Academic Publishers, Dordrecht, ISBN 978-94-010-7083-6*

investigate and describe our experience with the ultrasound and CT characteristics and their correlations in retinoblastoma. We present a constellation of clinical ultrasonic features and correlated CT findings which, taken together, point toward the diagnosis of retinoblastoma. Where possible, we also investigate histopathologic correlations of both the ultrasonic and the CT characteristics. Furthermore, we compare the ultrasonic distinction between the presence or absence of internal acoustic quiet zones with the CT distinction between nonhomogeneous and homogeneous calcification.

Materials and methods

24 patients with a total of 29 eyes affected with a diagnosed retinoblastoma were studied in the Ophthalmic Ultrasound Laboratory at the University of California Medical Center in San Francisco upon referral for this diagnosis and form the basis of this review. All patients were examined between 1974 and 1984 and ranged in age from 3 months to 12 years with a mean age of 2 years. The Sonometrics 150 A/B-mode instrument with the 10 MHz transducer was used, employing the immersion technique with the patient in the supine position. The Kretztechnik 7200 MA instrument with the 8 MHz transducer was used for A-mode analysis using the contact technique. 16 of the 24 patients with a total of 18 affected eyes were also studied with CT. 19 of the 24 patients underwent an enucleation, yielding a total of 19 eyes on which pathological examination was performed and reported. The ultrasound and CT studies and reports as well as the pathological reports and specimens were retrospectively abstracted and correlations were tested with Kendall-Tau B correlation coefficients using a significance limit of $p \leq 0.05$.

Results

Significant statistical correlations from the ultrasound examination of these eyes were noted. Axial length of the eye correlated positively with high-amplitude foreign body type echoes in the ultrasonic texture of the tumour $(r = 0.44, p \leq 0.01)$. Age correlated inversely with the presence of acoustic shadowing of both the orbital fat echo complex and the scleral echo by the tumour on ultrasound $(r = -0.48, p \leq 0.01)$.

A-mode and B-mode sonographic characteristics were statistically correlated with themselves and with the reported histopathologic findings. The ultrasonic appearance of a tumour so large that it extends to the posterior aspect of the lens echo correlated positively with the ultrasonic finding of acoustic shadowing strong enough to involve the sclera as well as the orbital fat ($r = 0.42$, $p \leqslant 0.03$). We could not make the expected correlation of this with the histopathology because the pathologists do not routinely (never in our series) meaure the tumours this way. Ultrasonic echoes consistent with total retinal detachment correlated positively with histopathologic tumour involvement of the optic nerve beyond the lamina cribosa ($r = 0.57$, $p \leqslant 0.02$). The echographic presence of high amplitude foreign body-type echoes within the internal texture of the tumour correlated positively with the pathological finding of multiple foci of viable tumour ($r = 0.52$, $p \leqslant 0.03$). Finally, an A-mode correlation was noted with pathology: increasing axial length as measured by A-mode correlated negatively with the presence of Flexner-Wintersteiner rosettes within the tumour ($r = -0.47$, $p \leqslant 0.04$).

CT characteristics were also evaluated and correlated. There was a negative correlation between a patient's age and a nonhomogeneous pattern of calcification on CT ($r = -0.70$, $p \leqslant 0.004$).

Some ultrasonic characteristics of retinoblastomas were correlated with CT characteristics. The non-specific detectability of an intraocular tumour (but not of a retinoblastoma specifically) by CT was correlated positively with acoustic shadowing of the orbital fat echo complex on ultrasound ($r = 0.54$, $p \leqslant 0.03$). The specific presence of a calcified lesion on CT was positively correlated with the ultrasonic presence of an echo complex consistent with retinal detachment ($r = 0.67$, $p \leqslant 0.01$). However, it is interesting that there was not direct association between areas of acoustic quieting within the tumour on ultrasound and a nonhomogeneous appearance of tumour calcification on CT.

There were many other important non-correlations observed statistically in our study. Areas of internal acoustic quieting within the tumour (Sterns' "cystic" appearance) were not correlated significantly with the pathologic finding of calcification, necrosis, Flexner-Wintersteiner rosettes, pseudorosettes, fleurettes, or haemorrhage within the tumour. Acoustic shadowing of the orbital fat echo complex alone or also including shadowing of the scleral echo as well was not significantly associated with pathologic findings of seeding of the tumour into the vitreous, choroidal extension of the tumour, optic nerve involvement of the tumour to or beyond the lamina cribosa, necrosis within the tumour, rosettes, pseudorosettes, or fleurettes or dystrophic calcification.

In terms of important histopathological non-correlations involving CT, a nonhomogeneous appearance of tumour calcification (as opposed to a homogenous appearance) on CT was not found to be associated with pathologic finding of choroidal extension by tumour haemorrhage or necrosis within the tumour, Flexner-Wintersteiner rosettes, pseudorosettes, or fleurettes.

Discussion

Certain pathologic features are highly predictive of prognosis and it would be ideal if an imaging system could detect these. These pathologic features include the presence of Flexner-Wintersteiner rosettes, which indicates approximately a six-fold better prognosis than the absence of rosettes does. Tumours composed of fleurettes have a better prognosis than tumours with no fleurettes. On the other hand, massive choroidal invasion, seen on the pathology examination in 37% of our cases, has connotated a 65% mortality rate. If the optic nerve is not invaded by tumour, the mortality is 8%. When the optic nerve is invaded to the lamina cribosa only, the mortality is 15%, and if invasion has spread posterior to the lamina cribosa, the mortality reaches 44% (Yanoff et al., 1982). In the pathology of our series, 53% of eyes did not show tumour involvement of the optic nerve, 37% of eyes showed involvement only to the lamina cribosa, and the remaining 11% demonstrated involvement posterior to the lamina cribosa. Unfortunately, neither CT nor ultrasound are very good at directly detecting any of these pathologic changes, but significant differences in the capabilities of these two imaging systems to exist.

An intraocular calcific density is considered to be the hallmark of CT diagnosis of retinoblastoma. Calcification, in fact, is the radiographic criterion which distinguishes retinoblastoma from the several types of pseudoretinoblastoma (Katz et al., 1984). In our series, 18 affected eyes were evaluated by both CT and ultrasound. One eye (6%) showed no evidence of an intraocular mass at all on CT, although the tumour was detected by ultrasound. While this single case does not provide a clear mandate for ultrasound over CT as it is felt that the relative sensitivity of CT and ultrasound has not yet been determined (Katz et al., 1984), it does serve as an example in which ultrasound had the greater sensitivity (Figs. 1, 2). Of the remaining 17 eyes, 3 additional cases (17%) showed non-specific, non-calcified intraocular masses on CT (Figs. 3, 4). In these cases, therefore, CT had not provided differentiation between non-calcific retinoblastoma and the various forms of pseudoretinoblastoma such as degenerative retina with thick subretinal fluid as is seen in PHPV and in long-standing rhegmatogenous retinal detachment, exudate intraretinally and subretinally as is seen in Coats' disease, or thick inflammatory subretinal exudate and membranes as is seen in endophthalmitis (Katz et al., 1984). Ultrasound, on the other hand, provides alternative diagnostic criteria because it is also sensitive to retinoblastoma features beside calcification. In view of the relative frequency of non-calcific retinoblastomas, this difference in the capabilities of CT and ultrasound becomes significant. Our prevalence of histopathologically calcific retinoblastomas (79%) is slightly lower than the incidence of calcific retinoblastomas in the

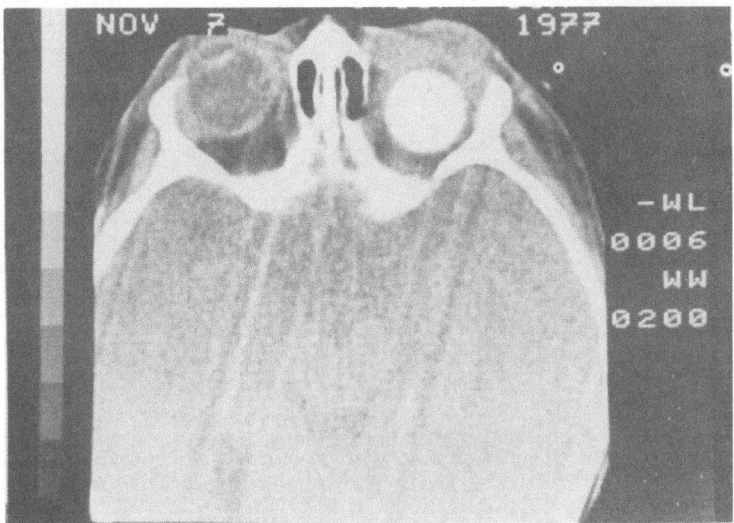

Fig. 1. Negative CT scan of remaining eye of a patient with bilateral retinoblastoma. Note orbital implant after enucleation of opposite eye.

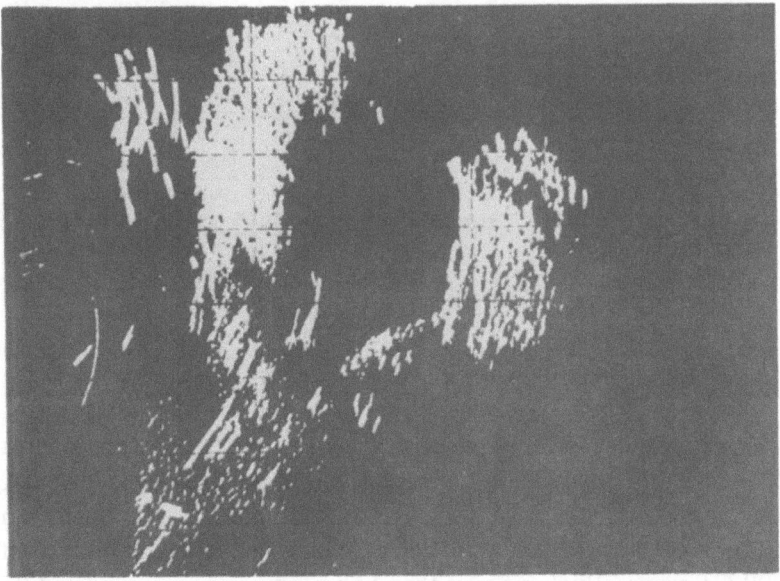

Fig. 2. Positive ultrasound of remaining eye described in Fig. 1.

202

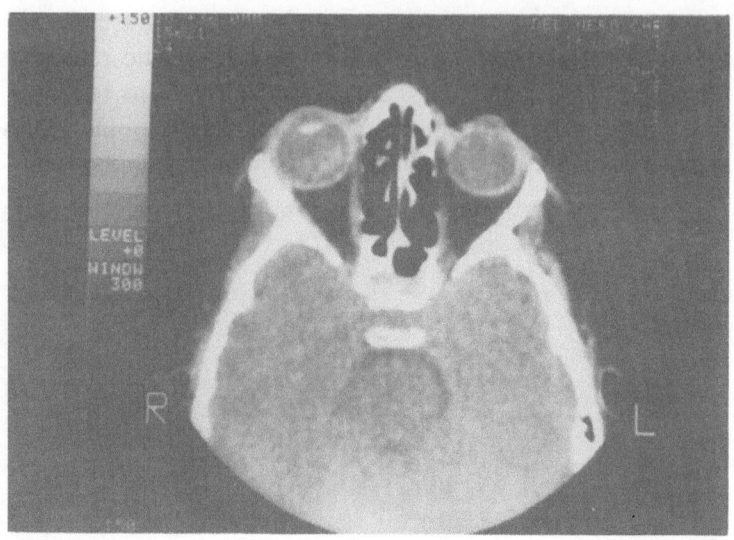

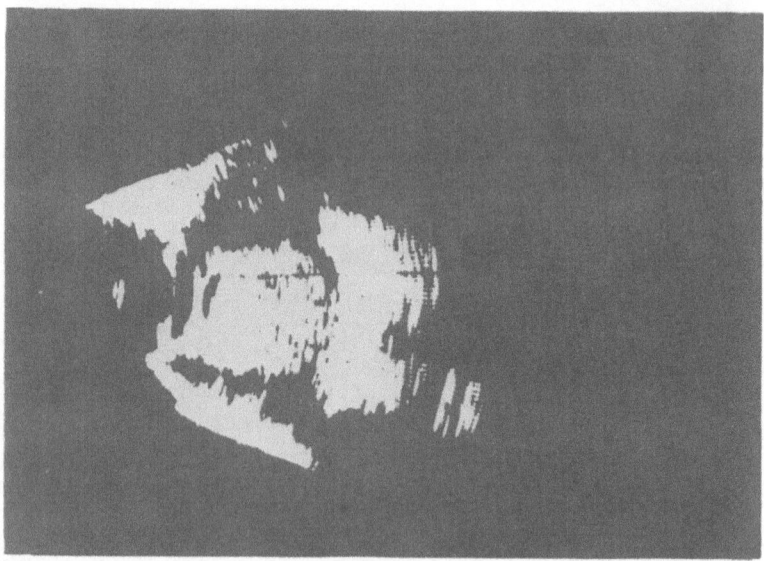

Fig. 4. The same eye in Fig. 3 contained a retinoblastoma ultrasonically.

literature. Bullock, Campbell, and Waller, for example, reported a 95% prevalence of calcification detection on pathology using histochemical techniques (Bullock et al., 1977). Char, Hedges, and Norman report detection of calcium flecks in 87% of retinoblastomas evaluation with GE 8800 CT scans, a higher figure than had been previously reported (Char et al., 1984).

Thus, the absence of tumour calcification on CT makes CT a relatively non-specific test for non-calcific tumours. There has been an effort, however, to subdivide tumours which do evidence calcification on CT. Char, Hedges, and Norman have noted two patterns of calcification in retinoblastomas: nonhomogeneous (Fig. 5) and homogeneous (Fig. 6). They point out that smaller tumours tend to be homogeneous (Char et al., 1984). In an effort to extend this work, we attempted to determine if either of these categories could be used to predict tumour histopathology. We

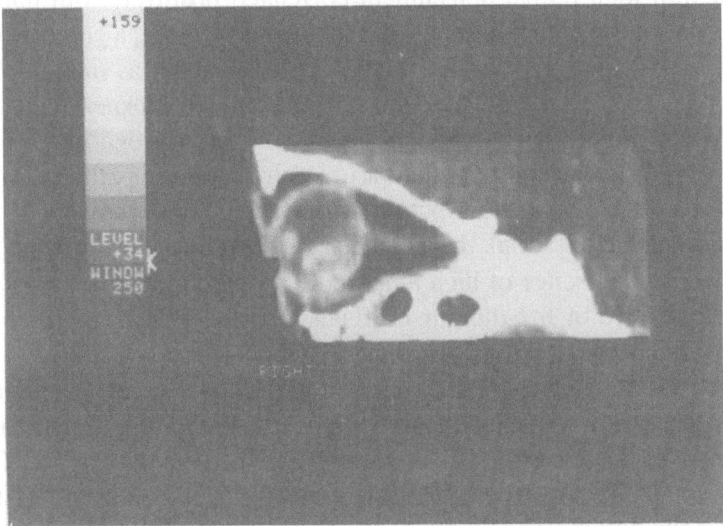

Fig. 5. Example of "non-homogeneous" CT calcification pattern seen in retinoblastoma.

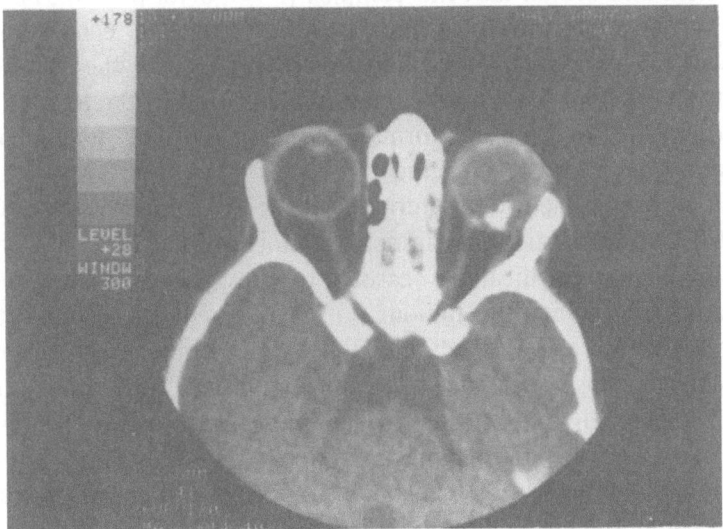

Fig. 6. Example of "homogeneous" CT calcification pattern seen in retinoblastoma.

204

found that none of the aforementioned predictive pathologic categories correlated with this breakdown of CT calcification. We did find, however, a negative correlation between age and a nonhomogeneous calcification pattern on CT ($r = -0.70, p \leqslant 0.004$).

Ultrasound, by contrast, may offer greater insight into tumour histopathology. We evaluated the correlation of ultrasonic echo patterns with pathologic features and found a correlation with some of the prognostically valuable pathological characteristics. We found that ultrasonic echoes consistent with total retinal detachment correlated positively with tumour involvement of the optic nerve beyond the lamina cribosa, a grave prognostic finding ($r = 0.57, p \leqslant 0.02$). Increasing axial length as measured in the A-mode correlated negatively with the presence of Flexner-Wintersteiner rosettes, whose presence connotates a six-fold better prognosis ($r = -0.47$, $p \leqslant 0.04$). While we do not attempt to imply that these pathologic features directly caused these echo patterns, the association provides a clinical index of suspicion about the presence of these prognostically important features. The presence of high amplitude, foreign body-type echoes in the acoustic texture of the tumour correlated positively with multiple foci of viable tumour on pathology ($r = 0.52, p \leqslant 0.03$).

Acoustic shadowing of the sclera and orbital fat echo complex correlated positively with the ultrasonic appearance of a tumour so large that it extends to the posterior aspect of the lens echo ($r = 0.42, p \leqslant 0.03$). We could not make the expected correlation of this with the histopathology because the pathologists do not routinely (never in our series) measure the tumours this way. The patient's age correlated inversely with shadowing of the sclera and orbital fat echo complex ($r = -0.48, p \leqslant 0.01$). Interestingly, acoustic shadowing of the sclera and orbital fat echo complex, or even of the orbital fat alone, did not correlate with the prognostically significant pathologic findings of choroidal invasion by the tumour, rosette, pseudorosette, or fleurette formation, seeding of the tumour into the vitreous or optic nerve involvement.

An ultrasonic picture of internal acoustic quiet zones (Sterns, Colman, and Ellsworth's "cystic" appearance) did not correlate directly with pathologic findings of calcification, necrosis, rosettes, pseudorosettes, fleurettes, or haemorrhage into the tumour. Of final note is the finding that the presence of internal acoustic quiet zones did not directly correlate with a nonhomogeneous appearance of calcification on CT as described by Char, Hedges, and Norman despite the similarity of these two "Swiss-cheese" appearances on the different imaging systems.

These differences in the capabilities of ultrasound and CT have known physical underpinnings. The radiologic detection techniques depend directly upon the measurable fundamental physical density of a structure (photon capture, scatter). Ultrasonic detection techniques depend directly upon the velocity changes of sound in a structure (density, elasticity, scatter). Multiple fragmented structures, as well as attenuation in a large tumour produce the acoustic shadowing, for example, a feature radiologic techniques do not detect.

Our results expand those of Basta, Israel, Gourley, and Acers who concluded that the echographic findings in retinoblastoma depend primarily on the degree of calcification and are not influenced independently by other specific pathologic characteristics (Basta et al., 1981). While we do not propose causation, we have notes valuable correlations between ultrasonic features and pathological characteristics other than calcification. In our study we have a larger and more varied series of eyes than that of Basta, et al. who used 11 eyes, all of which were without internal acoustic quiet zones (the "cystic" appearance of Sterns et al. (1974)). It is perhaps this difference in population which has led to our differing results. In addition, we have made ultrasound-CT-histopathology correlations from our series.

Thus, we conclude that, while the relative sensitivities of ultrasound and CT in diagnosing retinoblastoma have not yet been determined, ultrasound may be more valuable in ascertaining subtle tumours and, in the case of non-calcific retinoblastomas (21% of those seen in our series), ultrasound may be the preferred test as it has greater specificity.

Acknowledgements

Marvin Zielinski, COT, Sharon Humphrey, RDMS, and Ann Welling, RDMS, were technicians in the Ultrasound Laboratory, University of California, San Francisco, during this study. Nancy King typed the manuscript, which was processed on an IBM PC-XT, with Wordstar Software.

The authors have no financial, commercial, or proprietary interest in either the Sonometrics 150 A/B-mode instrument or the Kretztechnik 7200 MA A-mode instrument.

Statistical analysis was provided by Richard P. Juster, Ph.D. at the University of California, San Francisco Computer Center.

Pathological examinations were performed in the Eye Pathology Laboratory, Department of Ophthalmology, University of California School of Medicine, San Francisco, by J. Brooks Crawford, M.D., and Edward L. Howes, M.D.

This study was supported, in part, by an unrestricted grant from Research to Prevent Blindness, Inc.

References

Arrigg PG, Hedges TR, Char DH. 1983. Computed tomography in the diagnosis of retinoblastoma. Br J Ophthalmol. 67: 588—591.

Basta LL, Israel W, Gourley RD, Acers TE. 1981. Which pathologic characteristics influence echographic patterns of retinoblastoma. Ann Ophthalmol 13: 585—588.

Bullock JO, Campbell RJ, Waller RR. 1977. Calcification in retinoblastoma. Invest Ophthalmol Visual Sci 16: 252—255.

Char DH, Hedges TR, Norman D. 1984. Retinoblastoma CT diagnosis. Ophthalmology 91: 1347—1350.

Danziger A, Price HI. 1979. CT findings in retinoblastoma. Amer J Radiol 133: 695—697.

Howard GM, Ellsworth RM. 1965. Differential diagnosis of retinoblastoma. A statistical survey of 500 children. Am J Ophthalmol 60: 610—617.

Katz NNK, Margo CE, Dorwart RH. 1984. Computed tomography with histopathologic correlation in children with leukokoria. J Pediatr Ophthalmol Strabismus 21: 50—56.

Koch A, Gerke E, Hopping W. 1983. Echography in retinoblastoma. Graefe's Arch Clin Exp Ophthalmol 221: 27—30.

Margo CE, Zimmerman LE. 1983. Retinoblastoma: the accuracy of clinical diagnosis in children treated by enucleation. J Pediatr Ophthalmol Strabismus 20: 227—229.

Ossoinig KC, Till P. 1969. Methods and results of ultrasonography in diagnosing intraocular tumours. In: KA Gitter, AM Keeny, LK Sarin and D Meyer (eds) Ophthalmic Ultrasound: Proceedings of the Fourth International Congress on Ultrasonography in Ophthalmology. The C.V. Mosby Company, St Louis.

Ossoinig KC, Blodi FC. 1974. Preoperative differential diagnosis of tumours with echography, Part III. Diagnosis of intraocular tumours. Curr Concepts Ophthalmol 4: 296—313.

Shields JA. 1983. Diagnosis and Management of Intraocular Tumours. St Louis. The C.V. Mosby Company.

Sterns GK, Coleman DJ, Ellsworth RM. 1974. The ultrasonographic characteristics of retinoblastoma. Am J Ophthalmol 78: 606—611.

Yanoff M, Fine BS. 1982. Ocular pathology. Philadelphia. Harper and Row.

Highly reflective intraocular solid lesions

F. BIGAR

Summary

High-reflective lesions are found in various intraocular conditions such as retinoblastoma, retinoma, choroidal haemangioma, osteoma etc. using standardized A-Scan echography. Additional particular echographic findings and the clinical appearance are helpful in further differentiating the high-reflective lesions.

Introduction

In this contribution highly reflective, solid intraocular lesions are subdivided in 3 groups. The first covers children and deals with retinoblastoma. The second group of high reflective lesions occurs in adults and consists of a series of lesions which have to be thought of to be within the differential diagnosis of malignant melanoma of the ciliary body and the choroid. Lesions such as choroidal haemangiomas, metastatic carcinomas to the choroid, disciform macular degenerations, and choroidal ostomas are enumerated. In the third group secondary degenerative ossifications in phthisical eyes are mentioned.

Group I lesions: retinoblastoma

The first solid intraocular lesion of high reflectivity to be mentioned is the *retinoblastoma*. In presence of clear media and endophytic growth the pink tumour surface can easily be evaluated and the clinical diagnosis made rather reliably. If, however, the tumour is covered by seeding in the vitreous, or exists in the presence of pseudohypopyon, echography becomes particularly indicated. The main acoustic feature of retinoblastoma

Department of Ophthalmology, University Hospital, 8091 Zürich, Switzerland.

J. M. Thijssen (ed.) Ultrasonography in ophthalmology.
© 1988, *Kluwer Academic Publishers, Dordrecht, ISBN 978-94-010-7083-6*

208

is the extremely high reflectivity (95—100% of the display height of the Kretz 7200 MA at "tissue sensitivity") and in addition the shadowing on the sclera and orbital structures (Ossoinig et al., 1981).

The strong reflectivity is caused by small calcium deposits dispersed within the tumour which behave like small foreign bodies. In A-scan echography there is a short chain of single high spikes followed by lower spikes due to the strong sound attenuation (Fig. 1). In B-scan echography the shadowing of the retinoblastoma on the orbital structures behind the tumour can easily be demonstrated whereas the normal, highly reflective,

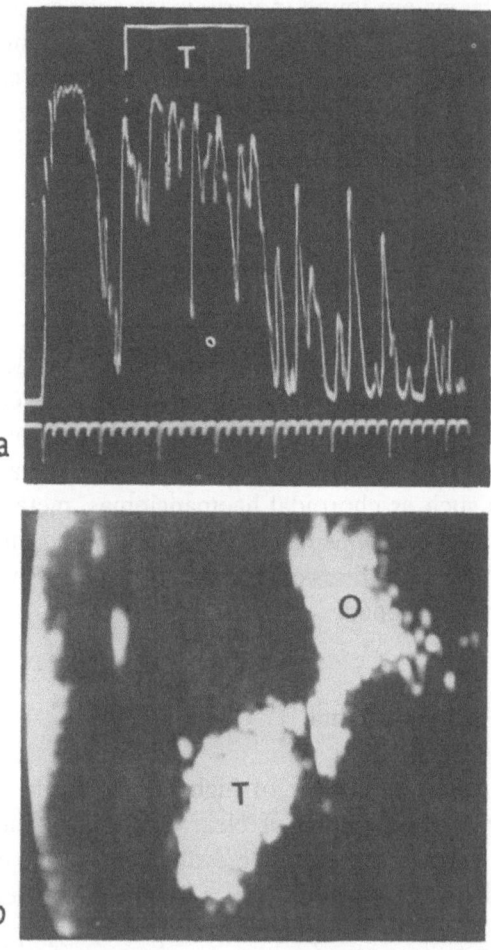

Fig. 1. Echograms in retinoblastoma. (a) A-scan echography at tissue sensitivity. Sound beam is directed to calcified tumour areas: short chain of high reflective tumour spikes (T) followed by signals of decreasing height due to strong sound attenuation. (b) B-scan echogram with acoustic shadowing of retinoblastoma (T) on orbital structures. The orbit (O) is displayed laterally of the tumour.

orbital structures next to the tumour are normally displayed. Other lesions causing leucocoria, such as persistent hyperplastic primary vitreous, Coats' disease, retrolental fibroplasia etc., show a different acoustic behaviour from that of retinoblastomas. These lesions display membranous structures and do not cause shadowing except for late stages of phthisical eyes which are discussed in the third group.

Group II. Adult intraocular lesions

The second group of highly reflective lesions concern those in adults. Despite modern diagnostic techniques such as biomicroscopy, binocular indirect ophthalmoscopy, fluorescein angiography, and the P_{32}-test, the differential diagnosis of malignant melanomas of the choroid and the ciliary body can still constitute diagnostic problems. Standardized echography complements the other examination techniques.

Whereas malignant melanomas have a low to medium reflectivity, most other lesions which have to be taken into account are of high reflectivity (Ossoinig and Blodi, 1974): Choroidal haemangiomas appear as an oval or round mass with a smooth, dome-shaped surface and are most usually of orange-red color. Quite often choroidal haemangiomas are hidden behind a secondary retinal detachment — making the use of ultrasound even more important.

Choroidal haemangiomas show a very high reflectivity with a spike height of 95—100% of the display height. The large and smooth surfaces of the vascular spaces represent large acoustic interfaces producing the high reflective signals. The interfaces are mostly regularly arranged: the internal acoustic structure, therefore, is regular.

Metastatic carcinoma to the choroid appears as a yellow lesion with evenly spaced brown pigment clumps. Most frequently this tumour has an irregular internal structure. High and low spikes show marked variation in changing the sound beam direction. But most areas of the tumour are of high reflectivity. Tumour cells are arranged in thick sheets and represent irregularly distributed acoustic interfaces (Fig. 2).

Disciform degeneration of the macula is mostly a bilateral condition which can however occur in an asymmetric manner. These degenerations produce typically 2 or 3 narrowly spaced high spikes representing the surfaces of the retina, the pigment epithelium and the choroid. Although echograms of disciform-like lesions differ significantly from malignant melanomas, such tumours should not be ruled out on the basis of a single examination. Follow-up examinations are necessary to prove the absence of growth or possibly regression of the lesion in order to safely rule out an

210

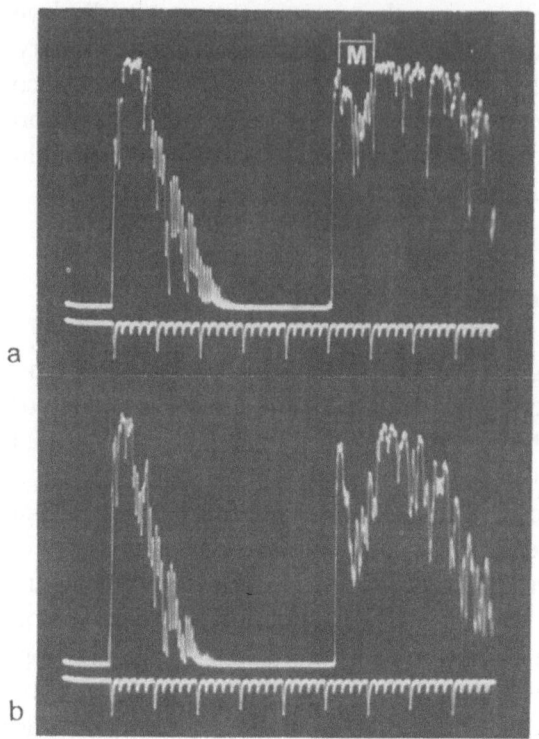

Fig. 2. Echograms in metastatic carcinoma to the choroid. (a) A-scan echogram at tissue sensitivity. Highly reflective lesion (M). (b) A-scan echogram at reduced system sensitivity with irregular internal structures.

atypical small malignant melanoma. It should be stressed that macular degenerations with production of collagenous tissue between the retina and the choroid can simulate echographically a malignant melanoma (Fig. 3). The newly formed collagenous tissue of considerable amount appears rather homogeneous and explains the echogram with an internal reflectivity of 65% (Fig. 4).

Choroidal osteomas

This rather rare, mostly unilateral, juxtapapillary tumour occurs predominantly in otherwise healthy young females (Gass et al., 1978). The typical ophthalmoscopic appearance of a slightly elevated tumour with well defined geographic borders and a yellow-white color can be absent in early stages and may simulate a choroidal haemangioma or a malignant melanoma. At the final stage, choroidal osteoma can resemble metastatic carcinomas or amelanotic melanomas. The clinically suspected diagnosis of choroidal osteomas is easily confirmed by echography or computerized

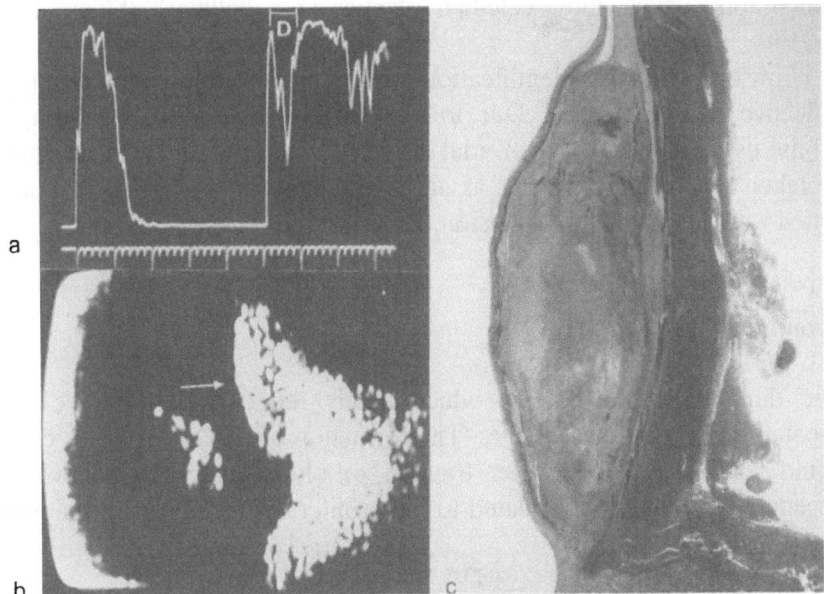

Fig. 3. Echograms and histology of productive senile macular degeneration. (a) A-scan echogram with a solid prominence of 3 µsec (D) and medium internal reflectivity of 65%. (b) B-scan echogram with vitreous haemorrhage and solid prominence of the posterior ocular wall (arrow). (c) Light-microscopic section of productive senile macular degeneration at low magnification: the retina is separated from the choroid by new formed collagenous connective tissue which is more than 10 times thicker than the normal retina. The proliferating tissue consists partly of parallel-arranged bundles and partly less dense connective tissue. At low magnification the structure of proliferating connective tissue appears homogeneous and explains the medium acoustic reflectivity.

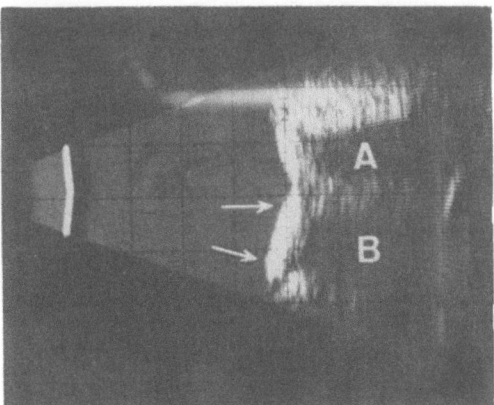

Fig. 4. B-scan echogram of choroidal osteoma. Arrows are pointing to slightly elevated juxtapapillary choroidal mass of high reflectivity. *B*: Absence of orbital echoes due to acoustic shadowing posterior to the lesion. *A*: V-shaped pattern of optic nerve stands out against the other shadow by a row of signals between A and B.

212

tomography which show calcified plaques as a hallmark (Spiess et al., 1979).

Ultrasound allows identification of a slightly prominent and highly reflective choroidal mass. Due to acoustic shadowing of the lesion, the orbital tissue behind the choroidal lesion appears as a defect. Care should be taken not to diagnose this as an enlargement of the optic nerve associated with the juxtapapillary lesion.

Group III. Ossifications

The third group of eyes in which highly reflective lesions are often encountered are phthisical eyes. The formation of osseous spicules can be found in phthisical eyes after traumas or old retinal detachments. The degenerative changes are related to the proliferation and transformation of

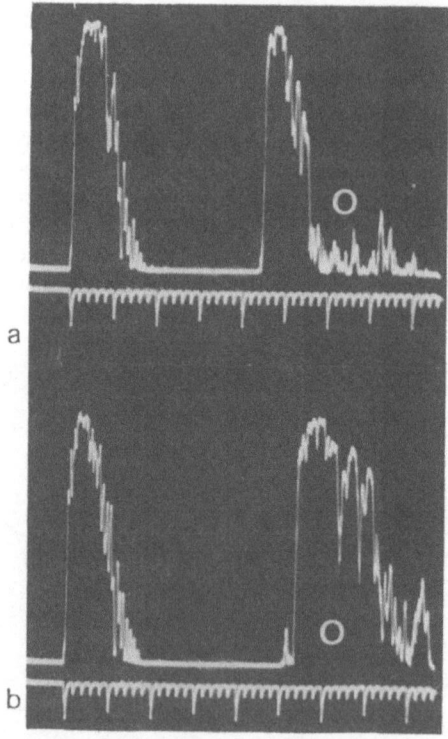

Fig. 5. A-scan echograms of choroidal osteoma. (a) Echogram of choroidal osteoma with sound beam directed toward slightly elevated mass. Shortening of the axial length (4 μsec), high signals due to retina and osseous choroidal tumour followed by decreasing and low orbital signals (O) due to strong acoustic attenuation. (b) Sound beam directed besides juxtapapillary osseous tumour. Larger vitreous length and high orbital signals (O).

retinal epithelial cells. Highly reflective lesions with acoustic shadowing on the sclera and orbital structures within a phthisical eye are signs of bone formation.

References

Gass JDM, Guerry K, Jack RL, Harris G. 1978. Choroidal osteoma. Arch Ophthalmol 96: 428—435.
Ossoinig KC, Blodi FC. 1974. III. Diagnosis of intraocular tumours. In: FC Blodi (ed) Current concepts in Ophthalmology. Mosby Saint Louis 4: 296—313.
Ossoinig KC, Cennamo G, Green RL, Weyer NL. 1981. Echographic results in the diagnosis of retinoblastoma. In: JM Thijssen and AM Verbeek (eds) Ultrasonography in Ophthalmology. Docum Ophthal Proc Series 29, Junk, The Hague, pp. 103—107.
Spiess H, Bigar F, Bosshard C. 1979. Kombination von Computertomographie und Echographie in der Ophthalmologie. Therap Umschau 36: 991—999.

A case report of pigment epithelium hamartoma: echographic and clinical findings

G. GRACIS, R. SPOLAORE AND F. L. CATANIA

Summary

The authors describe a case of a young patient with pigment epithelium hamartoma of the left eye with pre-retinal membranes located near the optic disk.

The differential diagnosis is also reported with complete echographic evaluation and with fluorescein and indocyanine green angiography. Our findings suggest that the echographic differential diagnosis is quite possible between pigment epithelium hamartoma and choroidal melanoma, haemangioma, retinoblastoma. However this differential diagnosis is quite difficult in comparison with metastatic lesions.

Case report

Clinic case: male child ten years old.
Medical record: no previous illnesses.
Ocular anamnesis: his vision had been deteriorating for the past 15 days (told by the parents).

V.A.R.E.: 10/10
V.A.L.E.: 2—3/10
IOP R.E.: 18 A
IOP L.E.: 12 A

Fundus right eye: normal.
Fundus left eye: a pale pink optic disk masked by preretinal vessel near to an irregular retinal prominence; this has a gray and deep halo and is situated in the lower nasal quadrant. The neoformation appears far from the optic disk. The macular region has become stretched with the fibroglial bridles that extend to the bottom (Fig. 1).

Civil Hospital S. Maria dei Battuti, Department of Ophthalmology, Conegliano Veneto (Treviso), Italy.

J. M. Thijssen (ed.) Ultrasonography in ophthalmology.
© 1988, *Kluwer Academic Publishers, Dordrecht, ISBN 978-94-010-7083-6*

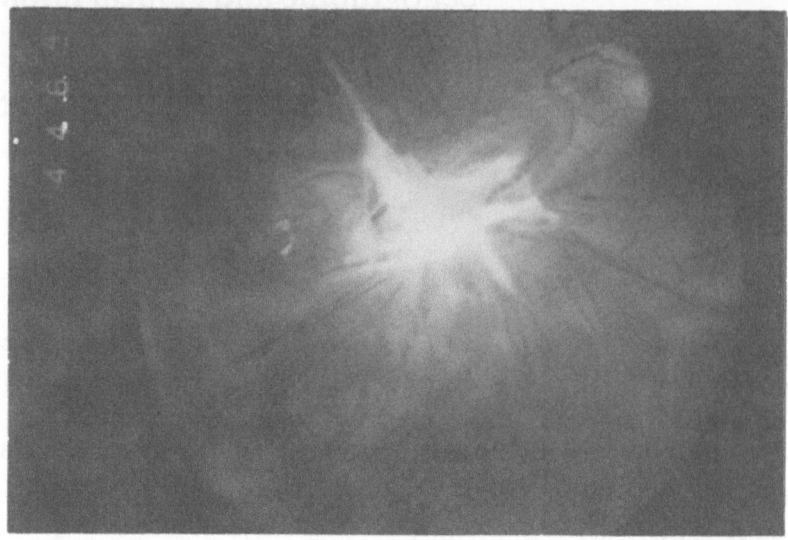

Fig. 1. An irregular retinal prominence with a gray and deep halo situated in the lower nasal quadrant.

A mode echography (Kretz Technik, 7200 MA)

At tissue sensitivity (72 dB) on the neoformation surface a very high peak was obtained followed by medium high peaks that decreased and then raised, "V mode". This aspect of the echogram is similar to that of intra-ocular metastasis of a carcinoma. "Shadowing" was not present (Fig. 2).

B-mode echography

B-mode echography appeared not very peculiar. It was done at the Oph-thalmic University Clinic of Ferrara with Sonometrics (Fig. 3) and (Fig. 4) equipment. The echogram after 10 months did not show extensive changes of growth.

Fluorescence angiography (Fig. 5): The filling time was normal. In the initial stages we remarked tortuousness of vascular net situated in the retinal raising. This net presents leakage in the late stages and it is surrounded by a deep masking that remains in the next stage as well. The optic disk is also hyperfluorescent. The aspect of the neoformation is not inflammatory and is compatible with P. E. Hamartoma. After two months the fluorangiography appeared to be unchanged.

Green indocyanine retinal angiography did not yield additional informa-tion. Echographic differential diagnosis:

(1) Choroidal melanoma has the following characteristics:

    A Scan: more regular echogram decreasing with a variable K angle, low/medium reflectivity (5—60%), spontaneous movements, growth with time, shadowing.

    B Scan: often mushroom shaped, choroidal excavation, acoustic vacuole.

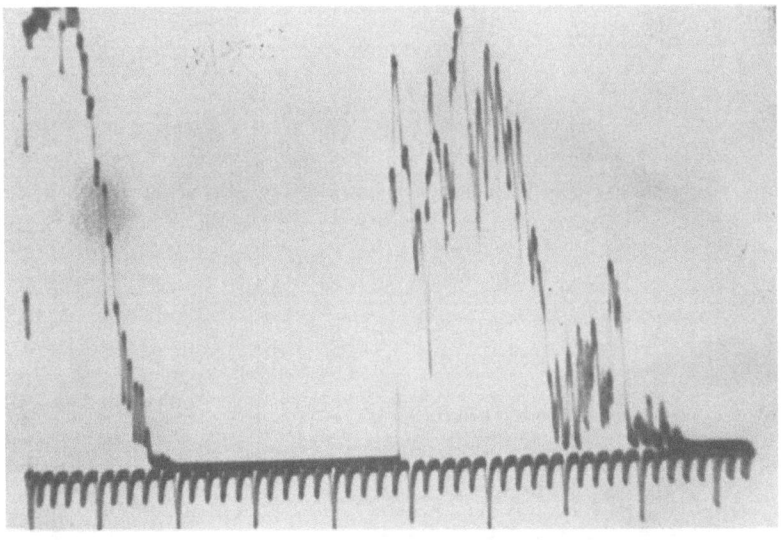

Fig. 2. A-mode echogram at 72 dB: the aspect "V mode" is clear.

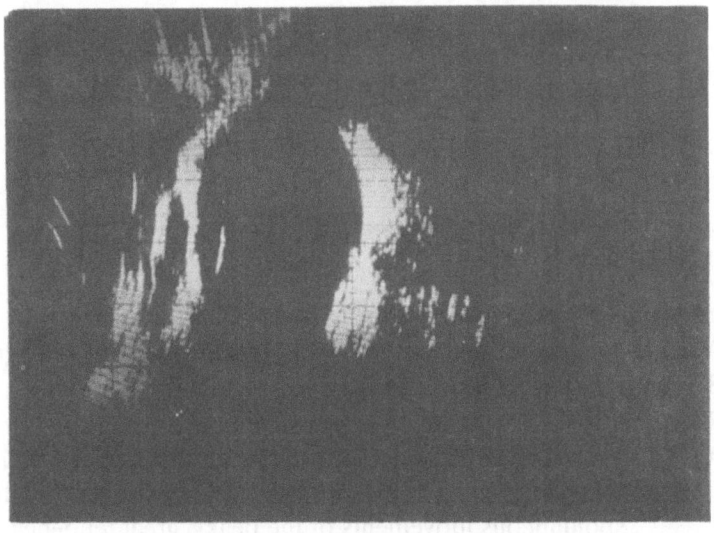

Fig. 3. B-mode is not very peculiar (contact B-mode).

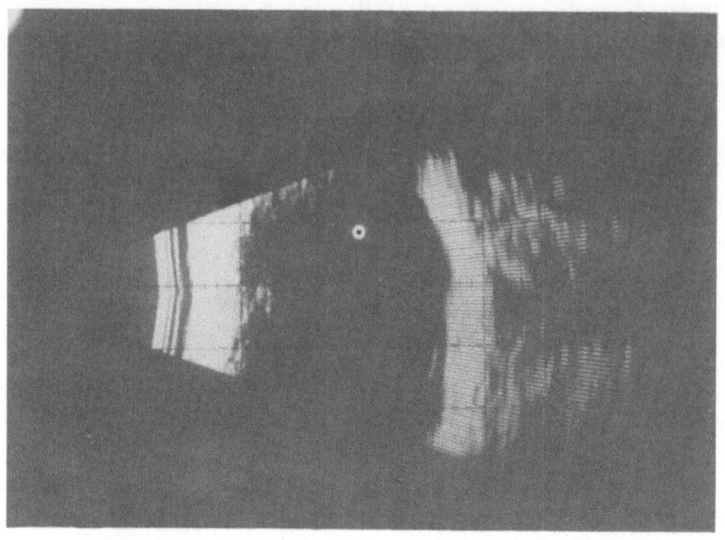

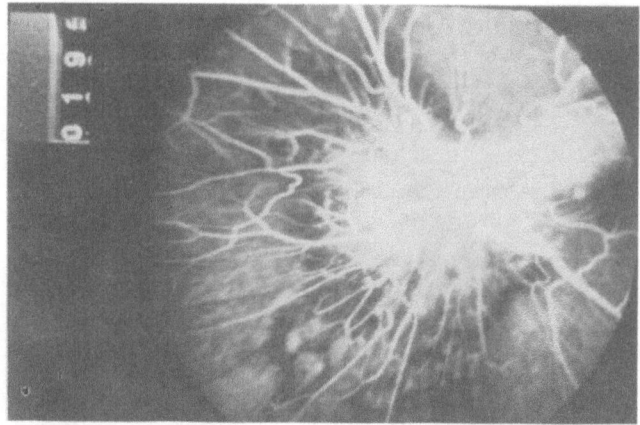

Fig. 5. The vascular net of neoformation presents leakage in the late stages and it is surrounded by a deep masking.

(2) Choroidal haemangioma has the following characteristics:
   A Scan: very high reflectivity (95—100%), does generally not grow.
   B Scan: flat shape, high reflectivity.
(3) Retinoblastoma has the following characteristics:
   A Scan: Irregular acoustic structure caused by necrotic zone; high reflectivity (70—90%) with maximal peaks also (calcification): spontaneous movements of the peaks, great tendency to grow, shadowing.
   B Scan: Irregular shape, high reflectivity, shadowing.

(4) More difficult is the differential diagnosis with metastatic carcinoma that has the following characteristics:

A Scan: high reflectivity (60—80%) with "V" aspect, small tendency to grow.

B Scan: subretinal echogenic mass with indistinct edges, medium attenuation, not much raising.

A rational doubt can raise when we have an intraocular neoformation in a adult subject, monolateral, with not very transparent dioptric means and uncertain anamnesis for visual acuity of this eye.

Conclusion

The hamartoma we observed in this patient confirms the statistics of this disease, as it affects a male child and his left eye. The hamartoma appears well separated from the optic disk (the optic disk is only deformed): this allows us to exclude an optic nerve pathology. The echogram allows us to exclude a melanoma, a haemangioma and a retinoblastoma also (no shadowing and no growth). The echogram is easily mistaken with the echogram of the choroidal metastatic carcinoma. Anamnesis, follow up and fluorangiography also permit the diagnosis of carcinoma.

References

Buffet JR, Bacin F, Audovin MC. 1979. Une technique simple d'angiographie en infra rouge au vert d'indocyanine. Bul Soc ophthal, France 79: 209.

Caballero Presencia A. 1982. Juxta-papillary hamartoma of the pigment epithelium and retina: review and report on two cases. J Fr Ophthal 5/12, pp. 787—792.

Cardell BS, Starbuck MJ. 1961. Juxtapapillary hamartoma of retina. Br J Ophth 45, pp. 672—677.

Coscas G, Sterkers M, Gaudric A, Guentel G. 1981. Aspects angiographiques de certaines tumeurs rétiniennes bénignes (hamartomes). Bull Soc Ophth/Fr 2, 81, pp. 187—191.

Craandijk A, Beek CA van. 1926. Indocyanine green fluorescence angiography of the choroid. Brit J Opht 60, pp. 377—385.

Dark AJ, Richardson J, Howe JW. 1978. Retinal hamartoma in childhood. J Pediatr Opth, Strabismus 15, pp. 273—277.

Flood TP, Orth DH, Haberg TM, Marcus DF. 1983. Macular hamartomas of the retinal pigment epithelium and retina. Retina 9/3, pp. 164—170.

Friberg TR, Gulledge SL. 1982. Hamartomas of the retina and pigment epithelium. Ophthal 17/2, pp. 56—60.

Gass JDM. 1973. An unusual hamartoma of the pigment epithelium and retina simulating choroidal melanoma and retinoplastoma. Trans Am Opth Soc 71, pp. 171—185.

Gass JDM. 1974. Differential diagnosis of intraocular tumours. Mosby, Saint-Louis.

Hartley Bowen J, Christensen FH, Klintworth GK, Sydnor CF. 1981. A clinicopathologic study of a cartilaginous hamartoma of the orbit. A rare cause of proptosis. Ophthalmol 88/12, pp. 1356—1360.

Harwig M, Laqua H. 1984. Clinical picture and follow up of astrocytic hamartoma of the retina and optic disk. Klin Monatsbl Augenheilkd 184/2, pp. 115—120.

Jabbour O, Payeur G. 1983. Malformation congénitale de l'épithelium pigmentaire et de la rétine. J Fr Opht 6, 20, pp. 149—154.

Kroll AJ, Ricker DP, Robb RA, Albert DM. 1981. Vitreous haemorrhage complicating retinal astrocytic hamartoma. Surv Ophthal 26/2, pp. 31—38.

Laqua M, Wessing A. 1979. Congenital retina-pigment epithelial malformation, previously described as hamartoma. Am J Opthal 87, pp. 34—42.

Mazzeo V, Giovannini A, Ravalli L, Costantini G. Echography and cardio-green angiography in eight cases of coroidal haemangiomas. Doc Ophthal, Proceeding Series 38, pp. 69—77.

McLean EB. 1976. Hamartoma of the retinal pigment epithelium. Am J Opht 82, pp. 227—231.

Patrinely JR, Font RL, Campbell RJ, Robertson DM. 1983. Hamatomatous adenoma of the non-pigmented ciliary epithelium arising in iris ciliary body coloboma. Light and election microscope observations. Ophthalmol 90/12, pp. 1540—1547.

Quentel G, Coscas G. 1984. Angiographie en Fluorescence infrarouge au vert d'indo-cyanine. Bull Soc Opht, France 5 IXXXIV, pp. 559—563.

Theobald GD, Floyd GG, Kirk HG. 1958. Hyperplasia of the retinal pigment epithelium. An J Ophth 45, pp. 235—240.

Vogel MH, Zimmerman LE, Gass JDM. 1969. Proliferation of the juxtapapillary pigment epithelium simulating malignant melanoma. Doc Opht 26, pp. 461—481.

Weleber RG, Zonana G. 1983. Iris hamartomas (lisch nodules) in a case of segmental neurofibromatosis. Am J Ophthal 96/6, pp. 740—743.

Choroidal haemangioma, king size or normal size by ultrasound?

A case report

H. C. FLEDELIUS[1] AND E. SCHERFIG

Summary

A case of presumed choroidal haemangioma is presented for reasons of the striking difference between the usual clinical assessment and echographic findings. By ultrasound, the tumour looked both thicker and more extensive than otherwise expected.

Case history

After having experienced a visual shadow for 2 weeks, in a right eye previously known to have a slight anisometropic amblyopia, an 18-year-old female was admitted for solid retinal detachment. A 6-8 diopter prominence, with mottled pigment disturbances to be seen only in side-illumination, was described in the upper temporal quadrant, with an inferior wrinkled slope to include the macular region. Corrected visual acuity has probably been 6/18 throughout the observation time of $3\frac{1}{4}$ years, however depending on how careful refractioning was done at the serial controls. There was evidence of increasing hypermetropia of the eye, now +5.0 comb. with +1.5 cyl. 95°, while the other eye had 6/6 with −1.75 sph.

An early deep tumour-filling during fluorescein angiography is shown in Fig. 1; the retinal vessels over the tumour are unaffected. We had no opportunity of supplementing with the indocyanin green method described by Mazzeo et al. (1983). Fig. 2 shows CT-scan of the lesion.

The ultrasound features (Figs. 3 and 4) are those of a highly reflecting tumour with a prominence of 5—6 mm. This is at variance with the optical assessment, where a prominence of only 2—3 mm was expected. Regarding tumour location, there was ultrasound evidence of a fundus lesion also on the nasal side of the optic nerve head.

---

[1] Eye Department, County Hospital, DK-3400, Hillerød, Denmark.

J. M. Thijssen (ed.) Ultrasonography in ophthalmology.
© 1988, *Kluwer Academic Publishers, Dordrecht, ISBN 978-94-010-7083-6*

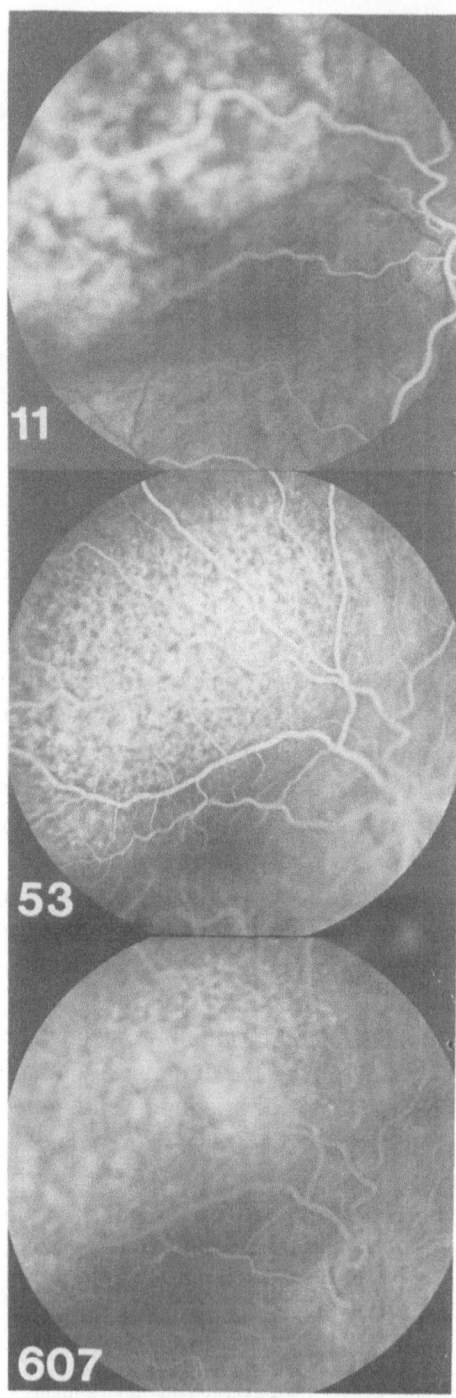

Fig. 1. Fluorescence angiography, 11, 53, and 607 seconds after injection. Tumour vessels without leakage are seen behind the unaffected retinal vessels, with the optic disc near the right border of all pictures.

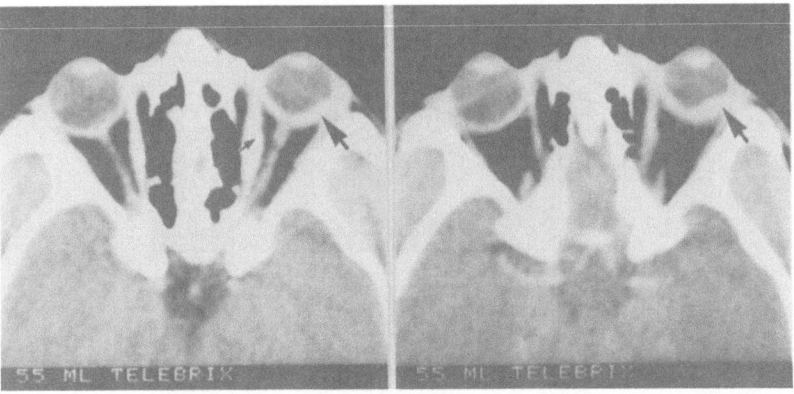

Fig. 2. Two CT-scan levels showing the intraocular tumour (arrows) confluent with a thick posterior eye wall. On the left picture a thickened medial rectus muscle is indicated by small arrow.

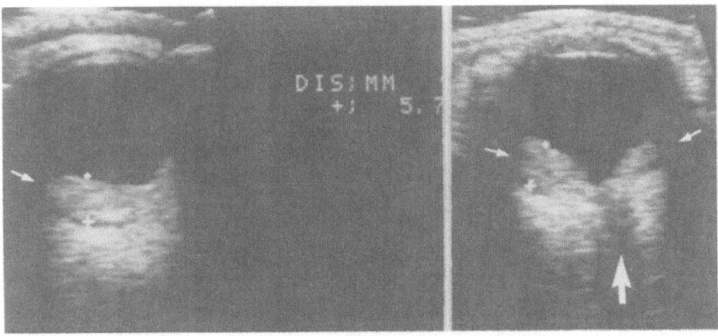

Fig. 3. Tumour thickness of 5.7 mm demonstrated (a) and extension of the tumour also to the medial side of the fundus (b). Tumour is indicated by small arrows, optic nerve shadow by thick arrow. Aloka scan 7.5 MHz.

Although made known with the risk of having a malignant lesion, the patient refused enucleation. To establish a diagnosis transvitreal choroido-retinal biopsies were performed. They showed retinal tissue over eosino-philic fluid with detritus and some blood cells, but a definite histopathology diagnosis was not forwarded.

Discussion

Suspecting choroidal melanoma, experienced clinicians twice advocated enucleation in the present case, a view founded mainly on periods with assumed increase in tumour prominence and reduction in visual acuity. In retrospect, however, the intraocular tumour has been pretty stable over 3½ years. Hypermetropia has increased, but visual acuity level is retained. Alternatively, a metastatic lesion had been suspected, but there was no

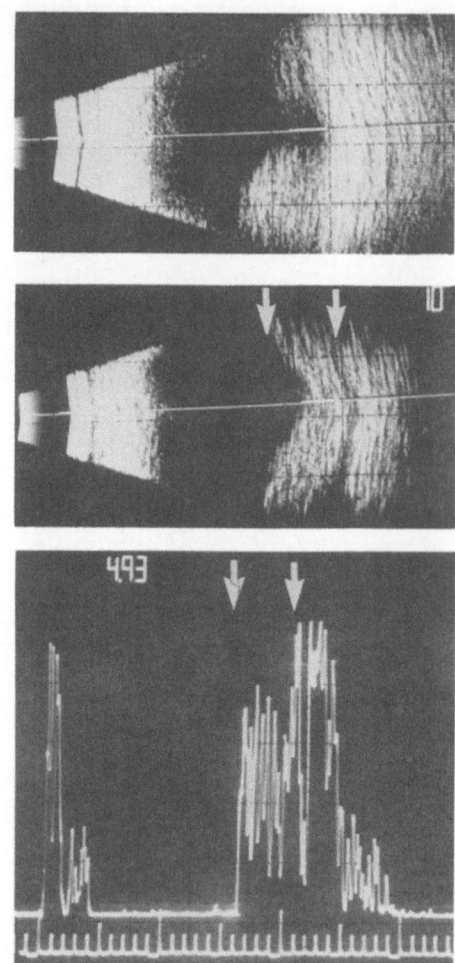

Fig. 4. Ocuscan 400 A and B-scan pictures showing the same features as in Fig. 3. On the A-scan (c) a tumour thickness of 4.9 mm is demonstrated (tumour between arrows). A 10 dB reduction of sensitivity setting was required to show the posterior tumour limit against remaining backwall plus orbital tissue echoes (b) cf. the confluent echoes (a).

support in general examination, nor in laboratory tests (except slightly abnormal liver values occasionally) or scintigraphic examinations.

In addition to the rather flat intraocular tumour (estimated thickness 2—3 mm), CT-scan indicated a thickened eye wall and a thick rectus muscle, but there was no clinical or ultrasound evidence of extraocular disease. Neither did two chorioretinal biopsies give any clear answer. A small amount of subretinal eosinophilic fluid with detritus was described, however only in one of the specimens. If there had been a subretinal pool of fluid with for instance synchysis-like particles, the high ultrasound reflectivity of the lesion might have been explained thereby, but fluorescence angiography was in far better accord with a solid vascularized lesion of the choroid.

Enucleation having been refused, we have no definitive pathology of the tumour. This leaves the case quite open, eventually with choroidal haemangioma as our best guess, a possibility not contradicted by the biopsy answer (although the pathologist cautiously hinted that the surgeon might have missed the tumour). We have presented the case anyhow, because of the discrepancy between ultrasound presentation and optical assessment. All who saw the ultrasound pictures said that these could hardly be from the eye they knew so well from repeated optic evaluation and CT-scans. By ultrasound the tumour presented with a prominence of 5—6 mm, and extended also into the nasal fundus. Choroidal haemangiomas being rare, there are not many examples in ultrasound literature, and clinically the diagnosis is difficult. The acoustic presentation of the present tumour gave us associations to haemangiomas of the orbit, so well known to all who perform ophthalmic diagnostic ultrasound. Orbital haemangiomas present as very extensive tumours on the screen; the internal echoes have very high amplitudes from the start, and with only slight reduction throughout the lesion.

Echographically, the size of any lesion on the screen depends on the sound velocity within the boundaries of the lesion. Regarding sound velocity we generally presume tissue values between 1450—1650 m/s, and there is no immediate reason to believe that haemangiomas should be much different. However, we feel that the present intraocular lesion — similar to what might be suggested from some orbital haemangiomas from literature — is depicted as a bigger tumour on the screen than anatomically founded (so to say: as king size, not normal size). A theoretical parallel is what intraocular silicone oil does to the sound, making the eye appear longer on the screen (Verbeek et al., 1981).

We feel that the above question is of importance for the concept of ultrasonic tissue differentiation in general.

References

Mazzeo V, Giovannini A, Ravalli L, Costantini G. 1983. Echography and Cardio-green angiography in eight cases of choroidal haemangioma. In: JS Hillman and MM LeMay (eds) Ophthalmic Ultrasonography Doc Ophthal Proc Series, Vol. 38, Junk, The Hague, pp. 69—75.
Verbeek AM, Bayer AL, Thijssen JM. 1981. Echographic diagnosis after intraocular silicone oil injection. In: JM Thijsen and AM Verbeek (eds) Ultrasonography in Ophthalmology Doc Ophthal Proc Series Vol. 29, Junk, The Hague, pp. 59—66.

Orbital and periorbital tumours

The orbital involvement in some paraorbital lesions

B. ILIĆ, S. TOŠOVIC AND S. DJURIĆ

Summary

The orbital participation in periorbital processes we consider as a very attractive field of diagnostic use of ultrasound for many reasons:

— These processes are usually treated by other specialists — ENT, maxillofacial surgeon, neurosurgeon — and the ophthalmologist is required to establish a correct diagnosis.
— Diagnostic and therapeutic approach should involve a team, and simultaneous applications of other diagnostic techniques beside the ultrasound (plain X-ray, CT-scan etc.). Without a team work, diagnostic errors and, consequently, inappropriate treatment may be expected.
— Lesions of the orbital bone wall necessitate identification of the primary lesion site — in or out of the orbit.

In this paper the cases of malignant tumours of the periorbital region affecting the orbit, benign neoformations, inflammatory syndromes with subperiostial abscessus rising from neighbourhood and some less frequent lesions due to trauma have been analysed.

Introduction

The immediate orbital neighbourhood consisting of important regions (intracranial space, paranasal sinuses, pterygopalatineal fossa) exposes the orbit to the penetration of various pathological processes which occur in its surroundings and some of those processes indirectly affect the orbit. These facts are well known and have been emphasised many times by those who are involved in the diagnostic and therapeutic procedures in such cases. On the other hand, the orbital pathological processes express

University Clinical Center, Hospital for Eye Diseases, 2, Pasterova ul., 11000, Beograd, Yugoslavia.

J. M. Thijssen (ed.) Ultrasonography in ophthalmology.
© 1988, *Kluwer Academic Publishers, Dordrecht, ISBN 978-94-010-7083-6*

themselves by more or less the same signs — proptosis, displacement, motility problems, visual impairment and signs of inflammation. All of these signs may not be present in every case and so the orbital syndrome may be inflammatory or noninflammatory, acute or chronic.

Apart from some rare cases, there are no specific clinical signs according to which we could determine the origin of the process. In practice, processes rising from the orbital soft contents and paraorbital lesions invading the orbit present in a similar manner. We can roughly divide the paraorbital lesions into those rising from the frontal and ethmoidal sinuses, the maxillary sinus, supraorbital region, chiasma region, cavernous sinus, from the orbital wall itself, the eyeball and metastatic lesions.

Our aim was to try to determine the role of echography in the detection and localization of those lesions, starting from the fact that this is a border area where orbitologists of different specialities meet — ophthalmologists, maxillofacial surgeons, neurosurgeons, ENT specialists and others. Some of our cases merit presentation because of accompanying diagnostic problems, the complexity of diagnostic and therapeutic approaches demanding multidisciplinary team work.

Case reports

Patient M.Z. was referred to us because of a lacrimal gland tumour. On echography we easily found a cystoid formation in the upper temporal orbital angle. That formation was clearly seen on plane X-rays. However, computed tomography (C.T.) did not reveal the lesion. We asked for another CT in correct coronal section and that time a mucopyocele of atypical localization was discovered. (Fig. 1). The patient was referred to the ENT Clinic for operation.

The acute inflammatory orbital syndromes are frequently found in childhood and usually referred as "cellulitis".

Owing to our excellent collaboration with the ENT Clinic, those children are now sent for echography before all other diagnostic and therapeutic procedures. It is relatively easy to discover the disorder, usually near the ethmoidal wall, as a sonolucent zone representing a subperiosteal ecudate. Often, but not always, we find echoes of the entire neighbouring ethmoidal cell, as a sign of ethmoidal involvement (Fig. 2 and 3). It is really an ethmoidal periostitis with collateral oedema of the soft orbital contents. Thus, the localization and the nature of the primary process are determined precisely and, if necessary, an ultrasonically guided puncture may be performed.

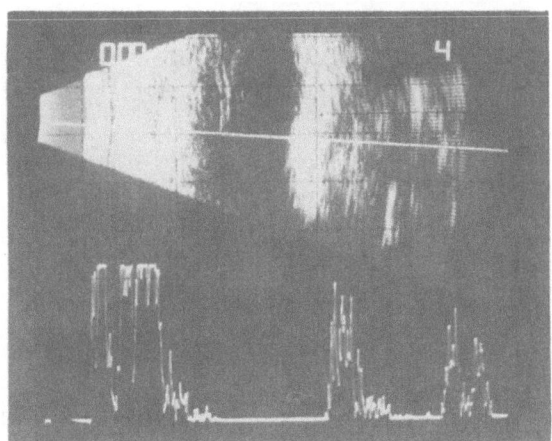

Fig. 1. A well outlined superotemporal lesion rising from the frontal sinus with was not initially found by CT.

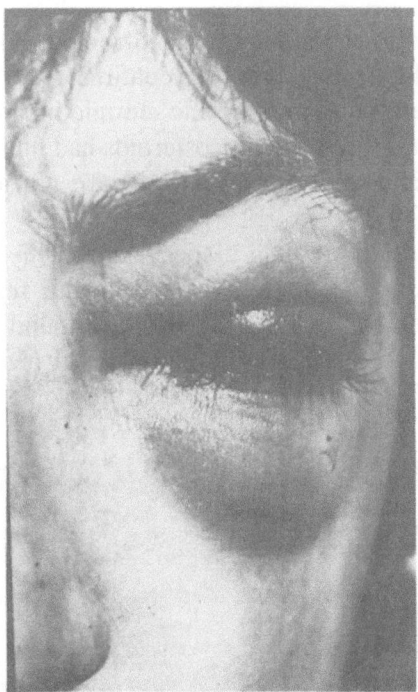

Fig. 2. A typical ethmoidal periostitis with oedema of the orbital contents.

The extremely inadequate term "cellulitis" is, owing to the successful collaboration with the ENT Clinic now almost out of use.

The localization of the original process is not always easy to determine. Patient R.S. was referred to us because of apex syndrome. Echographically

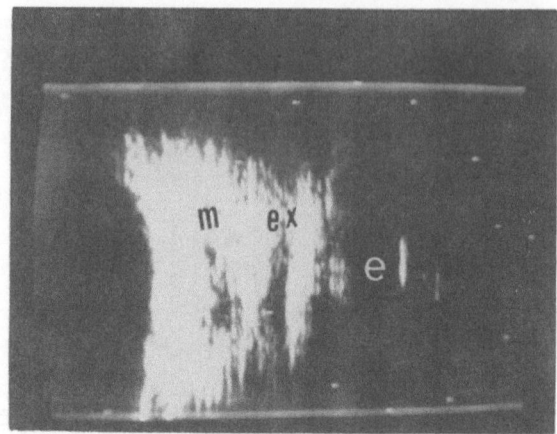

Fig. 3. Echography of the inflammatory syndrome (Fig. 2) demonstrates a strong echo of the ethmoidal wall with separation of the periosteum by exudate (ex), the ethmoidal cell (e) and the cross section of the medial rectus (m).

we found a solid lesion invading the orbit from all sides except superiorly, with a defect of the orbital floor. CT confirmed our diagnosis, but ENT surgery demonstrated only nonspecific chronic inflammation. No tumour elements were found (Fig. 4). Corticosteroids had limited effect and we are following this patient and at this time we are not able to reach a final diagnosis.

The apical region represents a specific problem for ultrasound diagnosis, since all normal anatomy structures in this region are oriented by their acoustic interfaces parallel to the ultrasound beam, and so they cannot be distinctly visualised. The pathological processes in this region have clear and rich clinical signs, but their ultrasonic presentation is often

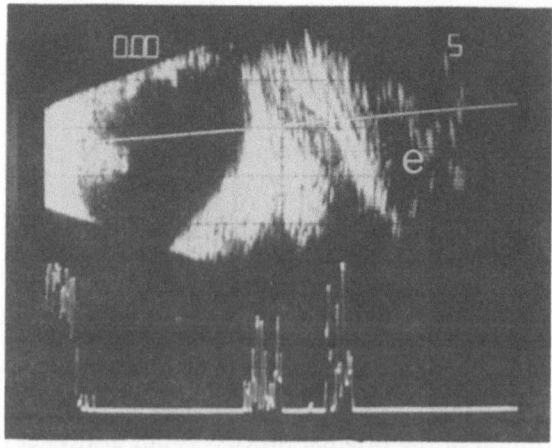

Fig. 4. The ethmoidal lesion invading the orbit.

very poor. Their relation with normal structures is difficult or impossible to determine, demanding other diagnostic methods, first of all computed tomography.

On the contrary, some paraorbital changes, such as caroticocavernous fistula, completely outside the orbit, have such very distinct clinical and echographic characteristics that is impossible not to recognize them.

Tumours of the orbital wall may cause certain diagnostic difficulties. R.M., a young girl, was referred to us because of a sudden proptosis, suggesting an orbital haematoma. On echography we found a cystoid, well outlined, polyseptal lesion and decided to perform a puncture. The result was a complete failure (Fig. 5). CT revealed a distinct tumour of the temporal orbital wall with bone involvement.

Choroidal malignant melanoma invading the orbit is not strictly a paraorbital lesion, but it deserves to be represented because of its clinical and echographic characteristics (Fig. 6).

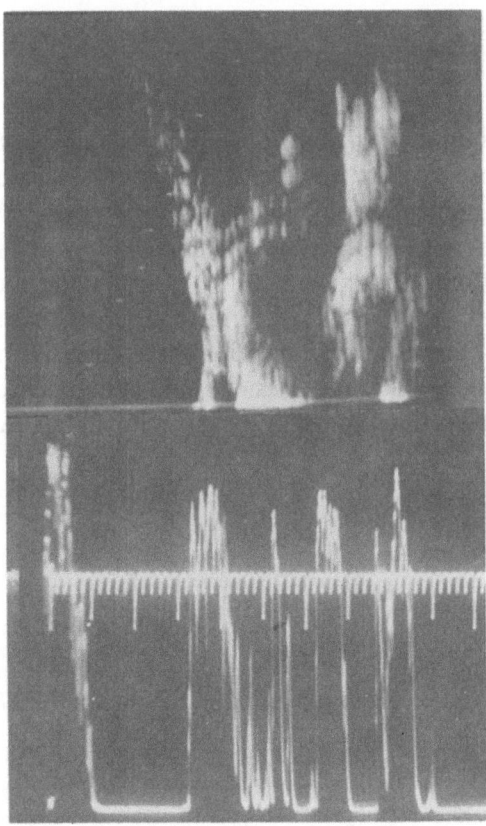

Fig. 5. A polyseptal cystoid formation near the temporal wall. The misdiagnosed solid lesion rising from the bone wall.

234

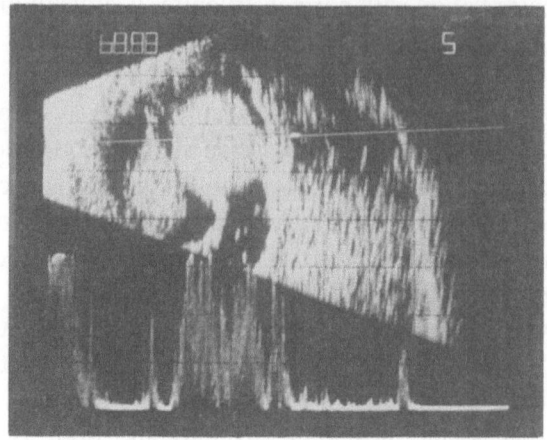

Fig. 6. Malignant melanoma of the choroid invading the whole orbit.

Conclusion

We have tried to indicate the difficulties which sometimes occur in the diagnostic and treatment procedures of orbital syndromes caused by paraorbital processes, by presenting a number of our cases. A well established and co-ordinated multidisciplinary approach in all these cases is absolutely necessary in order to avoid unpleasant surprises. The contribution of echography in these cases is considerable, because using this method we are able to exclude a primary orbital process, and, as a rule, refer the patient for further investigation in the most rational direction.

The localization of a primary lesion is the maxillary, frontal or ethmoidal sinuses, the orbital wall or in the anterior cranial fossa can be made with fair confidence.

References

Henderson JW. 1980. Orbital Tumours, Thieme-Stratton, New York.
Ilic B, Nagulic I. 1980. Apex Orbitae — a special problem in Ultrasound Diagnosis. In: A Kurjak (ed) Recent Advances in Ultrasound Diagnosis, Vol. 2, Excerpta Medica, pp. 515—519.
Ossoinig KC, Blody FC. 1974. Preoperative Differential Diagnosis of Tumours with Echography, Part IV, Diagnosis of Orbital Tumours. In: FC Blody (ed) Current Concepts in Ophthalmology, Vol. 4, Mosby, St Louis, pp. 313—341.
Ossoinig KC. 1978. The Role of Clinical Echography in Modern Diagnosis of Periorbital and Orbital Lesions. In: GF Bleeker (ed) 3rd Int Symp on Orbital Disorders, Junk, Amsterdam, pp. 496—540.

Savic D, Djuric D. 1982. Sinusitisi. In: Frontalni i etmoidalni sinusi, Decje Novine, Beograd, pp. 98—104.

Savic D, Djuric D. 1982. Maligni tumori. In: Frontani i etmoidalni sinusi, Decje Novine, Beograd, pp. 130—138.

Silva D. 1968. Orbital Tumours, Am J Ophthalmol 65: 318—339.

Till P. 1975. Echography in Rhinogenic Orbital Conditions. In: GM Bleeker (ed) Proc 2nd Int Symp on Orbital Disorders, Modern Problems in Ophthalmology, Vol. 14, Karger, Basel/New York, pp. 273—277.

The possibilities of application of ophthalmic ultrasound equipment in some head and neck diseases.

K. JANEV, O. KUBATI, D. ZORIC AND Q. HAXHIU

Summary

In this chapter we present three cases of head and neck diseases where, for diagostic purposes, ultrasound of high frequency was applied. The first case was a malignant melanoma of the infraorbital region of the skin whose echograms were similar to malignant melanoma of choroid. On the A-scan there was no first high spike of the tumour as with MM of choroid. We interpreted it as an absence of capsule of the tumour and the participation of retinal detachment in the first high spike of MM of choroid. Our second case was an example of Mikulicz disease with very characteristic echograms, which we then compared with those of mumps. The third case was a young man with a tumefaction in the region of the neck. Our echographic presumption that it was a chronic inflammation, was proved correct in the operating room and after bacteriological examination.

Introduction

Ophthalmology was one of the first medical disciplines in which diagnostic ultrasound was introduced (Vanysek et al., 1955). The practical use of ultrasound in ophthalmology today has a distinct place in relation to other branches of medicine. Due to the specific nature of the eyeball, ultrasound with very high frequency from 8 to 10 MHz or higher, which gives exceptionally good resolution, is used in ophthalmology. Crystals vibrating at the frequency from 2.5 to 5 or up to 7 MHz enabling good penetration but weak resolution are used in other medical disciplines.

Another advantage of ophthalmic ultrasound is that it uses two ultrasound methods, both A- and B-scan, respectively. While in most of the other medical disciplines the A-scan has been abandoned and replaced by the B-scan, the A-scan has however been retained and used in ophthalmol-

Department of Ophthalmology, Medical Faculty of the University, Pristina, Yugoslavia.

J. M. Thijssen (ed.) Ultrasonography in ophthalmology.
© 1988, *Kluwer Academic Publishers, Dordrecht, ISBN 978-94-010-7083-6*

ogy alongside with the B-scan. Moreover, with the A-scan a pathological lesion can be localized more precisely and a better tissue differentiation can be made than with the B-scan (Ossoinig, 1975). Therefore, in working with both scans we are more certain and closer to a correct diagnosis.

In our everyday practice we have ventured to move away from the eye and orbit and begun to examine some patients from the departments of E.N.T. and facio-maxillary surgery. We present two cases from this pioneer practice.

Materials and methods

Case No. 1. A 52-year-old patient in the Department of Facio-maxillary surgery with a semipigmented tumour in the infraorbital region. The tumour appeared about two years ago and has since grown slowly. Clinically, it could be malignant melanoma of the skin which had probably grown from pigmented naevus bellow (Fig. 1a). Echography: On the A-scan echogram we obtained spikes of low reflectivity, rather regularly distributed with the initial spike being of the same height as the other spikes, which was a sign that the tumour had no front capsule (Fig. 1b). On the B-scan we could see a lesion very well outlined in all directions, except for the side of the skin from where it had started. The echogram was similar to the echogram of malignant melanoma of the choroid (Fig. 1c). The inner echoes were almost of a homogeneous grey level but they were brighter than echoes of malignant melanoma of choroid. In the operating room the tumour of the size of a wallnut was removed. It had a fairly homogeneous internal structure, which was infiltrated by pigment. At histological examination, the tissue of the tumour was found to be composed of atypical polygonal cells located in alveolar formations and partially filled by small particles of pigment. Among the cells there were numerous thin, fibrous membranes (Fig. 1d). The histological diagnosis: Malignant melanoma of the skin.

Case No. 2. A 25-year-old man admitted to the E.N.T. Department because of a swelling of an unknown etiology in the neck region (Fig. 2a). The swelling appeared two months before, causing pain from time to time, without changing its size. Echography: On the A-scan echograms a lesion with vague border could be seen. Between those borders, in the front part, there were spikes coming from the low reflective space with small angle kappa, then, a few spikes with somewhat stronger reflectivity appeared, followed by a chain of equally low spikes which were a result of extremely low reflectivity (Fig. 2b). This part of the lesion looks like a cyst with some débris inside which yields very little reflection. The B-scan showed more

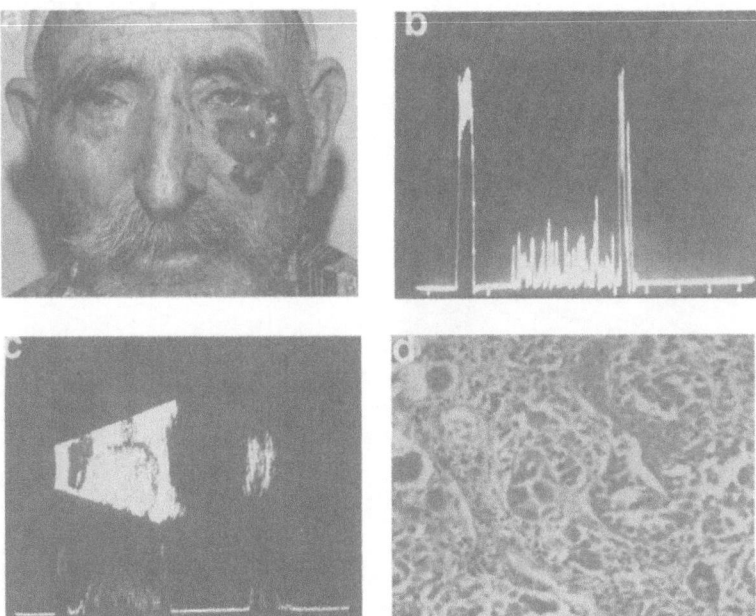

Fig. 1. (a) Patient with malignant melanoma of the skin which has probably started from the naevus below the tumour. (b) A-scan of malignant melanoma of the skin. There is no initial high spike because of the absence of capsule in the front part of the tumour. Some irregularity of inner spikes results from a large amount of connective tissue. (c) B-scan of the same tumour. The echogram looks like malignant melanoma of choroid but the position is reversed, because this one started from the skin. Atypical, polygonal cells in alveolar formations, between which a lot of thin, fibrous membranes appear.

clearly what we had discovered on the A-scan. In the front section of the lesion we could see a low reflective part, slowly decreasing, further on the zone reflected somewhat stronger, followed by a space resembling an incomplete cyst containing some opacities (Fig. 2c). According to the criteria of Ossoinig of the reflectivity of recent and long standing abscess in the orbit, we assumed that it was a chronic long standing inflammation with pus. Our assumption was proved correct by surgery. A content with specific etiology, partially purulent, was removed by incision.

Discussion

The works of Ossoinig about the diagnostic possibilities of ultrasound in periorbital diseases and with some tumours which are far from the orbit are well-known (Ossoinig, 1977; Nasr et al., 1985). We have continued this practice in diagnosing tumours and some other diseases using the Ophthalmoscan (Biophysic Medical Inc.) with crystal vibrations at 8 or

240

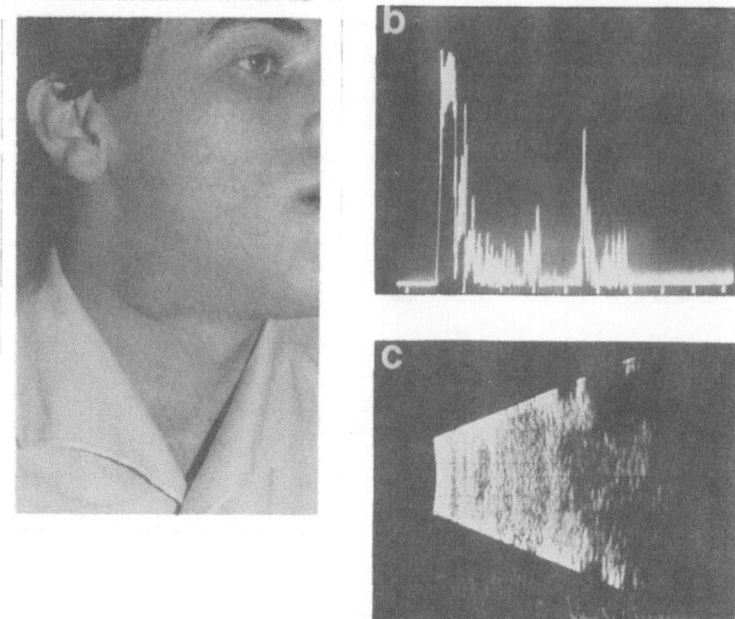

Fig. 2. (a) A young patient with a tumefaction in the neck region. (b) A-scan of tumefaction shows low reflective lesion in the front part followed by à cyst-like formation. (c) B-scan of the same patient. A zone of weaker reflectivity followed by an incomplete cyst.

10 MHz and applying the same criteria of reflectivity of tissues which are valid in ophthalmology.

In our first case with malignant melanoma of the skin, on the echogram of the A-scan there was no initial high spike of the tumour typical for malignant melanoma of choroid in the eye. It is because the initial high spike of malignant melanoma of the choroid stems more from the detached retina and less from the capsule of the tumour. With our case of malignant melanoma there was no capsule in the part of the skin where the tumour had started. The inner spikes of the echogram with malignant melanoma of the skin were higher and arranged somewhat differently as compared to the same tumour occurring in the eye as a result of histological difference between the two melanomas. The one in the skin has much more connective tissue than the other one in choroid. On the B-scan the malignant melanoma of the skin was very similar to that of the choroid, only the grey level contrast was reversed, because the tumour of the skin spreads in subcutaneous tissue while the tumour in the eye grows in the vitreous. A large amount of connective tissue accounted for the stronger reflectivity inside the tumour with malignant melanoma of skin.

The A- and B-scan echograms in our second case were more similar to the echogram of abscess of the orbit, which was proved in the operating room. This again means that existing criteria in ophthalmology can be applied to the examination of other diseases located as deep as the ultra-sound of such high frequencies can penetrate.

Conclusion

On the basis of our most recent experiences we can conclude that our instruments with crystals vibrating at frequencies from 8 to 10 MHz can be used in the differential diagnosis of some head and neck diseases, applying the same criteria which we have in ophthalmology.

References

Nasr AM, Ossoinig KC, Kersten RF, Blodi FC. 1985. Standardized echographic-histopatho-logic correlations in Liposarcoma. Amer J Ophthalm 99: 193—200.

Ossoinig KC. 1975. A-scan echography and orbital disease. Mod Probl Ophthalm 14: 203—235.

Ossoinig KC. 1977. Echography of the Eye, Orbit and Perorbital Region. In: PH Arger (ed) Orbit Röntgenology, Wiley, New York, pp. 224—269.

Vanysek J, Iserle J, Pacak M. 1955. Pokusy s electroakustickymi lokalisatory nitroocnih cizih teles. Prase Voj lék akad Hradec Králové 7: 12.

Diagnosis of orbital metastases with standardized echography

G. HASENFRATZ

Summary

According to large series metastatic and secondary tumours represent an important and prevalent form of orbital pathology and are a major group of orbital neoplasms. In a review of 38 cases (Jan. 83—Jan. 86) the echographic findings with Standardized Echography of metastatic haematogenic tumours and of secondary tumours from contiguous structures of the orbit will be presented. The acoustic criteria to achieve this very important diagnosis and the differentiation to other primary orbital tumours will be discussed.

Introduction

Though generally infrequent, among orbital neoplasms, metastatic tumours (tumours which spread in the orbit via the bloodstream from a primary tumour distant from the orbit) and secondary tumours (tumours which invade the orbit from contiguous anatomic structures) have to be considered a major group and a prevalent form of orbital pathology (Jakobiec et al., 1985). According to different surveys the incidence for orbital metastases ranges from 1% (Moss, 1962), 2.3% (Silva, 1968), 7.3% of orbital tumours/10% of orbital neoplasms (Henderson, 1980) to 12% (Ferry and Font, 1974). When adding the secondary tumours the incidence becomes even higher and both types of lesions constitute approximately 2% (Moss, 1962), 10% (Jakobiec, 1985) and up to 20% (Henderson, 1980) of orbital neoplasms. Moreover, as pointed out in these surveys metastatic carcinoma in the orbit is probably not nearly as rare as a review of the literature would indicate. Since only part of the patients which suffer from generalized metastatic disease are believed to be seen and examined by ophthalmologists (Henderson, 1980; Divine and Anderson, 1982;

Augenklinik der Universität München, Mathildenstr. 8, D-8000 München 2, FRG.

J. M. Thijssen (ed.) Ultrasonography in ophthalmology.
© 1988, *Kluwer Academic Publishers, Dordrecht, ISBN 978-94-010-7083-6*

Ferry, 1978). This aso stays true most likely for malignant tumours of the sinuses and the nose that invade the orbit.

The difficulties to diagnose metastatic and secondary tumours in the orbit only on the basis of clinical signs and symptoms are obvious and well known. The clinical features of such lesions depend from the source and type of neoplasm and from the site of first orbital involvement. Diplopia, swelling of the eye lids, blepharoptosis, proptosis, decrease of vision and pain are symptoms which are not typical for the lesions discussed here but are indicating any expanding lesion in the orbit. Sudden onset of symptoms are reported to be common but may be misleading (Henderson, 1980). Even by histopathology it may cause diagnostic problems, since the histo-pathologic features may vary widely and may be different to the primary tumour by the time the tumour reaches the orbit. In regard to this fact and when looking at the figures of incidence for these lesions the demand for a useful and reliable diagnostic method becomes evident. Particularly if the ophthalmologist is not aware of a history of a primary tumour elsewhere in the body it may be impossible to diagnose orbital metastases and secon-dary tumours without additional diagnostic methods or without orbital biopsy. That this latter fact is not a rare instance has been described in the literature and is documented in our series as well (Ferry, 1978; Font and Ferry, 1976). Ophthalmic echography — and in our opinion particularly the method of Standardized Echography — today has to be considered the diagnostic method of choice for non invasive and rapid screening of the orbit and detecting any orbital pathology. Moreover, for differentiation of a given orbital lesion echography this method is superior to other diag-nostic methods (Ossoinig, 1977, 1978, 1979, 1982, 1983; Ossoinig and Blodi, 1974, Blody, 1977).

Material and method

At the University Eye Hospital Munich the echographic examinations are performed with the method of Standardized Echography. This method is based on standardized A-scan and complemented by contact B-scan and — for orbital conditions — by Doppler sonography. For principles of instrumentation and examination techniques we refer to the literature (Ossoinig, 1977, 1978, 1979, 1982, 1983). The instruments we used were the 7200 MA (standardized A-scan; 8 MHz NF, Kretz-Technik), the Ocuscan 400 (contact B-scan; 10 MHz NF, Sonometrics) and the 1010-A (bi-directional Doppler; 4.1/9.6 MHz NF, Parks).

The study reviews the echographic findings of 34 cases examined between January 1983 and December 1985 (Table 1). In all cases the final clinical diagnosis — based on general clinical data (including echography) and/or on histopathologic findings — was that of a metastatic or secondary tumour of the orbit. Histopathologic diagnosis was made by orbital biopsy/ surgery in 15 cases (44%), in the remaining 19 cases (56%) histopathologic diagnosis was performed on specimens from the primary tumours. In the latter cases the diagnosis of an orbital involvement was accepted as verified by clinical, echographic and roentgenologic data. Since therapy concentrated on the primary neoplasm these patients were treated in departments for internal medicine or ENT and because of age and/or more advanced general metastatic disease orbital biopsy, orbital surgery or orbital radiation therapy was not performed. In 9 of these cases no echographic follow-up examinations could be performed.

Two groups of different types of orbital neoplasms in this study could be divided: metastatic tumours (n = 22, 64.7%) and secondary tumours (n = 12, 35.3%). The two groups were subdivided into metastatic neoplasms located in the orbital fat tissues (n = 17, 50%) and those located in extraocular muscles (n = 5, 14.7%) and secondary lesions invading the orbit from adjacent sinuses and from the nose (n = 10, 29.5%) and secondary orbital malignant melanoma after enucleation of the globe because of choroidal melanoma (n = 2, 5.8%).

In 6 patients (17%) the orbital involvement caused first symptoms whilst the primary disease/tumour was silent clinically (Table 2; marked with * in Tables 3 and 6).

Table 1. Metastatic and secondary tumours of the orbit.

---

n = 34

1983—1985 University Eye Hospital Munich

I	Metastatic tumour	* orbit	n = 17 (50%) age: 33—83 yrs (m = 60.7)
II	Metastatic tumour	* muscle	n = 5 (14.7%) age: 31—69 yrs (m = 53.4)
III	Secondary tumour	* orbit	n = 10 (29.5%) age: 22—79 yrs (m = 60.1)
IV	Secondary malignant melanoma	* orbit	n = 2 (5.8%) age: 65/87 yrs

---

Table 2. Metastatic and secondary tumours of the orbit with silent primary tumour.

n = 6 (17%)

Diagnosis	Site of orbital involvement
1 undiff. carcinoma (histopath.: metastatic)	(inf. post.)
1 undiff. adenocarcinoma of the breast	(sup. ant.)
1 small-cell carcinoma of the lung	(muscle)
1 undiff. carcinoma of the maxillary/ethmoidal sinuses	(inf.)
1 squamous cell carcinoma of the frontal sinus	(sup. ant.)
1 squamous cell carcinoma of the maxillary sinus	(inf. ant.)

Results

Metastatic tumours

The clinical diagnoses together with the first echographic diagnoses are listed in Table 3. In all the cases listed under *A* (Table 3) echographically the location of the tumour was predominantly in the orbital fat tissue. If a bony defect was present (n = 6) no major extraorbital parts of the tumour could be found (1 nasopharyngeal carcinoma without direct connection to the orbit; 2 breast carcinomas; 1 plasmocytoma; 1 lung carcinoma; 1 undifferentiated carcinoma that was suspicious by histopathologic features to be metastatic). The tumours listed under *B* (Table 3) were confined to extraocular muscles (one muscle affected in 4 cases, three muscles affected in 1 case).

The echographic criteria as they were described in the echographic reports for those lesions finally summarized under metastatic tumours (A, Table 3) are listed in Table 4. According to the examination techniques of Standardized Echography the echographic criteria were achieved by means of the specific examinations, namely quantitative, topographic and kinetic echography. Basically nine acoustic criteria are evaluated (reflectivity, internal structure, sound attenuation; borders, shape, location; vascularity, mobility, consistency). When summarizing all these echographic features some more predominant and frequent criteria can be determined. Thus when looking at the metastatic lesions located in the orbital fat tissue two groups regarding reflectivity and internal structure can be distinguished. One type (Fig. 1) shows low or very low reflectivity and simultaneously a rather regular and homogeneous, in 1 case slightly heterogeneous, internal structure. The other type (Figs. 2 and 3) presents very irregular, sometimes V-shaped patterns of the internal echo signals

Table 3. Metastatic tumours of the orbit.

Diagnosis	First echographic diagnosis	
A *Orbital fat tissue*		
5 Generalized metastatic disease carcinoma of the breast	* Cons. with metast. lesion	(2×)
	Periorbital malignancy	(2×)
	Lymphoma/Pseudotu/Sarcoma	(1×)
3 Generalized malignant lymphoma (M. Brill-Symmers)	Lymphoma/Pseudotu/Sarcoma	(3×)
1 Plasmocytoma	Periorbital malignancy	
1 Generalized metastatic disease carcinoma of the lung	Cons. with metast. lesion	
1 Sarcoidosis (M. Boeck)	Lymphoma/Pseudotu/Sarcoma	
1 Fibrous histiocytoma	Lymphoma/Pseudotu/Sarcoma	
1 Generalized metastatic disease hypernephroma	Cons. with metast. lesion	
1 Adenocarcinoma/Ethmoidal sinus	Lymphoma/Pseudotu/Sarcoma	
1 Undiff. carcinoma (Histo: most likely metastatic)	* Periorbital malignancy	
1 Generalized metastatic disease malignant melanoma of the skin	Cons. with metast. lesion	
1 Nasopharyngeal carcinoma	Cons. with metast. lesion DD Mucocele	
B *Extraocular muscles*		
2 Generalized metastatic disease carcinoma of the breast	Cons. with metast. lesion to the muscle	(2×)
	DD Myositis	(1×)
1 Generalized metastatic disease carcinoma of the lung	* Haematoma to the muscle	
1 Generalized metastatic disease malignant melanoma of the skin	Cons. with metast. lesion to the muscle	
1 Generalized malignant lymphoma (M. Brill-Symmers)	Lymphoma/Pseudotu/Sarcoma to the muscle	

which were described mostly high reflective in our reports, but the reflectivity could not be assessed in 4 cases. When looking at the clinical diagnoses of the first group the primary tumours of these metastatic lesions were: 3 generalized malignant lymphomas (M. Brill-Symmers), 1 nasopharyngeal carcinoma, 1 plasmocytoma, 1 hypernephroma, 1 generalized sarcoidosis (M. Boeck), 1 malignant melanoma of the skin, 1 fibrous histio-

Table 4. Metastatic tumour of the orbit.

n = 17

Histopathology/orbit:		n = 7 (41%)
Histopathology/primary tumour:		n = 10 (59%)

Quantitative echography/topographic echography/kinetic echography

Reflectivity	very low	2		medium	2		
	low	6		high	4		
Structure	regular/homog.	8		irregular	4		
	regular/heterog.	1		V-shape	4		
Sound attenuation	none	11		medium	2		
	weak	2		strong	0		
Borders	sharp	0		poor	3		
	well	8		diffuse	6		
Shape	flat/oval	7	round/oval	5	diffuse	4	
Location	inf/ant	3	med/ant	1	sup/ant	7	lat/ant	4
	inf/post	0	med/post	3	sup/post	1	lat/post	4
	diffuse	2						
Bony defects	+ : 6 (CT +:6)		−: 11				
Muscle(s) affected	+ : 3		−: 11				
Vascularity	(+) : 1		−: 15				
Mobility	+ :3		−: 13				
Consistency	hard : 6	firm : 5	soft : 0				

cytoma (primary site: thigh). In the second group the primary tumours were: 5 breast carcinomas, 1 lung carcinoma, 1 adenocarcinoma of the ethmoidal cells (no direct extension to the orbit neither by Standardized Echography nor by CT was found), 1 undifferentiated carcinoma. When determining the borders of these lesions by standardized A-scan again two types could be found: in 8 cases the borders were described "well out-lined", in 9 cases the lesions were outlined "poorly or diffusely". Both groups correlated almost exactly to the groups that could be differentiated in regard to their reflectivity and their internal structure. Besides the metastasis from generalized sarcoidosis and from fibrous histiocytoma all

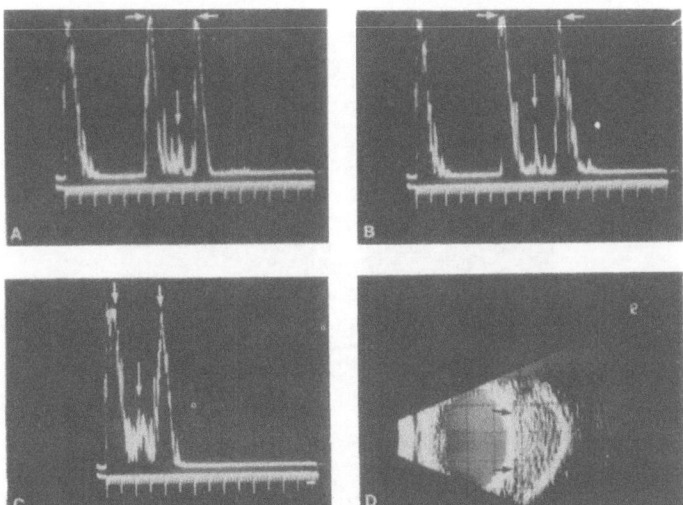

Fig. 1. Standardized A-scan echograms (transocular: A, B; paraocular: C) and contact B-scan echogram (D) of an orbital metastatic lesion in a case of generalized metastatic disease from malignant skin melanoma. Note the low reflectivity and only slightly hetero-geneous internal structure (long arrows) and the rather well outlining of the tumour (short arrows).

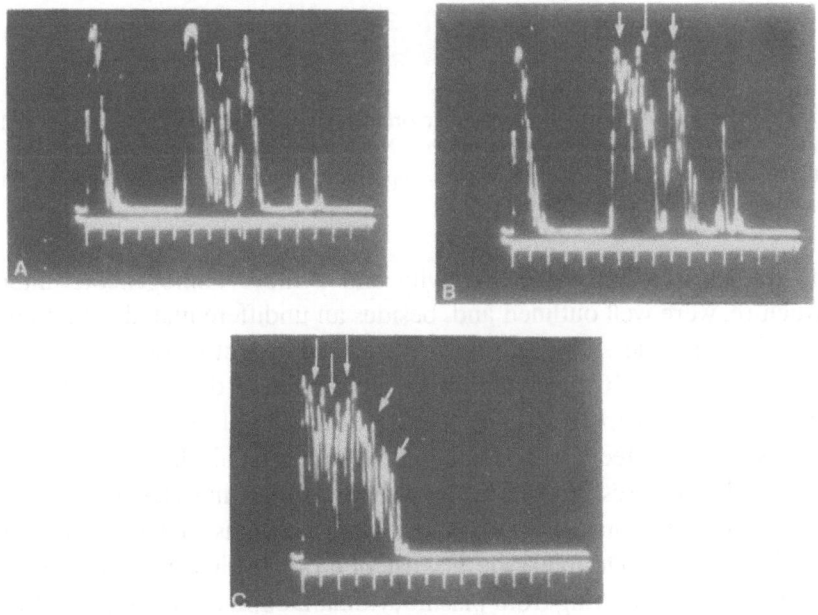

Fig. 2. Transocular (A, B) and paraocular (C) standardized A-scan echograms of an orbital metastatic lesion in a case generalized metastatic disease from breast carcinoma. Note the very heterogeneous internal structure (A, B: two different sections with very irregular height of the internal echo signals; long arrows), the V-shaped appearance of the signals (C: first 20 microsec, long arrows) and the diffuse border of this lesion (C: short arrows).

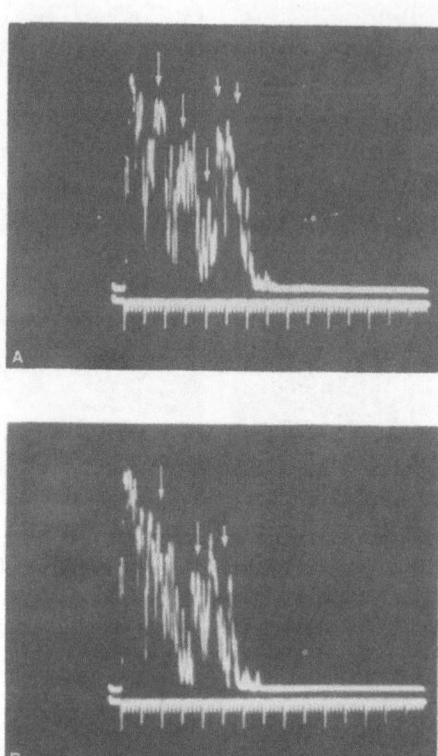

Fig. 3. Paraocular A-scan echograms of an orbital metastatic lesion in a case of generalized metastatic disease from breast carcinoma. Note the very heterogeneous and irregular internal structure with a slight V-shaped appearance in one section (A) and the diffuse borders of the lesion (short arrows).

the lesions that had low reflectivity and a more homogeneous internal structure, were well outlined and, besides an undifferentiated carcinoma of the orbit (that was suspicious to be metastatic by histopathologic features), the metastases with irregular structure had poor or diffuse borders. There was no typical shape nor a prevalent localization of any of the metastatic lesions. Bony defects were encountered echographically in 6 cases (see above). In 3 cases a thickening of extraocular muscles was detected additionally. The majority of tumours had no signs of vascularity (standardized A-scan, Doppler). In the case of a rather big orbital tumour in an elderly woman suffering from plasmocytoma Doppler-sonography revealed localized vascularity which was believed to be due to enlarged vessels on the tumour surface. Most of the tumours were not mobile and of firm to hard, sometimes very hard consistency. In few reports there were no remarks about kinetic echographic criteria.

The echographic features for the metastatic lesions located only in extraocular muscles (B, Table 3) are listed in Table 5. In contrast to normal extraocular muscle patterns achieved with standardized A-scan the reflectivity in these cases was mostly low whilst still regular and homogeneous to slightly heterogeneous. There was no predominant muscle harbouring the metastases. We did not find vascularity in any of the cases, the infiltrated muscles appeared to be firm and were mostly markedly thickened (Fig. 4).

Secondary tumours

The clinical diagnoses together with the first echographic diagnoses are listed in Table 6. In this group of tumours all the lesions which had orbital and extraorbital parts (C, Table 6), and two malignant melanomas of the orbit after enucleation of the globe, because of malignant choroidal melanoma (time intervals 2 and 6 yrs) (D, Table 6), are summarized. The main acoustic criteria (Table 7) we found for secondary tumours invading

Table 5. Metastatic tumour to extraocular muscle(s).

n = 5				
Histopathology/muscle:			n = 1	(20%)
Histopathology/primary tumour:			n = 4	(80%)

Quantitative echography/topographic echography/kinetic echography

Reflectivity	very low	0	medium	1
	low	4	high	0
Structure	regular/hom.	3	irregular	0
	regular/heterog.	3	V-shape	0
Sound attenuation	none:	5		
Borders	: location in extraocular muscle			
Shape	: location in extraocular muscle/flat-oval			
Location	sup. rect. m.	3	lat. rect. m.	2
	inf. rect. m.	1	med. rect. m.	1	CT: +:3
Vascularity	− : 5			
Mobility	− : 5			
Consistency	hard	0	firm	5	soft	0

252

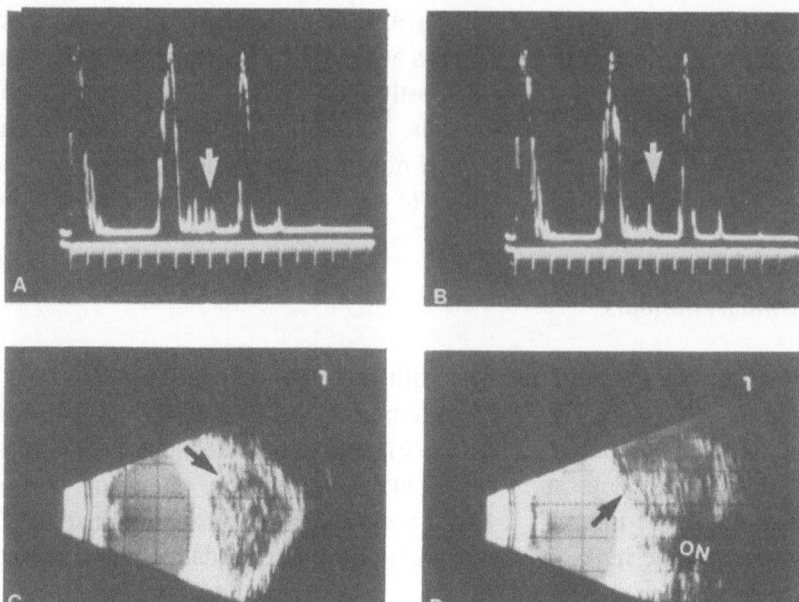

Fig. 4 Transocular A-scan echograms (A, B) and contact B-scan echograms (C: transversal section/12:00/middle orbit; D: longitudinal section/12:00) of a metastatic lesion in a case of generalized metastatic disease from breast carcinoma affecting only the superior rectus muscle. Note the low reflectivity (A, B: arrows), the pronounced thickening with slight displacement of the optic nerve (ON).

Table 6. Secondary tumours of the orbit.

Diagnosis	First echographic diagnosis
C From sinuses/nose/lid	
2 Squamous cell carcinoma frontal sinus	* Periorbital malignancy
3 Nasopharyngeal carcinoma	Periorbital malignancy
1 Esthesioneuroblastoma	Cons. with periorbit. malignancy DD Lymphoma
1 Squamous cell carcinoma maxillary sinus	* Periorbital malignancy
2 Undifferentiated carcinoma maxillary/ethmoidal sinus	* Periorbital malignancy
1 Basalioma	Cons. with metast. lesion
D After enucleation/choroid. MM	
2 Orbital malignant melanoma	Orbital melanoma cons. with orbital melanoma

Table 7. Secondary tumour of the orbit.

n = 10

Histopathology/orbit:	n = 5 (50%)
Histopathology/primary tumour:	n = 5 (50%)

Quantitative echography/topographic echography/kinetic echography

Reflectivity	very low	0			medium	3	
	low	0			high	6	
Structure	regular/hom.	1			irregular	6	
	regular/heterog.	0			V-shape	4	
Sound attenuation		none	7		medium	1	
		weak	2		strong	0	
Borders		sharp	0		poor	3	
		well	2		diffuse	5	
Shape	flat/oval	2	round/oval	1	diffuse	7	

Location	inf/ant	3	med/ant	2	sup/ant	2	lat/ant	0
	inf/post	4	med/post	2	sup/post	2	lat/ant	0
	diffuse	1						

Bony Defects	+ : 9	(CT:9)	− : 1
Muscle(s) affected	+ : 2		− : 8
Vascularity	+ : (1)		− : 9
Mobility	+ : 0		− : 10

Consistency	hard	9	firm	1	soft	0

the orbit by direct extension from contiguous anatomic structures (*C*, Table 6) were a predominant high reflectivity with irregular, and in 4 cases a V-shaped pattern of the internal echo signals (Figs. 5 and 6). Only one tumour — an esthesioneuroblastoma with primary location in the nose — had a more regular and homogeneous appearance. Other important echographic features we found in this type of lesion were mostly poor or diffuse borders and in all cases but one (lidbasalioma) multiple bone defects in the orbital wall at the site of invasion from the adjacent sinus. All the tumours were of hard, at least of very firm consistency, they were not mobile and no vascularity could be found. Particularly the presence of multiple bone

254

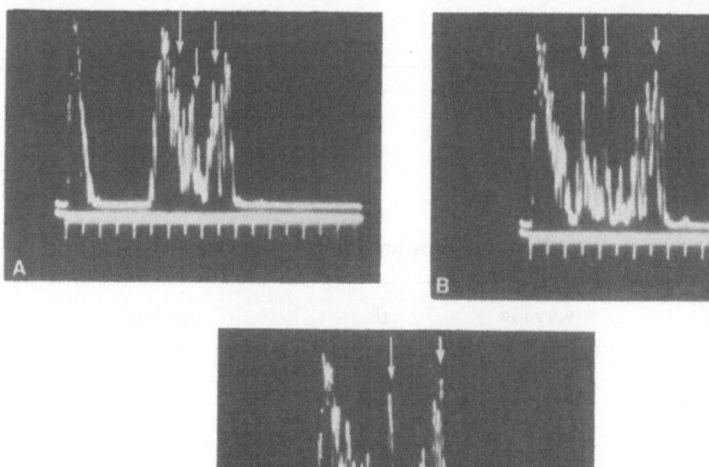

Fig. 5. Transocular (A) and paraocular (B, C) A-scan echograms of a squamous cell carcinoma of the frontal sinus invading the orbit secondarily. Note the irregular internal structure (A: slightly V-shaped type, long arrows), the echo signals caused by bony remnants within the tumour mass (B, C: long arrows) and the poor outlining of the lesion (short arrows).

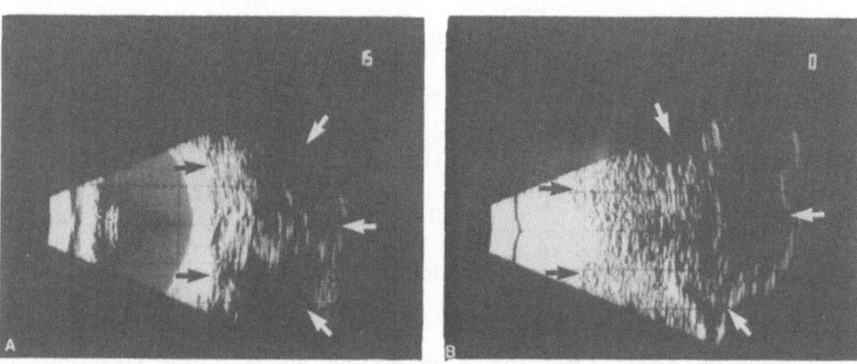

Fig. 6. Contact B-scan echograms (A: transocular; B: paraocular) of the same lesion like in Fig. 5. The majority of the tumour mass is located extraorbital (white arrows).

defects in our feeling is a key criterion for secondary orbital tumours originating from carcinomas of the sinuses and the nose.

The echographic findings (Table 8) in the two orbital malignant melanomas (*D*, Table 6) which occurred 2 and 6 yrs after enucleation of eyes harbouring a malignant melanoma of the choroid (no extraocular extension of the melanomas had been described in histopathology of these eyes)

Table 8. Secondary orbital malignant melanoma (choroidal malignant melanoma as primary tumour).

n = 2

Histopathology/orbit: n = 2

Quantitative echography/topographic echography/kinetic echography

Reflectivity	low	2
Structure	regular/heterog.	2
Sound attenuation	none	1
	weak	1
Borders	well-outlined	2
Shape	flat-oval	1
	round-oval	1
Location	orbit	
Vascularity	+ :	2
Mobility	− :	2
Consistency	hard	1
	firm	1

could be diagnosed with Standardized Echography due to the well known echographic features for intraocular melanomas and which were present in these orbital lesions too: low reflectivity, regular or slightly heterogeneous internal structure, and positive signs of vascularity (standardized A-scan, Doppler).

Discussion

Echographic findings with the method of Standardized Echography in metastatic and secondary tumours of the orbit have been described in a number of studies (Ossoinig, 1977, 1978, 1982; Ossoinig and Blodi, 1974; Divine et al., 1982; Till and Hauff, 1981). In summary the main echographic criteria for orbital metastases have been described as highly reflective with a (mostly) V-shaped arrangement of the internal echo signals. The borders of these lesions are characterized by indistinct surface signals indicating poor or diffuse outlining, by firm to extremely hard consistency and by the lack of mobility ("frozen globe") and vascularity. These echographic criteria were correlated to the mostly cellular and diffuse infiltration of the orbital tissue causing a decrease of the normally very high reflective orbital tissue pattern. The V-shaped appearance of the internal structure was described to be due to more densely packed tumour cells and foci of necrosis in the center of the lesion. When comparing our findings there was one group (primary tumours: 5 breast carcinoma, 1 lung carcinoma, 1 adenocarcinoma/ethmoidal cells/no direct extension into the orbit, 1 undifferentiated carcinoma) in which the echographic features mentioned above were present too. When looking at the pathology metastases from breast carcinomas (the most common source of orbital metastatic lesions) in particular are highly cellular and diffusely infiltrative tumours with central necroses. They are well stromatized with incited fibrouse response in the more peripheral parts of the tumour (Jakobiec et al., 1985). This histopathology is nicely illustrated by the standardized A-scan. Additionally in our series we had a second group of metastatic lesions (primary tumours/malignancies: 1 nasopharyngeal carcinoma, 1 plasmocytoma, 3 malignant lymphomas, 1 hypernephroma, 1 sarcoidosis, 1 malignant melanoma of the skin, 1 fibrous histiocytoma) which had lower reflectivity and a rather regular internal structure. These lesions had mostly well outlined borders. We feel that these A-scan characteristics are due to the special type of metastases where the orbital tissues are one site of occurrence of the systemic disease and where a purely cellular mass is located within the orbital fat. It may be mentioned that in all the cases of this latter group the general disease was known at the time of ophthalmologic/echographic examination. When looking at the first echographic diagnoses the predominant diagnostic classification was that of a tumour out of the "lymphoma, pseudotumour, sarcoma" group. Thus in cases where a general disease, for example generalized malignant lymphoma (M. Brill-Symmers) or systemic metastatic disease from malignant skin melanoma is present, the echographic diagnostician should include the differential diagnosis of a metastatic orbital lesion even if it presents low reflective and rather homogeneous. Follow-up examinations with careful measurements of the size are necessary and helpful. Additionally at least in cases where the general diagnosis is not yet substantiated a therapeutic trial of systemic corticosteroids under echographic control can be justified.

A separate and very interesting group of metastatic lesions in the orbit is the one where only extraocular muscles are harbouring the metastasis. We had 5 cases in our study and they presented with the typical change of the muscle pattern in standardized A-scan (Divine and Anderson, 1982; Ossoinig and Hermsen, 1983; Ossoinig, 1984). Dense cellular infiltration of muscle tissue either from inflammatory, lymphoblastic or malignant metastatic cells causes a decrease of the reflectivity due to more indistinct interfaces within the muscle or — like in metastatic infiltration — due to destruction of the connective tissue layers and septa. The internal structure of the affected muscle, particularly when metastatic infiltration is present, becomes more homogeneous. In contrast to other diseases of the muscles (myositis, haematoma, lymphoma, inflammatory pseudotumour) in metastatic infiltrations predominantly the muscle belly seems to be affected and there might be a more nodular appearance of the muscle (B-scan). Since clinical symptoms, as it is described for orbital metastases too, may occur very suddenly echographic differential diagnosis may be difficult when the patient is examined the first time. Any thickening of an extraocular muscle with low reflectivity should be followed-up carefully by standardized A-scan in rather short time intervals (2—5 dys) and we would recommend early biopsy in case the thickening increases. This becomes true particularly when other clinical symptoms indicating e.g. myositis are absent and/or therapy has been applied.

The most important diagnostic echographic criteria in secondary tumours invading the orbit from adjacent anatomic structures were the irregular, mostly high reflectivity, the irregular, sometimes V-shaped internal structure and the proof of mainly extraorbital location of the tumour mass (with typical location in the sinuses) through mostly multiple bony defects in the orbital wall. These very typical echographic features achieved particularly with standardized A-scan allowed the correct diagnosis of a periorbital malignancy in 9 out of 10 cases. It should be stressed that in approximately one third of these cases Standardized Echography detected the primary tumour located outside of the orbit and based on this echographic diagnosis the patients could be referred to ENT departments for adequate therapy.

Two malignant melanomas of the orbit occurring 2 and 6 years after enucleation of the globe because of malignant melanoma of the choroid could be diagnosed correctly. The echographic criteria leading to the diagnosis correlated closely to those well known for intraocular melanomas (low to medium reflectivity, homogeneous internal structure, vascularity). Particularly the proof of vascularity has to be considered very important and is an echographic key criterion. Since biopsy in cases where expanding lesions occur in the remaining orbital tissues after enucleation can be performed easily echography mainly has the task to measure the dimensions of such lesions and guide biopsy.

258

References

Blodi FC. 1977. Modern diagnostic methods for orbital lesions. In: GM Bleeker (ed) Proc of 3rd Int Symp on orbital disorders, Junk, The Hague, pp. 6—14.

Divine RD, Anderson RL. 1982. Metastatic small cell carcinoma masquerading as orbital myositis. Ophthalmic Surgery 13: 483—487.

Divine RD, Anderson RL, Ossoinig KC. 1982. Metastatic carcinoid unresponsive to radiation therapy presenting as a lacrimal fossa mass. Ophthalmology 89: 516—520.

Ferry AP, Font RL. 1974. Carcinoma metastatic to the eye and orbit: I. A clinicopathologic study of 227 cases. Arch Ophthalmol 92: 276—286.

Ferry AP. 1978. Tumours metastatic to the eye and ocular adnexa. In: FA Jakobiec (ed) Ocular and adnexal tumours. Chap 57. Aesculapius Publ Comp, Birmingham, Alabama.

Font RL, Ferry AP. 1976. Carcinoma metastatic to the eye and orbit: III. A clinicopathologic study of 28 cases metastatic to the orbit. Cancer 38: 1326—1335.

Henderson JW. 1980. Orbital tumours. Thieme-Stratton, New York.

Jakobiec FA, Rootman J, Jones JS. 1985. Secondary and metastatic tumours of the orbit. In: TD Duane (ed) Clinical Ophthalmology. Vol. 2, Chap 46. Harper & Row, Publ, Philadelphia.

Moss HM. 1962. Expanding lesions of the orbit. Am J Ophthalmol 54: 761—770.

Ossoinig KC, Blodi FC. 1974. Preoperative differential diagnosis of tumours with echography. Part IV: Diagnosis of orbital tumours. In: FC Blodi (ed) Current concepts in ophthalmology, Vol. 4, Mosby, St Louis, pp. 313—341.

Ossoinig KC. 1977. Echography of the eye, orbit, and periorbital region. In: PH Arger (ed) Orbit roentgenology. J Wiley & Sons, New York, pp. 223—269.

Ossoinig KC. 1978. The role of clinical echography in modern diagnosis of periorbital and orbital lesions. In: GM Bleeker (ed) Proc of 3rd Int Symp on orbital disorders, Junk, The Hague, pp. 496—540.

Ossoinig KC. 1979. Standardized echography: basic principles, clinical applications and results. In: RL Dallow (ed) Ophthalmic ultrasonography: comparative techniques. Int Ophthalmol Clin 19: 127—210.

Ossoinig KC. 1982. Bedeutung der standardisierten Echographie für die Diagnostik orbitaler und periorbitaler Krankheitsherde. In: OE Lund and K Riedel (eds) Automation und neuere Technologie in der Ophthalmologie. F Enke Verlag, Stuttgart, pp. 110—144.

Ossoining KC. 1983. Advances in diagnostic ultrasound. In: P Henkind (ed) Acta: XXIV Int Congr Ophthalmol, Lippincott, Philadelphia, pp. 89—114.

Ossoinig KC, Hermsen VM. 1983. Myositis of extraocular muscles diagnosed with standardized echography. In: JS Hillman and MM LeMay (eds) Ophthalmic Ultrasonography. Proc of the 9th SIDUO Congr Doc Ophthalmol Proc Ser 38, Junk, The Hague, pp. 381—392.

Ossoinig KC. 1984. Ultrasonic diagnosis of Graves' Ophthalmopathy. In: CA Gorman, RR Waller and JA Dyer (eds) The eye and orbit in thyroid disease. Raven Press, New York, pp. 185—211.

Silva D. 1968. Orbital tumours. Am J Ophthalmol 65: 318—339.

Till P, Hauff W. 1981. Differential diagnostic results of clinical echography in orbital tumours. In: JM Thijssen and AM Verbeek (eds) Ultrasonography in Ophthalmology. Proc of the 8th SIDUO Congr Doc Ophthalmol Proc Ser, Vol. 29, Junk, The Hague, pp. 277—282.

Echographic differential diagnosis of congenital cystic lesions of the orbit

R. ROCHELS

Summary

Typical A- and B-scan findings in congenital cystic lesions such as serous cyst, dermoid cyst, congenital cystic eye, cysts of the optic nerve, cystic lymphangioma, and meningo(encephalo)cele are demonstrated and characteristic combinations of criteria for each entity are outlined.

Introduction

The most common causes of congenital proptosis are neonatal sepsis and tumours; in the latter group rhabdomyosarcoma, metastatic neuroblastoma, undifferentiated sarcoma, and a variety of cystic tumours have to be considered. *Cystic orbital lesions* are most often congenital, even though they can manifest themselves years later (Howard, 1985). The differential diagnosis of these rare cystic lesions includes *serous cysts, dermoid cysts, congenital cystic eye* and *cysts of the optic nerve* in colobomatous malformations, *cystic lymphangiomas,* and *meningo(encephalo)celes.*

In standardized *A-scan ultrasonography* cyst-like lesions are characterized by regular internal structure, medium to extremely low reflectivity, well-outlined borders (wall-like delineation by very high, double-peaked surface spikes), variable consistency, roundish shape, and weak to no sound attenuation (Ossoinig, 1977). Bone defects are pathognomonic for meningo(encephalo)celes, and later in life, mucopyoceles (Hasenfratz and Ossoinig, 1984; Rochels et al., 1985).

In *B-scan ultrasonography,* cyst-like lesions are characterized by a more or less compressible roundish lesion with few homogeneously distributed internal echos and good sound transmission (Coleman et al., 1977; Poujol and Le Roy, 1984).

University Eye Hospital, Langenbeckstrasse 1, D-65 Mainz, FRG.

J. M. Thijssen (ed.) Ultrasonography in ophthalmology.
© 1988, *Kluwer Academic Publishers, Dordrecht, ISBN 978-94-010-7083-6*

Echographic findings

Serous cysts

In standardized A-scan sonography, a serous orbital cyst (Fig. 1A) is characterized by a regular internal structure, an extremely low reflectivity, a delineation by two very high, double-peaked surface spikes, a soft consistency, a roundish shape, and no sound attenuation (Ossoinig, 1977). In the B-scan, a well-outlined, non-echogenic lesion is found (Fig. 1B).

Dermoid cysts

Preseptal (Fig. 2) and intraorbital (Fig. 3) dermoid cysts have the following criteria: the A-scan shows a roundish, regularly structured lesion with low to medium reflectivity, bordered by two very high, double-peaked surface spikes. There is a strong correlation between the degree of reflectivity, the consistency of the dermoid (hard to soft) and the composition of its contents (Rochels et al., 1986). In large orbital dermoids another high double-peaked spike can sometimes be seen between the surface spikes; it

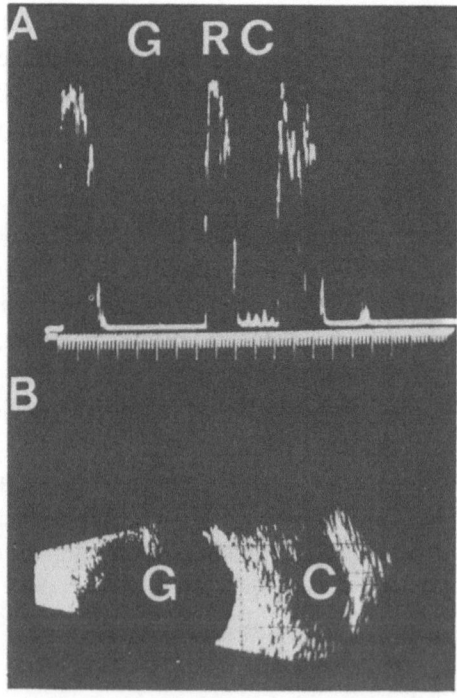

Fig. 1. Serous orbital cyst. A. A-scan: extremely low-reflective, well-outlined cyst (C); G: globe, R: rear-wall echospikes. B. B-scan: well-outlined, non-echogenic cyst (C); G: globe.

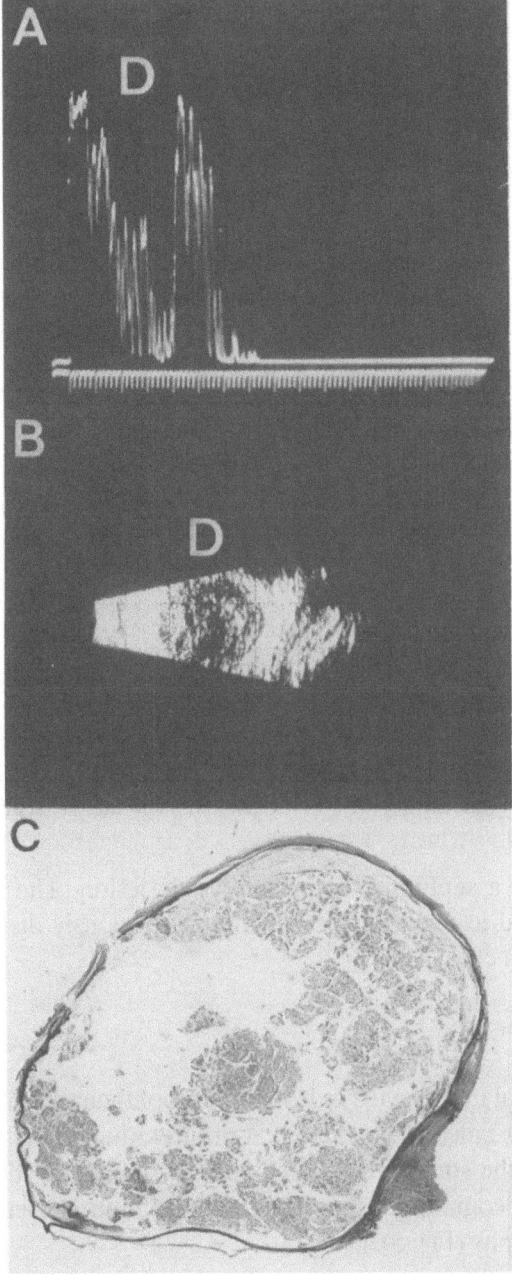

Fig. 2. Preseptal orbital dermoid. A. A-scan: well-outlined dermoid (D) with regular internal structure and medium reflectivity. B. B-scan: well-outlined dermoid (D) with few, homogeneously distributed internal echos. C. Histological specimen showing the capsule and the homogeneous contents of a preseptal dermoid.

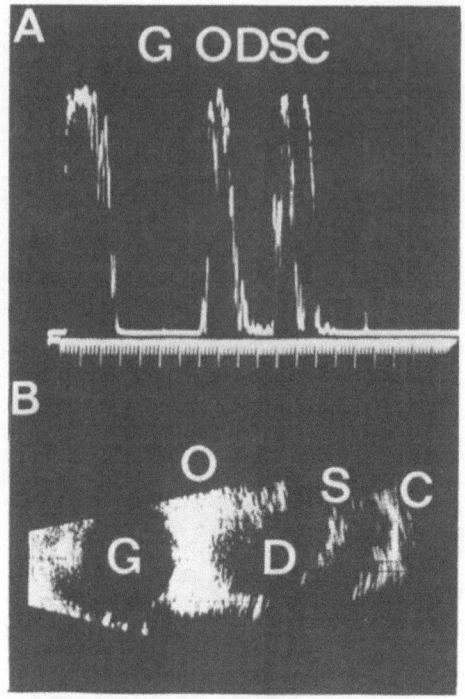

Fig. 3. Intraorbital dermoid. A. A-scan: low-reflective, well-outlined dermoid (D) with capsule (C) and an internal septum (S); G: globe, O: orbital echospikes. B. B-scan: well-outlined, non-echogenic dermoid (D) with capsule (C) and internal septum (S); G: globe, O: orbital echopattern.

correlates with a septum dividing this cystic lesion. The B-scan shows a sharply outlined lesion with very few, homogeneously distributed internal echos (Coleman et al., 1977).

Congenital cystic eye

In the congenital cystic-eye-syndrome (microphthalmus with cyst) the fetal optic fissure has failed to close, so that proliferating retinal tissue protrudes into the orbit; the small eye and the large cystic cavity (Fig. 4) are sometimes in broad communication. This malformation is easily diagnosed by B-scan sonography (Fig. 5).

Cysts of the optic nerve

Cysts of the optic nerve are another entity encountered in nonclosure of the fetal optic fissure: these colobomatous cysts may be large and are

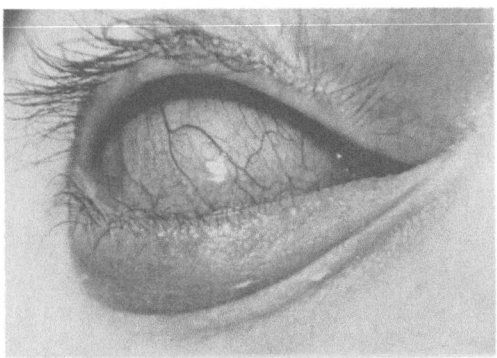

Fig. 4. Clinical aspect of the congenital cystic-eye-syndrome.

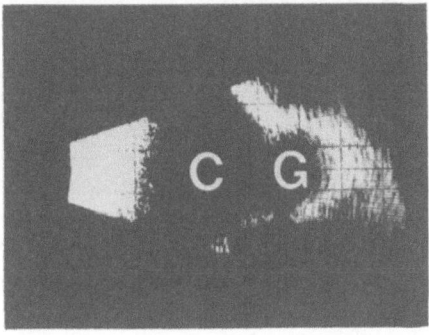

Fig. 5. Congenital cystic-eye-syndrome: B-scan showing a small (microphthalmic) globe (G) in broad communication with a large orbital cyst (C).

sometimes lobulated. The A-scan findings are identical with those of a serous cyst. The B-scan shows a well-outlined, non-echogenic lesion of the optic nerve (Fig. 6A). Small cysts next to the globe are diagnosed with B-scan sonography, too: it reveals a well-outlined, echofree area just behind the optic nerve head (Fig. 6B).

Cystic lymphangiomas

The A-scan criteria of cystic orbital lymphangiomas (Fig. 7A) are pathognomonic: an extremely heterogeneous internal structure with very high spikes from the septa and very low reflective areas from the homogeneous fluid in large cavernous spaces. This soft tumour has a weak sound attenuation, irregular borders and shape (Ossoinig, 1981). B-scan sonography (Fig. 7B) reveals a poorly-outlined lesion with heterogeneously distributed echogenic (septa) and non-echogenic (fluid-filled spaces) areas, resembling a "swiss cheese".

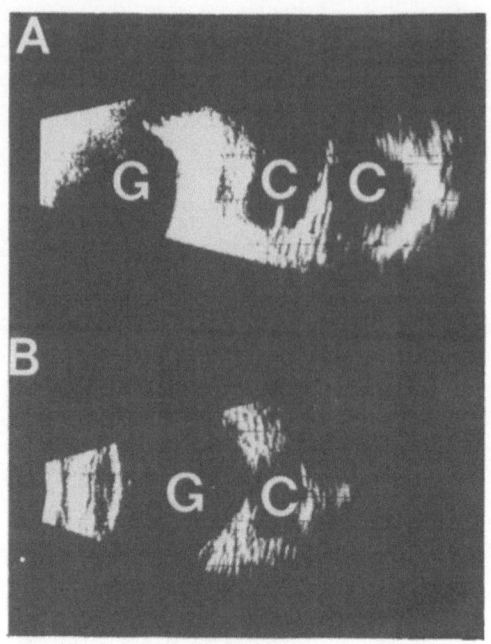

Fig. 6. Cysts of the optic nerve. A. B-scan: large, lobulated cyst (C) of the optic nerve, which is not shown in this section; G: globe. B. B-scan: small cyst (C) of the anterior part of the optic nerve; G: globe.

Meningo(encephalo)celes

Meningo(encephalo)celes (Fig. 8) are the result of a herniation of meninges with or without cerebral tissue through congenital dehiscences in the orbital walls. Besides the A-scan criteria of a cystic lesion (well-outlined borders, extremely low reflectivity, soft consistency, roundish shape) (Fig. 9A) the major echographic findings are the detection of a large, regularly outlined bone defect, and echospikes beyond the extension of the orbit. B-scan ultrasonography (Fig. 9B, C) is very useful in the pre-operative evaluation of the topography, a CT-scan (Fig. 9D) is nevertheless mandatory.

Discussion

Standardized A- (Ossoinig, 1977) and B-scan (Coleman et al., 1977) ultrasonography are well established in the diagnosis of orbital space-occupying *solid tumours*. The same holds true for the variety of *cystic lesions*: the B-scan clearly shows their extension and topography, whereas

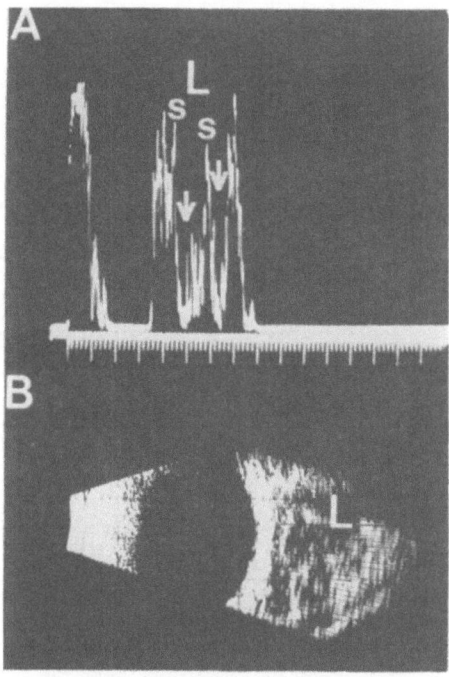

Fig. 7. Cystic orbital lymphangioma. A. A-scan: lymphangioma (L) with high spikes from the septa (S) and low-reflective areas (arrows) from fluid-filled cavernous spaces. B. B-scan: poorly-outlined lymphangioma (L) with the typical "swiss cheese" echopattern.

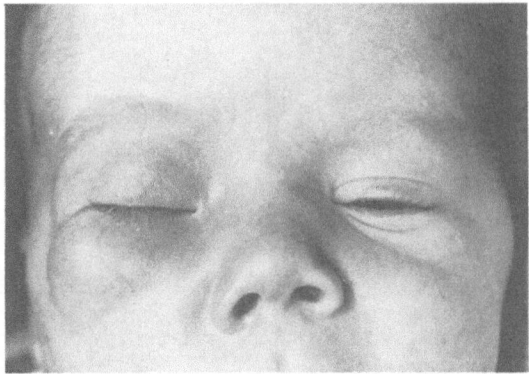

Fig. 8. Clinical aspect of a large posterior orbital meningoencephalocele with extension into the lower lid.

the A-scan can differentiate them. The common criteria of cystic orbital lesions are regular structure, well-outlined borders and roundish shape. In *serous cysts* additional findings are extremely low reflectivity, soft consistency, and no sound attenuation. In *dermoids* the reflectivity ranges

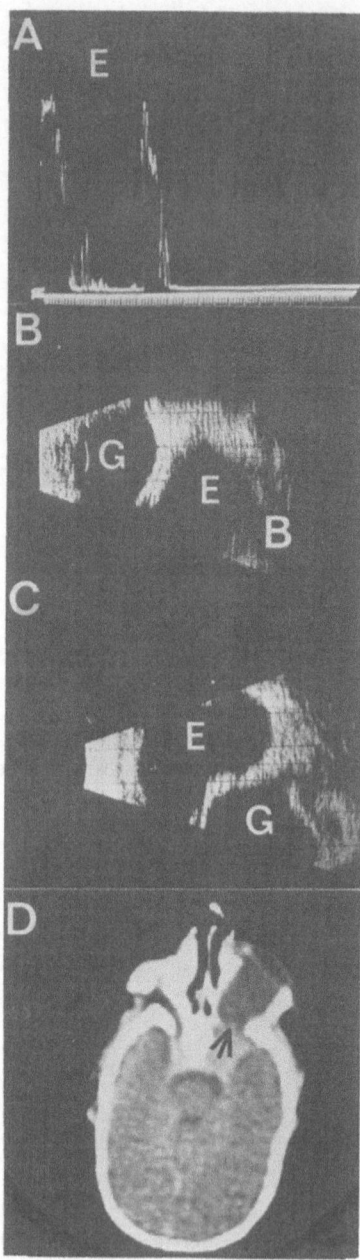

Fig. 9. Large, lobulated posterior orbital meningoencephalocele. A. Paraocular A-scan with the probe placed nasally on the upper lid: well-outlined, very low-reflective encephalocele (E) with echospikes beyond the extension of the orbit. B. Vertical transocular B-scan showing the extension of the encephalocele (E) behind and below the globe (G); B: bone defect in the posterior orbital wall. C. Horizontal transocular B-scan showing the inferior lateral palpebral extension of the encephalocele (E); G: globe. D. CT-scan: large bone defect in the posterior orbital wall (arrow).

from low to medium, the consistency from soft to hard; the sound attenuation is weak. The *congenital cystic eye* and *cysts of the optic nerve* are easily visualized with B-scan sonography, whereas *cystic lymphangiomas* are definitely characterized by the A-scan criteria of a mixture of very high spikes from the septa and areas of zero-reflectivity from the cystic, fluid-filled spaces. The leading features of *meningo(encephalo)celes* are the detection of a large, regularly outlined bone defect in the orbital walls and echos beyond the extension of the orbit.

References

Coleman DJ, Lizzi FL, Jack RL. 1977. Ultrasonography of the eye and orbit. Lea & Febiger, Philadelphia, pp. 307—312.

Hasenfratz G, Ossoinig KC. 1984. The diagnosis of orbital mucoceles and pyoceles with standardized echography. In: JS Hillman and MM LeMay (eds) Ophthalmic Ultrasound, Docum Ophthal Proc Ser Vol. 38, Junk, The Hague, pp. 407—415.

Howard GM. 1985. Cystic tumours. In: TD Duane and EA Jaeger (eds) Clinical ophthalmology, Vol. 2, chapt 31, 1—10, Harper & Row, Philadelphia.

Ossoinig K. 1977. Echography of the eye, orbit and periorbital region. In: PH Arger (ed) Orbit roentgenology, Wiley & Sons, New York, pp. 224—269.

Ossoinig KC. 1981. Echographic differentiation of vascular tumours in the orbit. In: JM Thijssen and AM Verbeek (eds) Ultrasonography in Ophthalmology, Docum Ophthal Proc Ser Vol. 29, Junk Publ, The Hague, pp. 283—291.

Poujol J, Le Roy M. 1984. Aspects échographiques des kystes orbitaires. Bull Soc Opht France 84: 35—38.

Rochels R, Geyer G, Bleier R. 1985. Echographische Diagnostik bei orbitalen Mukozelen. Laryng Rhinol Otol 64: 181—184.

Rochels R, Nover A, Hackelbusch R. 1986. Echographische Befunde und Differentialdiagnostik bei (peri-)orbitalen Dermoidzysten. Klin Mbl Augenheilk 188: 101—104.

Echographic patterns of an orbital myxoma and schwannoma

W. LIEB AND R. ROCHELS

Summary

A case of intramuscular orbital myxoma and of a schwannoma of the orbit were studied with B-scan and standardized A-scan echography as described by Ossoinig. The myxoma appeared as a well outlined process with medium internal reflectivity and areas of low internal reflectivity. Postoperatively the incompletely excised tumour was followed with echography as well as CT and MRI. The second tumour, a schwannoma had a very sharply defined shape, with a thick low to medium reflective outer wall and low internal reflectivity. This corresponds to the Antoni A and Antoni B patterns of the excised tumour.

Introduction

Standardized A- and B-scan sonography have proved to be very predicatory in the differential diagnosis of orbital mass lesions (Coleman et al., 1977; Ossoinig, 1975, 1978; Till, 1981); approximately seventy entities cannot only be detected, localized and measured, but also differentiated. In this paper, the echographic patterns of an orbital myxoma and a schwannoma (neurilemmoma) will be reported.

Case reports

Case 1: Orbital myxoma

A 27 year old man presented with a slowly progressive protrusion of his left eye, with vertical diplopia on upgaze. The visual acuity was 20/25 OU; there was a 10 mm Hertel difference. The other morphological and functional findings were within normal limits.

University Eye Hospital, Johannes Gutenberg-University, Langenbeckstr. 1, 6500 Mainz, FRG.

J. M. Thijssen (ed.) Ultrasonography in ophthalmology.
© 1988. *Kluwer Academic Publishers, Dordrecht, ISBN 978-94-010-7083-6*

A-scan sonography was performed using the 7200 MA Kretz Technik apparatus with an 8 MHz probe: A well outlined, regularly structured mass lesion with cystic spaces and medium sound attenuation was found (Fig. 1A, B). There were no signs of vascularity and late compressibility.

B-scan sonography was performed with the Ocuscan 400 (Sonometrics) at 10 MHz: A large well outlined mass lesion, with homogeneously distributed internal echos, and some echo-free areas were found (Fig. 1C, D). The lesion was located near the superior rectus muscle, whereas the other extraocular muscles and the optic nerve were not involved.

CT-scan confirmed the diagnosis of a solid tumour in the lateral superior portion of the left orbit, with displacement of the optic nerve (Fig. 2). Surgical excision was performed through a transfrontal craniotomy.

The histological examination revealed a semimalignant myxoma with infiltration of the superior rectus muscle (Fig. 3).

Case 2: Orbital schwannoma

An 80 year old woman had noticed a displacement of her left globe since 3 years. There was a 6 mm protrusion of the left eye, impeded elevation and abduction without diplopia. The visual acuity was 20/40 OU.

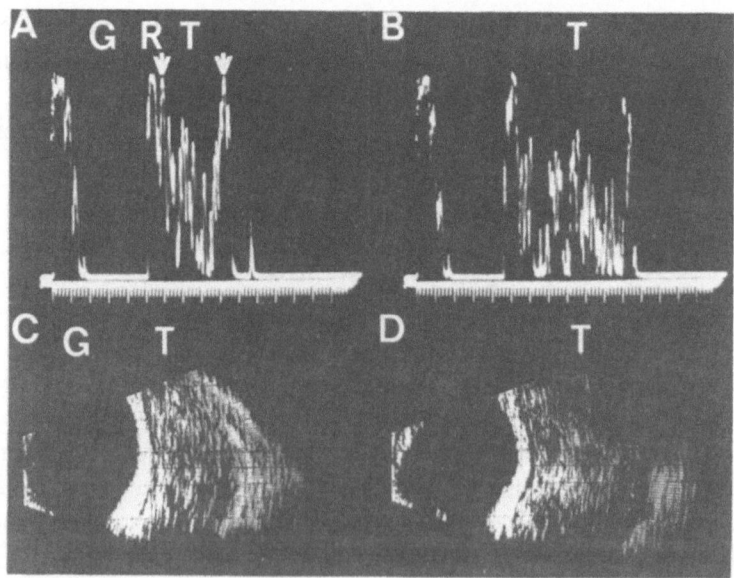

Fig. 1. (1A, 1B) Trans-ocular A-scan findings of a orbital myxoma. (G = globe, R = rear wall echo, T = tumour). (1C, 1D) Trans-ocular vertical and horizontal A-scan findings of an orbital myxoma.

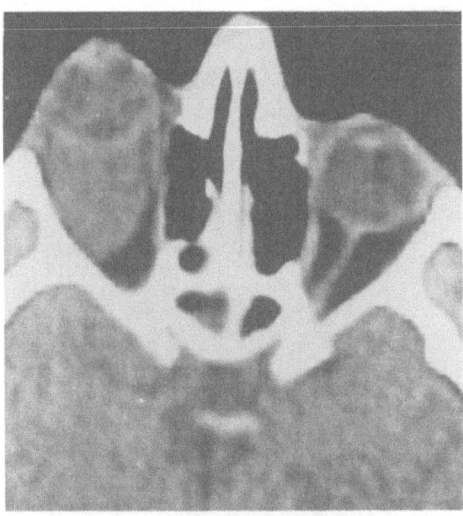

Fig. 2. CT-scan of the myxoma showing a well outlined mass in the left orbit.

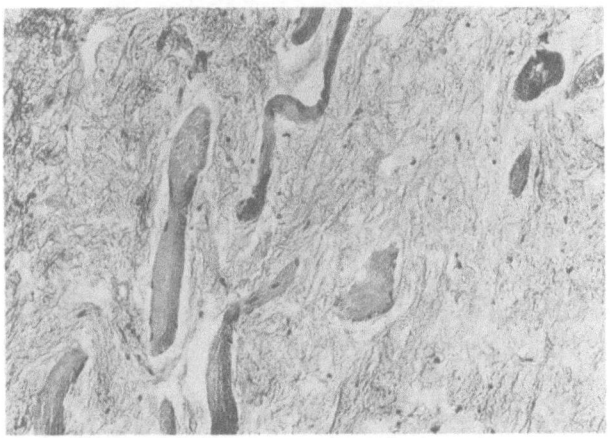

Fig. 3. Histologic section of the myxoma, between the muscle fibers there are areas of mucinous matrix, with reticulin fibers and stellate cells resembling precursor mesenchyme. (H&E × 63)

A-scan sonography showed a sharply outlined lesion with an extremely low reflectivity and a cystic center (Fig. 4A). B-scan sonography revealed a rather peculiar pattern of a solid, sharply outlined lesion with a cystic inner part (Fig. 4B, C). The A-scan showed no signs of vascularity.

The CT-scan displayed a well defined roundish mass, with a central hypodense zone (Fig. 5). The tumour was removed through a modified Krönlein approach. The gross specimen was 2.0 cm × 2.6 cm and hard, it showed cystic degeneration and haemorrhage in the center, surrounded by a solid parenchymal tissue and a thin capsule (Fig. 6).

272

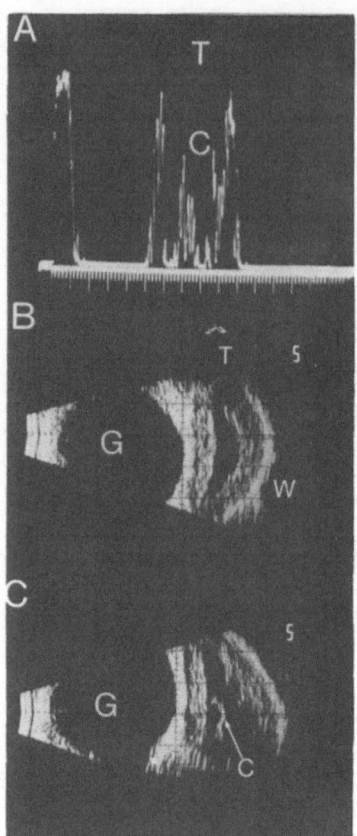

Fig. 4. A- and B-scan of an orbital schwannoma. A: Trans-ocular A-scan shows a sharply outlined low reflective tumour (T) with a cystic center part (C). B, C: Trans-ocular B-scans. A well outlined (W) tumour (T) with a thick two-layered outer and a cystic inner part (C).

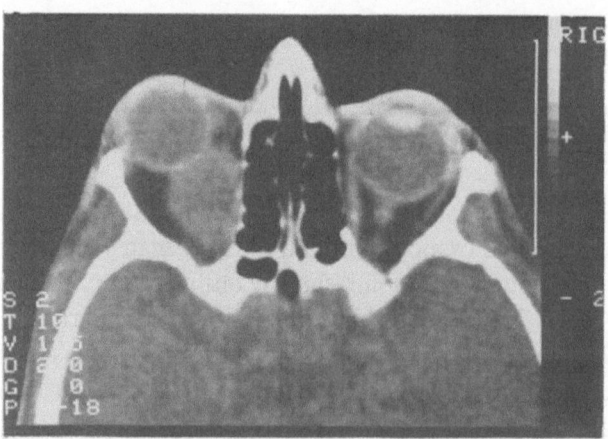

Fig. 5. Axial CT-scan of the schwannoma through the superior orbit demonstrates a solid, well encapsulated tumour in the superior nasal orbit. In the center of the tumour there is a hypodense zone.

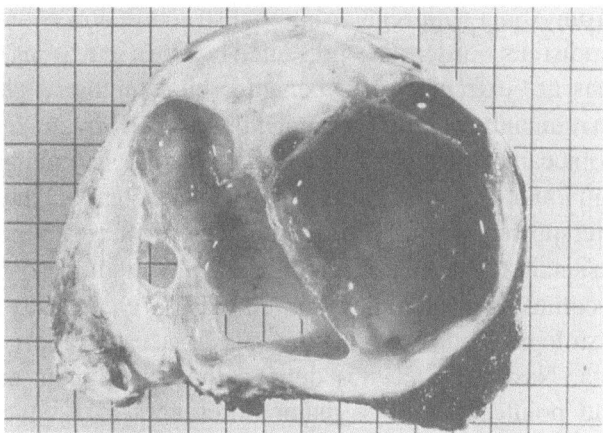

Fig. 6. Gross specimen of a large neurilemmoma (schwannoma) with cystic degeneration and haemorrhage in the center.

Histology showed a neurilemmoma with a distinct capsule, a peripheral solid and central cystic part, containing old haemorrhage. The solid portion displayed the typical highly cellular Antoni A pattern, with palisading of the spindle shaped cells.

More centrally close to the central cystic zone there were more loosely organized cells in an Antoni B fashion (Fig. 7).

Discussion

Krueger et al. (1967) reported the echographic findings of an orbital myxoma; it was a sharply defined tumour next to the optic nerve. A case of

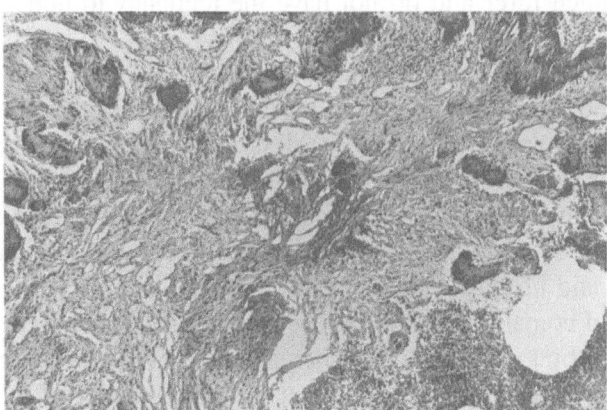

Fig. 7. Histology of the schwannoma (neurilemmoma): on the left rather solid and compactly arranged spindle cells with a basophilic nucleus, arranged in palisades. (Antoni A). In the middle Antoni B-pattern with stellate cells distributed in a mucinous matrix. At the right cystic area with haemorrhage. (H&E × 63)

orbital fibromyxoma with regular internal structure, low to medium reflectivity and indistinct borders was presented by Dorn and Srenger (1980).

Myxomas are extremely rare benign orbital tumours, which probably originate in remnants of embryonic mucinous tissue (Blodi, 1969; Henderson, 1973; Jakobiec and Jones, 1979). The main histologic findings in myxomas are a benign looking cellular pattern with a major component of a mucinous matrix, interspersed with a delicate framework of reticulin and collagen fibers, with small stellate cells resembling the precursor mesenchyme.

Liposarcomas, fibrosarcomas, and chondrosarcomas may display comparable histologic features of a myxoma. In a case report of an orbital liposarcoma, Nasr et al. (1985) defined the echographic criteria of this tumour and pointed out three major differences to a typical adult type cavernous haemangioma: The liposarcoma was softer, had areas of low reflectivity and was not sharply outlined in all sections. In our case we could find similar differences between the myxoma and the adult type cavernous haemangioma, Cappaert et al. (1983). In contrast to the case presented by Dorn and Srenger (1980) the tumour presented by us had a partially formed capsule and showed no signs of vascularity.

Comparing the echographic pattern with the histology, the low reflective areas corresponded to the areas of loosely arranged spindle-shaped cells lying in an edematous connective tissue stroma. The more highly reflective parts correlated with highly cellular myxoma parts and the muscular infiltration.

Schwannomas account for about 1% of all orbital tumours. They can be found anywhere in the orbit (Rootman et al., 1982). They arise from peripheral nerves and are relatively pure proliferations of Schwann cells. They are encapsulated by perineural cells. In contrast to neurofibromas, they are much rarer and do not have the tendency to undergo malignant transformation.

Ossoinig (1975) and Mazzeo et al. (1983) characterized these neurogenic tumours as highly reflective, variable in consistency, poorly outlined and mobile. Coleman et al. (1977) described neurilemmomas and neurofibromas as poorly encapsulated; Restori et al. (1978) and Restori (1979) saw neurilemmomas as a round echo free mass with medium amplitude echos within the lesion. Our case correlates well with the findings on gross pathology and histology. Like all schwannomas, the tumour had a distinct capsule and contained a solid parenchymal part with densely packed cells represented by low reflectivity, whereas, the more loosely Antoni B areas and the central haemorrhage appeared as cystic spaces.

From these observations no echographic criteria for the diagnosis of myxomas and schwannomas can be derived, however they show again that the criteria pointed out by Ossoinig (1978) allow in many cases histological correlation and differentiation of orbital lesions.

References

Blodi FC. 1969. Unusual orbital neoplasms. Am J Ophthalmol 68: 407—412.

Cappaert WE, Kiprov RV, Frank KE. 1983. Sector B-scan ultrasonographic "Hemangioma-like" pattern. Arch Ophthalmol 101: 74—77.

Coleman DJ, Lizzi FC, Jack RL. 1977. Ultrasonography of the eye and orbit. Lea and Febiger, Philadelphia.

Dorn V, Srenger Z. 1980. Zum echographischen Bild des orbitalen Cholesteatoms und des Fibromyxoms. Klin Mbl Augenheilk. 176: 140—146.

Henderson JW. 1973. Orbital tumours. Saunders Co., Philadelphia.

Jakobiec FA, Jones IS. 1979. Mesenchymal and fibro-osseous tumours. In: IS Jones and FA Jakobiec (eds) Diseases of the orbit. Harper & Row Publ, Hagerstown, pp. 461—502.

Krueger EG, Polifrone JC, Baum G. 1967. Retrobulbar orbital myxoma and its detection by ultrasonography. J Neurosurg 26: 87—91.

Mazzeo V, Scorrano R, Ravalli L, Spettoli M. 1983. Echographic patterns of peripheral nerve tumours. In: JS Hillman and MM Le May (eds) Ophthalmic Ultrasonography Doc Ophthalmologic Proc Ser, Vol. 38, Junk, The Hague, pp. 417—421.

Nasr AM, Ossoinig KC, Kersten RF, Blodi FC. 1985. Standardized echographic histopatho-logic correlations in liposarcoma. Am J Ophthalmol 99: 193—200.

Ossoinig KC. 1975. A-scan echography and orbital disease. Mod Probl Ophthalmol 14: 203—231.

Ossoinig KC. 1978. The role of clinical echography in modern diagnosis of periorbital and orbital lesions. In: Proc 3rd Int Symp on Orbital Disorders, Amsterdam 1978. Junk, The Hague, pp. 496—540.

Rootman J, Goldberg C, Robertson W. 1982. Primary orbital schwannomas. Brit J Ophthalmol 66: 194—204.

Restori M, Wright JE, McLeod D. 1978. B-scan and CT-scan imaging in the orbit. In: Proc of the 3rd Int Symp on Orbital Disorders, Amsterdam 1978. Junk, The Hague, pp. 43—48.

Restori M. 1979. Ultrasound in orbital diagnosis. Trans Ophthal Soc UK 99: 223—231.

Till P, Hauff W. 1981. Differential diagnostic results of clinical echography in orbital tumours. In: JM Thijssen and AM Verbeek (eds) Ultrasonography in Ophthalmology, Doc Ophthal Proc Series, Vol. 29, Junk, The Hague, pp. 277—282.

Lacrimal gland region disorders

L. RAVALLI AND V. MAZZEO[1]

Summary

The echographic patterns of different disorders which can originate in the lacrimal gland region are reported. The differential diagnoses among cystic, inflammatory and tumoural lesions will be discussed. Particular attention will be payed to the A- and B-scan characteristic of the adenoid cystic carcinoma.

Introduction

A normal lacrimal gland cannot be demonstrated by echography (Mazzeo et a1., 1981; Motolese et al., 1985), therefore any anomaly which is found in its region has to be considered pathological.

The pathological forms that are typical of the gland can be divided into inflammatory, cystic and tumour. It is possible that some other lesions may arise in the region of the gland appearing as pathology of the gland-lymphomata, pseudotumours and dermoid cysts are comparatively frequent in that region.

Inflammatory diseases

Among the inflammatory lesions, acute dacryoadenitis is shown in A-scan as a poorly defined lesion with high reflectivity and low sound attenuation (minimum angle K) (Hackelbush et al., 1983). It appears better defined in B-scan and presents an intense density of internal echoes (Fig. 1). Chronic dacryoadenitis, in contrast, appears echographically as a lesion with low internal reflectivity and with regular acoustic structure. Pseudotumour and lymphoma are of difficult differential diagnosis. If the inflammatory fea-

NHS USL 31, Ophthalmology Department, University Eye Clinic[1] Ferrara, Italy.

J. M. Thijssen (ed.) Ultrasonography in ophthalmology.
© 1988, *Kluwer Academic Publishers, Dordrecht, ISBN 978-94-010-7083-6*

278

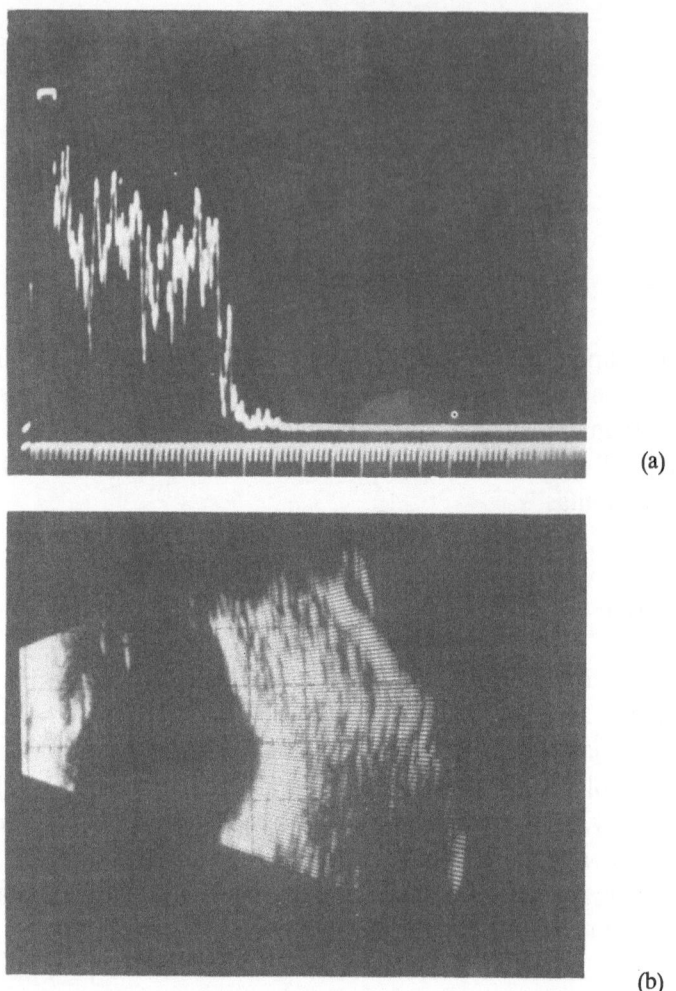

(a)

(b)

Fig. 1. Acute dacryoadenitis. (a) A-scan, parabulbar projection. Badly delimited lesion, medium to high reflectivity. (b) Contact B-scan, transbulbar projection. Lesion limits are visible, a high density of internal echoes is present.

tures that are typical of the pseudotumours are little emphasized (Mazzeo et al., 1981), they do not present echographic characteristics different from those that are found in the other regions. They show a low reflectivity specially on A-scan and a small angle K, while the limits of the lesions can be very variable, that is from being absent to be very evident. These pathologies present the appearance of a solid lesion on the B-scan, often infiltrating, with a remarkable acoustic homogeneity that appears by the absence or the scarcity of internal echoes. It is particularly difficult to diagnose if the echoformation has its starting point in the gland or in its region (Restori, 1979).

Cysts

The cysts that have their starting points in the gland (dacryops) are rare and, from the echographic point of view, they appear as well defined lesions, of regular form and with no internal reflectivity (Motolese et al., 1985).

Dermoid cyst that often appears just in the lacrimal gland area is more frequent in young people. It appears on A-scan as a formation clearly defined by maximal and bifid limiting echoes, with an internal reflectivity that changes according to the contents. We can sometimes observe that there are some high isolated peaks inside. It appears on B-scan as a round or oval structure very well defined with a variable internal texture.

Neoplasms

The most common neoplasms arising from the glands are the mixed tumours or pleomorphic adenoma, benign or malignant, and the cylindroma or adenoid cystic carcinoma. Because of the known similarity of the cytologic structure (Ossoinig, 1975) it has usually considered that it was possible to put the echographic tracing A-scan of the mixed tumour on that of the cavernous angioma, from which it differentiates because of the lower attenuation and mostly because of the location, since angioma is almost always found within the muscle cone. Then we deal with a very well defined lesion with a changeable reflectivity from an average level to a high one, with a low or average sound attenuation. It is sometimes possible to observe some small areas with a low reflectivity, probably due to cystic gatherings of bigger dimensions (Francois and Goes, 1978).

The mixed tumour appears on B-scan as a well defined lesion with good sound transmission and it is possible to notice a very coarse echo texture inside it. It is almost always necessary to reduce the amplification of equipment in these pathologies in order to define the tumour limits, that are otherwise poorly distinguished from the normal orbital tissue.

Adenoid cystic carcinoma is the most common malignant tumour starting from the gland.

The echographic characteristics of this tumour have not been codified yet because of the noticeable variability of the findings, probably justified by the histological structure variability. We observed, in two of the three cases we treated, that reflectivity was at a level between average and low with a moderate angle K. In both cases we examined it was possible to notice higher echoes distributed regularly and separated by spaces with a much lower reflectivity (Fig. 2).

280

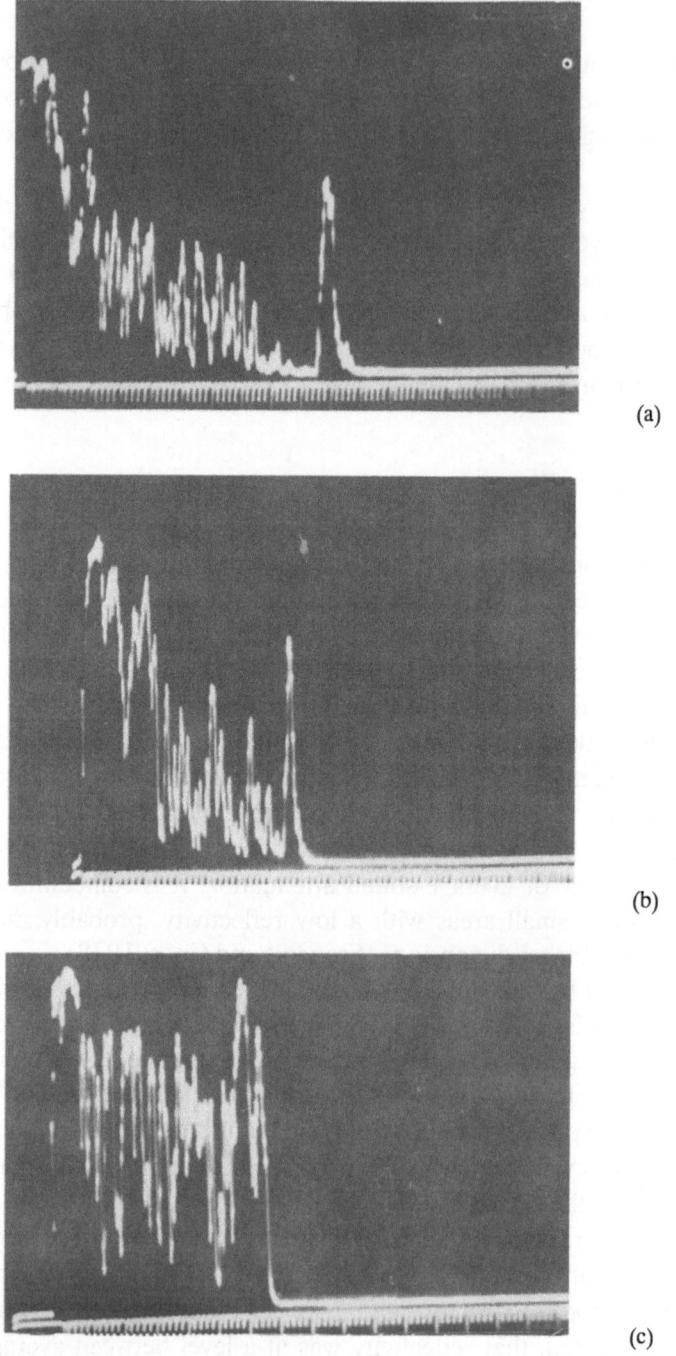

Fig. 2. Adenoid-cystic carcinoma. (a) and (b) low to medium internal reflectivity. The higher spikes are subdivided by areas of lower reflectivity. (c) high internal reflectivity. The high and broad spikes are densely packed and separated by areas of lower reflectivity.

Also Dagher and co-workers (1980) found a cystic adenoid carcinoma with a reflectivity going from a low level to an average one with a moderate degree of heterogenity. The third case presented, in contrast, an average to high level of reflectivity with high and long broadened echoes, but separated by small spaces with lower reflectivity and small angle K. Hackelbush and co-workers (1983) describe in these cases two kinds of findings. The normal cylindroma presents an alternating pattern of areas with high reflectivity and spaces, clearly cystic, characterized by high echoes separated by areas practically with no echo. In the cubiform variant the echo pattern is characterized only by high reflectivity, with sound attenuation.

Also Motolese and Colleagues (1985), who studied from the echographic point of view six cases of adenoid cystic carcinoma, found a variable internal reflectivity from low to high level, with a regular internal structure, sharp margins and an average attenuation. It is possible to observe a lesion in the typical region with the B-scan.

Conclusion

We observe that it is often difficult or impossible to make a certain diagnosis among the various kinds of tumours starting from the lacrimal gland, but we also observe that echographic investigation is always necessary to differentiate the forms that are clearly encapsulated from those that are diffused or badly delimitated. In the latter type treatment by adequate medical or chemical therapy will be helpful, while a complete excision of the lesion in the clearly delimitated forms is preferable (Dagher et al., 1980).

References

Dagher G, Anderson RL, Ossoinig KC, Baker JD. 1980. Adenoid cystic carcinoma of a lacrimal gland in a child. Arch. Ophthalmol 98: 1098–1100.

Francois J, Goes F. 1978. A-scan ultrasonography and diagnosis of unilateral exophthalmos. In: 3rd International Symposium on Orbital Disorders. Junk, The Hague, pp. 24–41.

Hackelbusch R, Rochels R, Knieper P. 1983. Korrelation echographisches and histologischer Befunde bei Erkrankungen der Tränendrüse. Ophthalmologica, Basel, 186: 113–124.

Mazzeo V, Ravalli L, Scorrano R. 1981. L'ecografia nei tumori dell'orbita. In: A Rossi (ed) Clinica dei tumori dell'occhio e dell'orbita. Sate Ferrara, pp. 453–504.

Motolese E, Esposti P, Patacchini E. 1985. La ecografia nelle formazioni cistiche. In: D Frezzotti (ed) Patologia, Clinica e Terapia delle malattie dell'orbita. Tipografia Senese, Siena, pp. 242–246.

282

Motolese E, Esposti P, Patacchini E. 1985. L'ecografia nei tumori della ghiandola lacrimale. In: R. Frezzotti (ed) Patologia, Clinica e Terapia delle malattie dell'orbita. Tipografia Senese, Siena, pp. 336—341.

Ossoinig KC. 1975. A-scan echography and orbital disease. In: GM Bleeker et al. (eds) Orbital disorders. Mod Probl Ophthal 14. Karger, Basel, pp. 203—235.

Restori M. 1979. Ultrasound in orbital diagnosis. Trans Ophthal Soc UK 99: 223—225.

Extraocular muscles and optic nerve

The echobiometric measurement of the extraocular muscles in normal subjects

A. REIBALDI[1], G. ASSENNATO[2], T. AVITABILE[1] AND
M. G. UVA[1]

Summary

There is a need for a more detailed study of the thickness of extraocular muscles which is fundamental in the diagnosis of many orbital diseases. Often the limit noticed with echography between physiological and pathological value of the muscle thickness is almost indefinite.

For some time we have used for comparison the McNutt and Ossoinig tables which report percentile values obtained by a case report of 100 cases.

After having examined, in preliminary work, the results obtained from 100 normal eyes, we proceeded to carry out a wider study (c400 cases) taking into account further factors such as: sex, weight, height, use of convergence, which could ultimately influence the distribution of the related values. This report presents the results of our study.

Introduction

The usefulness of the measurement of the extraocular rectus muscles with standardized technique and equipment (Kretz 7200 MA) introduced by Ossoinig (1974) is well known both in the diagnosis of orbital diseases (myositis, haematoma, etc.) and also systemic diseases, especially Graves' orbitopathy which has been the subject of our previous studies (Reibaldi et al., 1975, 1983, 1985, etc.).

We have previously used as reference values the McNutt (1975) tables, obtained by a case report of 102 eyes of normal subjects and considering as upper limits of normal the values above the 90th and 95th percentile.

In the literature there are some recent tables (Tane and Komatsu 1982) also obtained by a small case report (102 eyes) but without a standardized equipment.

---

[1] Clinica Oculistica, University of Catania, Catania, Italy; [2] Medicina del Lavoro, University of Bari, Bari, Italy.

J. M. Thijssen (ed.) Ultrasonography in ophthalmology.
© 1988, *Kluwer Academic Publishers, Dordrecht, ISBN 978-94-010-7083-6*

As no study had been made on European populations and considering that values may differ between different ethnic groups, in a recent study we developed our own tables (Avitabile et al., 1985).

We measured the muscles of 100 eyes of normal subjects, the same sample size as the other Authors but on plotting histograms we found some deviations from normal that could not be correlated to sex, age, weight, height, hours of reading etc., owing to the small number of cases studied.

In the present study we enlarged the case report in order to circumvent such limitations.

Subjects and methods

At the Echographic centre of the Eye Clinic of Bari University (Italy) we measured the four extraocular muscles of 408 eyes of 204 patients (see Table 1) with no history of ocular or general diseases which could affect muscle size.

The technique used was that standardized by Ossoinig (1974) and previously described (Avitabile et al., 1985).

We measured the muscle when the maximal thickness was displayed as the widest defect bordered by steeply rising high surface signals.

All the measurements were performed by the same examiner and repeated five times for each muscle and the mean of the 5 measurements was taken.

Results

In the second table we report the means and standard deviation (s.d.) for each muscle of right and left eyes.

We then calculated for each muscle the value in microseconds of the 90th and 95th percentile (see Table 3).

We report for each muscle one value which is the mean of the right and left eye since their values were almost identical. We have calculated percentiles because especially for lateral and superior rectus a Gaussian distribution was not shown as indicated by skewness and kurtosis indexes. In Table 4 we report, (in microseconds) the 90th and 95th percentiles of the difference between the value of a muscle of right and left eye.

In this way we can easily know the probability that a difference in muscle sizes between right and left eye lies within normal subjects.

By means of correlation coefficients we appreciated that there was no difference in muscle thickness when compared to sex, age, weight, height and number of hours of reading or close work per day.

Table 1. Characteristics of the study population.

		123 males
Number of subjects: 204		
		81 females
Number of eyes: 408		

Age: (yrs)	mean 51.75 s.d. 17.69 range 14—89	Height: (cm)	mean 163.29 s.d. 8.83 range 137—190
Weight (kg)	mean 70.07 s.d. 12.65 range 43—119	Reading or near working hours/day	mean 2.42 s.d. 2.67 range 0—10

Table 2. Rectus muscles size in normals (value in microseconds).

	Right eye			Left eye		
Muscle	N.	Mean	S.D.	N.	Mean	S.D.
Superior	204	5.4	0.65	204	5.38	0.64
Lateral	204	5.1	0.52	204	5.02	0.51
Inferior	204	5.2	0.31	204	5.02	0.40
Medial	204	5.7	0.75	204	5.70	0.77

Table 3. Rectus muscles sizes in normal population.

Muscle	Percentile	Value (microseconds)
Superior	95	6.7
	90	6.0
Lateral	95	6.0
	90	5.4
Inferior	95	5.9
	90	5.7
Medial	95	7.0
	90	7.0

288

Table 4. Difference in rectus muscle sizes between eyes.

Muscle	Percentile	Value (microseconds)
Superior	95	0.84
	90	0.66
Lateral	95	0.83
	90	0.50
Inferior	95	1.00
	90	0.66
Medial	95	1.00
	90	0.66

Discussion

The present literature contains only a few reports on the measurement of the extraocular muscles in normal subjects for use as a standard. We have reviewed the studies of McNutt who in 1975 studied 102 eyes of 52 Caucasian patients in the U.S.A. and of Tane and Komatsu who measured in 1982 the muscles of 104 eyes of 52 healthy persons in Japan with non-standardized equipment.

Considering that no study of this kind had been made in Europe and considering that physiological parameters may differ between races we have calculated muscle thickness in our population in Southern Italy. In this study we have measured the muscles of 408 eyes in order to have a large case report, improving on one of our previous studies (Avitabile et

Table 5. Comparison of our results of rectus muscle sizes and those of other authors.

Muscle	Percentile	Value in microseconds*		
		McNutt 1975	Reibaldi 1986	Tane 1982
Superior	95	6.1	6.7	5.9
	90	5.8	6.0	
Lateral	95	6.8	6.0	6.9
	90	6.5	5.4	
Inferior	95	5.9	5.9	6.0
	90	5.6	5.7	
Medial	95	6.9	7.0	6.8
	90	5.4	7.0	

* The data of Tane were in millimeters and we have considered 1 microsecond equals 3/4 mm.

al., 1985), and to analyse a possible correlation between muscle size and sex, age, weight, height, hours of reading and close working per day. Our results differed from those of McNutt who found that superior rectus varied inversely with height and medial rectus directly with hours of reading as we did not detect any correlation with these parameters.

Considering that we did not find a Gaussian distribution for some muscles, we suggest that one should consider the 95th percentile as the upper limit of normal population. In Table 5 we compare our results with those of other authors.

From this Table a good agreement is shown between our and other authors' values especially for some muscles (inferior and medial).

As regards the differences in sizes between the right and left eye our data are significantly lower than those of other authors as shown in Table 6.

The higher homogeneity in our case study could be attributed to either a better selection of the study population or to a higher reliability in the analytical measurements.

References

Avitabile T, Uva MG, Fiordalisi F. 1985. I nostri valori ecobiometrici normali per la misurazione dei muscoli retti. I Congr S.I.E.O., Ferrara.

McNutt LC. 1975. Ultrasound of Graves' orbitopathy. (Seminar) Department of Ophthalmology, University of Iowa, Iowa City.

Table 6. Comparison of our results of the differences in rectus muscles sizes and those of other authors.

Muscle	Percentile	Value in microseconds*		
		McNutt 1975	Reibaldi 1986	Tane 1982
Superior	95	2.0	0.84	1.9
	90	1.4	0.66	
Lateral	95	1.5	0.83	2.4
	90	1.2	0.50	
Inferior	95	2.0	1.00	2.1
	90	1.9	0.66	
Medial	95	1.8	1.00	2.1
	90	1.5	0.66	

* The data of Tane were in millimeters and we have considered 1 microsecond equals 3/4 mm.

McNutt LC, Kaefring SL, Ossoinig KC. 1977. Echographic measurement of extraocular muscles. In: DN White and RE Brown (eds) Ultrasound in Medicine. Vol. 3A, Plenum, New York, pp. 927–932.

Ossoinig KC. 1974. Preoperative differential diagnosis of tumours with echography. I Physical principles and morphologic background of tissue echograms. In: FC Blodi (ed) Current Concepts in Ophthalmology. Vol. 4, Mosby, St Louis, pp. 264–280.

Ossoinig KC. 1979. Standardized echography: basic principles, clinical applications and results. Int Ophthalm Clinics 19: 127–285.

Reibaldi A, Bracciolini M. 1975. L'ecografia orbitaria nella diagnosi dell'esoftalmo endocrino, Comunicazione alle Giornate Endocrinologiche Pugliesi, Bari.

Reibaldi A, Scuderi GL, Avitabile T. 1983. Attuali possibilita' diagnostiche ecografiche nella oftalmopatia di Graves. Atti VIII Conv Societa' Oftalmologica Siciliana, Taormina-Giardini Naxos, pp. 303–306.

Reibaldi A, Avitabile T, Uva MG, Tritto M. 1985. Utility of ultrasound in monolateral endocrine exophthalmus. 5th International Symposium on Orbital Disorders. Amsterdam.

Reibaldi A, Avitabile T, Uva MG. 1985. Consuntivo di 15 anni di diagnostica ecografica nella patologia orbitaria di natura endocrina. Convegno su Occhio e Patologia Endocrina, Rimini.

Tane S, Komatsu A. 1982. Echographic measurements of extraocular muscles in normal persons and in patients with thyroid orbitopathy. Acta XXIV Int Congress of Ophthalmology, San Francisco, pp. 120–131.

Echographically determined changes of the optic nerve in hypertensive retinopathy (Stage IV)

A. STANOWSKY

Summary

Standardized A-scan echography of 2 patients with hypertensive retinopathy IV and pronounced papilledema showed changes as follows in the
optic nerve area:

1. Expansion of the overall diameter of the optic nerve with meninges.
2. Expansion of the subarachnoidal space around the optic nerve.
3. "Mobile optic nerve" phenomenon.
4. Positive abduction test.

These findings are characteristic of intracranial hypertension; they show
that papilledema in hypertensive retinopathy IV cannot be caused by
vascular changes in the ocular area alone.

Introduction

Papilledema is characteristic of hypertensive retinopathy IV (Keith et al.,
1939). Distinguishing it from a choked disc can be clinically difficult
(Walsh and Hoyt, 1969).

Opinions vary on the causation of papilledema in hypertensive retinopathy IV and include both vascular factors in the ocular region itself (Ford
and Murphy 1939, Fishberg and Oppenheimer, 1930) and extraocular
factors as well, in particular an increase in intracranial pressure (Elschnig,
1895).

Our question was whether echographical examination of the optic nerve
can help to clear up this pathogenesis; our starting point was the reflection
that if papilledema in hypertensive retinopathy IV is caused by increased
intracranial pressure an expansion of the subarachnoidal space around the

University Eye Clinic Tübingen, Ophthalmology III: Diseases of the Posterior Eye, 7400
Tübingen, FRG.

J. M. Thijssen (ed.) Ultrasonography in ophthalmology.
© 1988, *Kluwer Academic Publishers, Dordrecht, ISBN 978-94-010-7083-6*

292

optic nerve should be present (Hayreh, 1964). This can be confirmed with standardized A-scan echography (Ossoinig, 1981).

Material and method

Up to now we have echographically examined 2 patients with hypertensive retinopathy IV. The examinations were done with the Kretz Technik (7200 MA) A-scan and the Ocuscan (400) B-scan units. After anaesthesia with Proxymetacain-HCl the patient was asked to look straight ahead. The probe was then placed on the temporal conjunctiva and moved posteriorly until the optic nerve was displayed. The patient was then asked to abduct the eye, first by 30° (a small fixation light was used) and then maximally. Both eyes were examined in this way. The A-scan unit had been set according to Ossoinig's standardized guidelines (Ossoinig, 1979). We used a 9.5 MHz probe for the B-scan.

Case reports

Patient 1.

In this 43-year-old woman patient a hypertonus of renal origin was diagnosed 10 years ago. Blood pressure was 240/110 mmHg at the time of examination.

Visual acuity was 20/600 in both eyes. The anterior segments of both eyes were normal. Both fundi showed an advanced papilledema with a circinata figure in the macula, cotton-wool spots and retinal haemorrhages.

The standardized A-scan showed a total optic nerve diameter (inner dura surface to inner dura surface) of 10.5 μsec in the right eye, 11.0 μsec in the left eye upon gaze straight ahead. The diameter of the optic nerve itself was 5.5 μsec in both eyes. The total diameter diminished by 1.5 μsec in both eyes following 30° abduction, 2.5 μsec upon maximum abduction. The "mobile optic nerve", that is, a shifting of the optic nerve in the enlarged subarachnoidal space during eye movements, was present (Fig. 1).

The B-scan indicated an expansion of the subarachnoidal space both when the eyes looked straight ahead and when they were abducted.

Patient 2.

This 41-year-old woman noticed a slight deterioration of vision in both eyes over 2 years with increasingly frequent headaches. She had not previously been under the care of a physician.

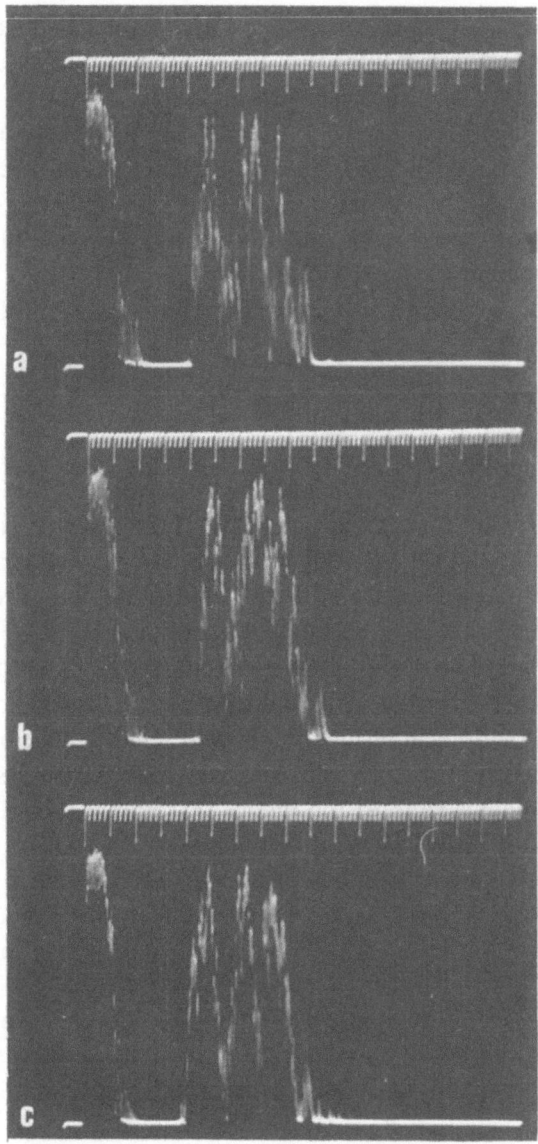

Fig. 1. Echographical findings of the right eye by (a) gaze straight ahead (b) 30° abduction and (c) maximal abduction (mobile optic nerve phenomenon positive).

The internal examination showed an essential hypertonia with a blood pressure of 220/110 mmHg. No underlying illness or indications of an intracranial tumour were found either neurologically or computer tomographically.

Visual acuity was 20/40 in both eyes. The anterior eye segments were normal. Both fundi showed a pronounced papilledema with a few lipoid deposits, scattered retinal haemorrhages, and cotton wool patches.

294

Standardized A-scan echography showed a total diameter of 9.0 µsec for the optic nerve and meninges of the right eye and 9.5 µsec for the left eye when both eyes looked straight ahead.

The optic nerve lay in the center of the subarachnoidal space; its diameter was 4.5 µsec in both the right and the left eye. The total diameter of the optic nerve diminished by 1.0 µsec in both eyes following a 30° abduction, 2.0 µsec after maximal abduction. The "mobile optic nerve" was barely perceptible (Stanowsky and Kreissig, 1984).

The B-scan showed no certain signs of an expansion of the subarachnoidal space.

Discussion

It is safe to assume that the papilledema of these 2 patients was caused solely by high blood pressure. This is indicated by the clinical development (regression of the papilledema following control of blood pressure) and the ophthalmological, neurological and internal findings.

Using echography (in particular the standardized A-scan) it was possible to show that the subarachnoidal space had enlarged around the optic nerve. The echographical results therefore resemble those of pseudotumor cerebri and attained the same values (Stanowsky and Kreissig, 1984). The examination findings support the theory that papilledema in hypertensive retinopathy IV originates from intracranial hypertension.

Our group of patients is of course too small for definitive conclusions. It should also be noted that this method cannot exclude vascular changes in the disc area or the retina which might foster the development of papilledema.

Nevertheless the thesis that papilledema in hypertensive retinopathy is exclusively a result of vascular factors in the eye area may well be said to have grown less probable as a result of these examinations.

References

Elschnig A. 1895. Über die pathologische Anatomie und Pathogenese der sogenannten Stauungspapille. Graefes Arch Ophthalmol 41: 179—293.

Fishberg AM, Oppenheimer BS. 1930. The differentiation and significance of certain ophthalmoscopic pictures in hypertensive disease. Arch Intern Med (Chicago) 46: 901—920.

Ford FR, Murphy EL. 1939. Increased intracranial pressure. Clinical analysis of the causes and characteristics of several types. Bull Hopkins Hosp 64: 369—398.

Hayreh SS. 1964. Pathogenesis of oedema of the optic disc (papilloedema). A preliminary report. Br J Ophthalmol 48: 522—543.

Keith NM, Wagener HP, Barker NW. 1939. Some different types of essential hypertension: their course and prognosis. Am J med Sci 197: 332—343.

Ossoinig C. 1979. Standardized echography, basic principles, clinical applications and results. In: RL Dallow (ed) Ophthalmic Ultrasonography: Comparative Techniques. (Int Ophthalmol Clin 19/4), Little, Brown & Co, Boston.

Ossoinig C et al. 1981. Echographic differential diagnosis of optic nerve lesions. Doc Ophthalmol 29: 327—335.

Stanowsky A, Kreissig I. 1984. Hat die echographische Untersuchung des Nervus opticus und seiner Meningen eine Bedeutung in der Diagnostik eines Pseudotumor cerebri? Fortschr Ophthalmol 81: 604—607.

Walsh FB, Hoyt WF. 1969. Clinical Neuro-ophthalmology. 3rd ed. Williams and Wilkins Co., Baltimore.

Echographic results in painful exophthalmos with ophthalmoplegia

P. FEDRIGA, M. BRODA, A. PARROZZANI AND T. SIBILLA

Summary

In this paper the authors have reported the echographic results obtained from a case of scleroderma which developed painful exophthalmos involving the III, IV, V, VI and VII cranial nerves.

The symptomatology, known as Painful Ophthalmoplegia, or the Tolosa — Hunt Syndrome is, in this case, accompanied by deficiencies of the VII cranial nerve and involvement of the maxillary sinus as in Wegener's Syndrome.

The orbital and paraorbital echography are described.

Clinical and echographical features regressed rapidly after cortisone therapy but revealed a tendency to recur during the five years of follow-up.

Introduction

Painful exophthalmos with ophthalmoplegia is known as the Tolosa — Hunt Syndrome and is attributed to inflammation of the orbital apex and cavernous sinus. The response to steroids is characteristic and relapses are common.

Wegener's granulomatosis is also referred to as an infrequent cause of exophthalmos induced by an orbital inflammatory pseudotumour with involvement of the maxillary sinus.

The echographic findings referred to were obtained from a case of scleroderma with both syndromes developing in an interlacing and overlapping fashion.

Case report

The patient, a 73 year old woman, had been diagnosed as having scleroderma six years previously.

Divisione Oculistica, Ospedale di Montebelluna, Montebelluna (TV), Italy.

J. M. Thijssen (ed.) Ultrasonography in ophthalmology.
© 1988, *Kluwer Academic Publishers, Dordrecht, ISBN 978-94-010-7083-6*

At our examination visual acuity was RE = 2/10 with lens; visual field: central scotoma and concentric constriction; visual acuity LE = 5/10 with lens.

The patient was examined for painful exophthalmos of the RE, ophthalmoplegia of cranial nerves III, IV, and VI, corneal hypoaesthesia as a result of the involvement of the trigeminal ophthalmic branch and unilateral paresis of VII cranial nerve.

The response to corticosteroid therapy was immediate and significant with resolution of almost all symptoms: only visual acuity remained blurred and visual field restricted.

With the recurrence of painful exophthalmos on follow-up, therapy included corticosteroid treatment on a number of occasions.

Echographic results

An A-Scan echographic examination revealed these finding:

(1) the orbital trace appeared more extended: scanning measurements from the base of the orbit to the apex were delimited by an isolated, high terminal peak (Figs. 1 and 2).
(2) the inner reflectivity appeared low and the peak mobility was poor.
(3) the same trace was obtained from the upper part of the unilateral maxillary sinus (Fig. 3).
(4) the echographic findings underwent few changes even during remission of the clinical features.

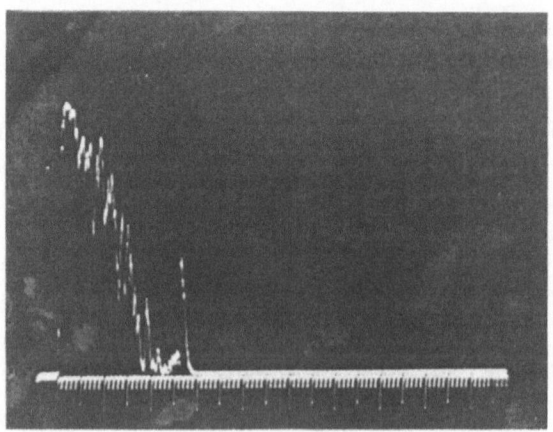

Fig. 1. Orbital echography without compression.

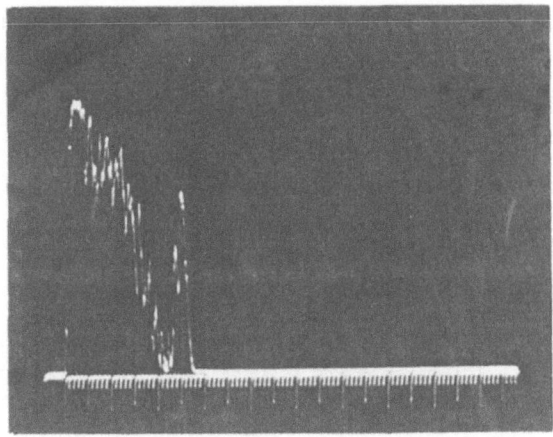

Fig. 2. Orbital echography with compression.

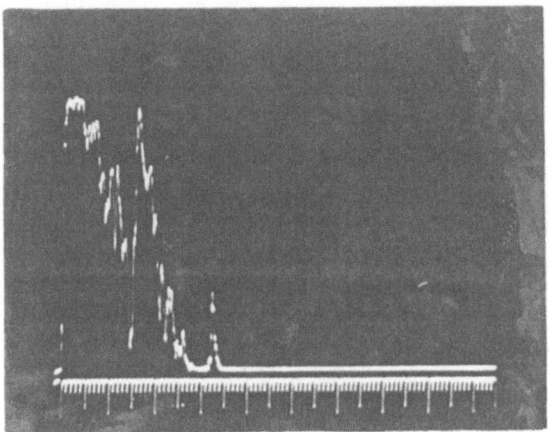

Fig. 3. Maxillary sinus echography.

Discussion

Though the clinical and echographic features of the inflammatory pseudo-tumour and the neurological effects are typical of the Tolosa — Hunt Syndrome, the concurrent paresis of the VII cranial nerve, the involvement of the maxillary sinus with restriction of the visual field and reduction of visual acuity point more to Wegener's granulomatosis. Only the echographic findings give a full picture.

The tracing reveals an inflammatory pseudo-tumour and granulomatosis located in the orbital apex and maxillary sinus.

These results induce us to consider both of the syndromes mentioned, in this case overlapping, as possible local manifestations of a more generalised affection.

Biometry

Proposal of a formula for evaluating the dioptric power of the posterior surface of the cornea*

M. CAMELLIN

Summary

The author carried out mathematical calculations to determine the radius of the corneal posterior surface, with the aim of determining the power of the cornea more exactly.

The knowledge of this value can be used to obtain a more accurate IOL power.

Introduction

The total power of the cornea (the anterior surface power plus the posterior surface power) is one of the variables involved in the formulas for the calculation of the intraocular lenses.

Nowadays, the total power of the cornea is still calculated on the basis of a fictitious refractive index. The fictitious index compensates for the negative power of the posterior surface, thus reducing the power of the corneal anterior surface itself (Contino, 1983; Davson, 1962; Duke-Elder, 1961; Heed, 1959; Helmholtz, 1962; Le Grand, 1964; Lo Cascio, 1955; Maione, 1957).

It has not been possible till now to evaluate the real power of the posterior surface in vivo.

Therefore, a geometric method has been worked out to calculate the power of the posterior surface; it is based on data obtained by ultrasonic pachymetry and ophthalmometry, and on a few assumptions on the geometry of the cornea itself.

By using this method, possible miscalculations in the evaluation of the power of IOL can be avoided.

---

* Paper awarded by SIEO (Società Italiana di EcoOftalmologia).
University Eye Clinic, Ferrara, Italy.

J. M. Thijssen (ed.) Ultrasonography in ophthalmology.
© 1988, *Kluwer Academic Publishers, Dordrecht, ISBN 978-94-010-7083-6*

304

Materials and methods

An ultrasound pachymetry and a keratometry are necessary. The data concerning the corneal thickness in predetermined positions are fundamental to the calculations. In order to obtain these, the topographical cornea pachymetry attachment of Merlin et al. (1986) is used. The calculations are based on the assumption that the cornea is a perfect sphere in the optical zone. The size of this spherical surface has been repeatedly determined in the literature (Helmholtz, 1962; Lo Cascio, 1955) as having a diameter of about 4 mm.

Geometric Calculations

Figure 1 shows the section of a cornea.

The circumferences relative to the anterior and the posterior surfaces of the optical zone have been arbitrarily prolonged.

OB = Radius of the anterior surface
BF = Chord; thickness is measured at the extremities of this chord
DE = Corneal thickness at the apex of the optical zone
AB = Corneal thickness at the periphery of the optical zone

This imaginary corneal section has been referred to a system of cartesian axes. The origin of the coordinates, and the center of the circumference which represents the anterior surface of the cornea coincide, while the center of the circumference of the posterior surface is assumed to be on the x-axis.

The radius of these circumferences, i.e. CD, has to be estimated.

Points A and D are calculated through trigonometry.

$$A: ((\overline{OB} - \overline{AB}) * \cos \text{alfa}; (\overline{OB} - \overline{AB}) * \sin \text{alfa})$$
$$D: ((\overline{OB} - \overline{DE}); 0)$$

since $\overline{BF}/(2 * \overline{OB}) = \sin \text{alfa}$, $\text{alfa} = \arcsin \overline{BF}/(2 * \overline{OB})$

In this way the coordinates of the points we required can be determined.

Given the point of coordinates (X_1, Y_1), the general formula of the circle, centred in C and of radius $\overline{CD}$, passing in that point is

$$(X - X_1)^2 + (Y - Y_1)^2 = \overline{CD}^2.$$

Since we assumed that the centres of the circumferences relative to the two corneal surfaces are on the same axis, the value of Y_1, ordinate of the

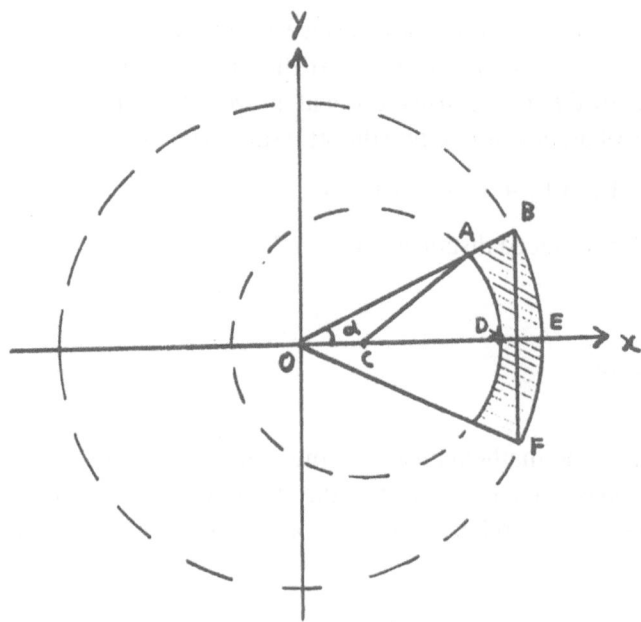

Fig. 1. Cross section of cornea, showing the geometrical assumptions.

centre of the circle relative to the posterior surface, is 0; consequently, it is possible to simplify the formula as follows:

$$(X - X_1)^2 + Y^2 = \overline{CD}^2.$$

By replacing the values of the coordinates of A and D to X and Y, and $\overline{OC}$ to X_1, we obtain a system of quadratic equations with two unknown quantities

$$\begin{cases} \overline{CD}^2 = (X_A - \overline{OC})^2 + Y_A^2 \\ \overline{CD}^2 = (X_D - \overline{OC})^2 + Y_D^2 \end{cases}$$

where the unknown quantities are: $\overline{CD}$, the radius of the posterior surface, and $\overline{OC}$, abscissa X identifying the centre of the circumference, also relative to the posterior surface. X_A and Y_A give the value of X and Y in A, whereas X_D and Y_D are the values of the coordinates in D (both A and D are points belonging to the circumference).

By solving the unknown quantity in one of the two equations, we can determine $\overline{OC}$, thus:

$$\overline{OC} = \frac{X_A^2 + Y_A^2 - (X_D^2 + Y_D^2)}{2 * (X_A - X_D)}$$

so the value of the radius of the posterior surface of the cornea is:

$$\overline{CD} = \sqrt{(X_A - \overline{OC})^2 + Y_A^2}.$$

If we know the posterior surface radius, we can easily determine the power of the posterior surface. At this stage we possess all the necessary data to evaluate the total corneal power by applying the Gullstrand's formula of association of two dioptric surfaces:

$$P_T = P_1 + P_2 - \delta * P_1 * P_2$$

where δ = reduced distance between the two surfaces.

Discussion

In spite of the mathematical exactness of the calculation a series of factors are involved. They can affect the accuracy of the final result. Two of these factors are relative to the geometrical assumptions made and which involve:

1. The sphericity of the optical zone.
   This has been repeatedly demonstrated in the literature (Lo Cascio, 1955).
2. The coaxiality of the rotation centres of the anterior and posterior surfaces.

This problem can easily be overcome by calculating the average of two pachymetric measurements in points which are diametrically opposed with respect to the optical centre.

The other factors relate to the variability of the parameters which are utilized to calculate the power of the cornea:

1. refractive index of the air (n)
2. refractive index of the cornea
3. refractive index of the acqueous
4. velocity of the ultrasound in the cornea.

Of these, only the ultrasound velocity in the cornea is still the subject of controversy. By now, however, this unknown quantity has been roughly evaluated. 1640 m/sec seems to be a reasonably accurate value.

Variations in the velocity may affect the measurement of the corneal thickness at the apex, as well as at the periphery of the optical zone; and, as a consequence, they may affect also the final result, which may vary by about 0.01 dioptres.

Moreover, we have to consider the variability of the data. The data are:

1. the anterior surface radius
2. the chord; measurements are taken at the extremities of the chord
3. apical thickness
4. thickness at the periphery of the optical zone

Table 1 gives a summary presentation of all possible errors. It also shows that errors are considered to occur all in the same direction: either towards an increase in the corneal power in relation to real power, or towards a decrease in the same. Moreover, as far as the chord is concerned, it should be remembered that, when using the topographical cornea pachymetry attachment of Merlin et al. (1986) the error is always towards a decrease in the length of the chord itself.

It must be noted, however, that the keratometric error is always present even when the fictitious refractive index is used; consequently the error of this method varies between −0.27 dioptres and +0.41.

Conclusions

By using this method to calculate the total dioptric power of the cornea in the formulas for the predictive evaluation of IOL, we are able to avoid approximations which could sometimes lead to mistakes. It will also be possible to continue research into certain aspects of corneal physiology of which still little is known.

References

Contino F. 1983. Ottica fisiopatologica. Florio edizioni scientifiche, 2° edizione, Napoli.

Table 1. Possible errors in the calculation of total corneal power.

Increase in relation to real power	Errors in the measurements	Decrease in relation to real power
0.14	−0.2 mm chord	—
0.30	−0.05 radius +0.05	0.29
0.13	+0.009 thickness at the apex −0.009	0.13
0.14	−0.009 thickness at the periphery +0.009	0.14
0.71 dt	amount	0.56 dt

308

Davson H. 1962. The eye, Visual Optics and the optical space sense. Academic Press, New York and London.

Duke-Elder S. 1962. System of ophthalmology. Kimpton, London, II, pp. 92—93.

Heed AF. 1959. Physiology of the eye. Mosby, St Louis, pp. 43—46.

Helmoltz H. 1962. Helmoltz's treaties on physiological optics. Dover, New York.

Kestenbaum A. 1963. Applied Anatomy of the Eye. Grune & Stratton, New York.

Le Grand Y. 1964. Optique Phisiologique. Revue d'Optique, Paris.

Lo Cascio G. 1955. Elementi di diottrica oculare, Istituto Editoriale del Mezzogiorno. Napoli.

Maione M. 1957. Manuale di ottica fisiologica. Vol. I, Edizioni Universitarie, Genova, I, pp. 133—136.

Merlin U, Camellin M, Mazzeo V. 1986. Dispositivo per la pachimetria corneale topografica; in corso di pubblicazione sulla rivista Clinica oculistica e patologia oculare, C.I.C., Roma.

Safir A. 1980. Refraction and Clinical Optics. Harper & Row, Hargestown, pp. 81—87.

Saraux H, Bias B. 1983. Phisiologie Oculaire. Masson, Paris.

Contact techniques in ocular biometry, influences of intraocular pressure and probe contact pressure

R. GUTHOFF

Summary

In an experimental study the influence of the intraocular pressure and the contact pressure of the transducer to the cornea is examined. The aim was to evaluate some of the advantages and disadvantages of applanation methods for ultrasound oculometrie. In conclusion the IOP and the probe contact pressure are only minor sources of error leading to maximal faults in IOL calculation of 0.75 dpt. More valid disadvantages of contact measurements seemed to be the stronger dependence on patients cooperation and problems in positioning the slit lamp mounted probe compared to handguided techniques.

Introduction

Ocular biometry had reached an excellent standard already several years ago due to the most fruitful work of the pioneers of ultrasound known to all of us (Buschman, 1963; Gernet, 1964; Nover et al. 1965; François and Goes, 1969; Binkhorst and Loones, 1976).

Recent developments in this field mainly dealt with automatisation and simplification of measuring procedures. (Lepper and Trier, 1984; Thijssen et al., 1984).

In the old-fashioned immersion technique there was a manually controlled probe, an analogue display and the examiner who had to decide which signal to choose for the measurement. This procedure has been replaced in many offices and hospitals by computer-assisted contact techniques, avoiding the inconveniences of the water bath.

Under those conditions any measuring procedure has to put some pressure on the eye to keep the probe in contact with the corneal surface. The manufacturers' advices how to use the instruments vary and some-

University Eye Clinic, Eppendorf, Martinistrasse 52, D-2000 Hamburg, FRG.

J. M. Thijssen (ed.) Ultrasonography in ophthalmology.
© 1988, *Kluwer Academic Publishers, Dordrecht, ISBN 978-94-010-7083-6*

times they are not precise at all. Our first results with this type of equipment have been a somewhat disappointing. We, therefore, tried to analyze at least one possible source of error.

Material and methods

We examined experimentally the influence of the intraocular pressure and the probe contact pressure on the results of axia length measurements. The equipment in use was a digitized A-scan manufactured by Cooper Vision and "with a fluid-filled contact probe" mounted on the Goldmann Tonometer of a Zeiss slit-lamp. The immersion measurements were performed with a 10 MHz transducer of the Kretz Technik (7200 MA) adapted to the Digital-A.

An enucleated eye was mounted up to the equator in a mould and fixed on the head rest of a slitlamp (Fig. 1). We connected the vitreous space via the pars plana with an irrigation system as used in vitreous surgery. With this device the intraocular pressure could be adjusted according to the height of the fluid level in the infusion bottle. The force which the transducer contacts to the eye was controlled by the spring balance of the tonometer.

All axial length measurements were performed under the following conditions:

There are three parameters to modify:

1. The intraocular pressure by lifting or lowering the bottle.
2. The force exerted on the eye by the transducer.
3. The time this force operates, in other words the tonography effect of the probe.

Results

In the first experiment (Fig. 2) we looked for the maximal effect we have to deal with. So we choose a constant high applanation pressure of 70 units of the Goldmann Tonometer setting. With an intraocular pressure of 10 mm of the water column we measured an axial length of 22.8 mm. Raising the water column from 10 to 70 cm the axial length increased by 1.4 mm up to 24.2 mm. This would have caused a difference in lens power calculation of at least 4 dioptres.

Therefore, without any doubt a relation exists between the intraocular pressure and the axial length estimated with contact measuring devices.

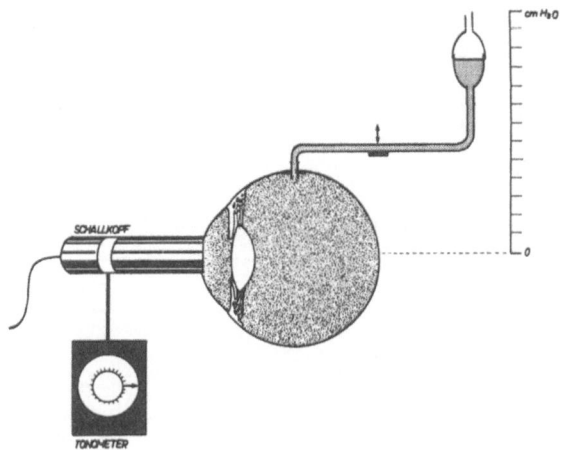

Fig. 1. Experiment setting to measure the correlation between intraocular pressure (IOP), applanation power and axial length of a human cadaver eye.

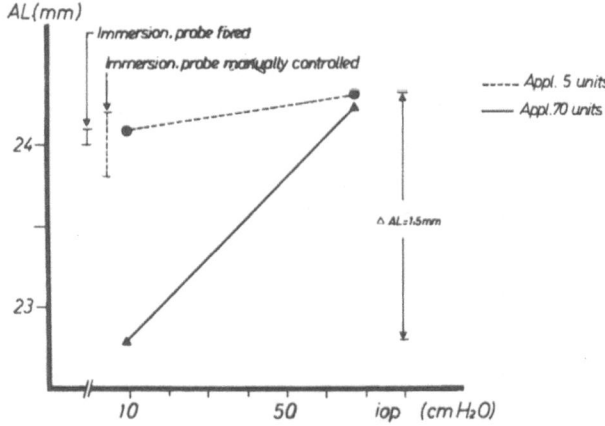

Fig. 2. Influence of intraocular pressure on axial length under extreme conditions to evaluate the maximal effect possible. With a tonometer setting of 70 units, the axial length increases by 1.5 mm raising the intraocular pressure from 10—70 cm of water column.

The diagram in Fig. 3 demonstrates these relations under more physiological conditions: with an applanation force of 20 units there is a maximal increase in the axial length of 0.4 mm. This is achieved when raising the intraocular pressure from 10 to 70 cm of water column as we have done in the previous experiment. What happens when we alter the applanation pressure and leaving the intraocular pressure uninfluenced? (Fig. 4). In this experiment we set the intraocular pressure at 15 cm of the water-column and performed axial length measurements with a step-wise elevation of the applanation power from 5—60 units. This led to an overall decrease of the axial length of about 0.3 mm.

312

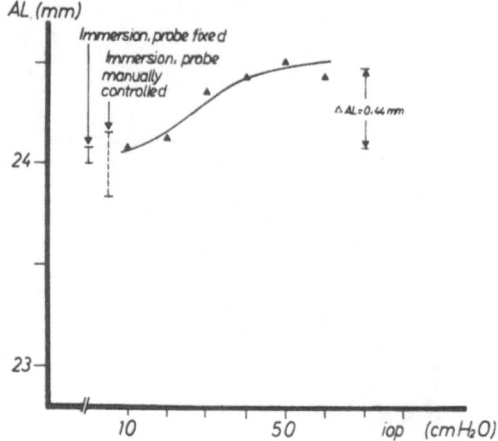

Fig. 3. Influence of intraocular pressure an axial length during a stepwise elevation of IOP and a constant applanation power of 20 units tonometer setting. Under these conditions axial length is increased by 0.44 mm as a maximum raising IOP from 10—60 cm of water-column.

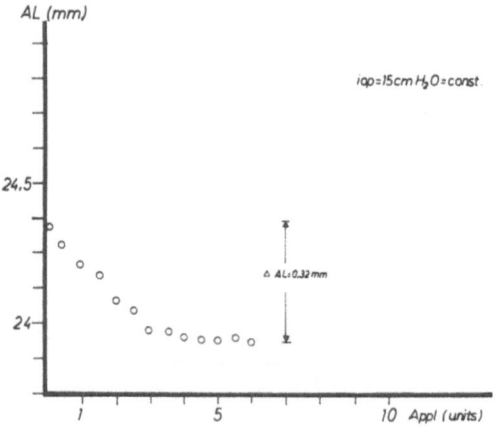

Fig. 4. Influence of applanation power leaving IOP unchanged. Stepwise elevation of applanation power from 2—60 units of tonometer setting leads to a decrease in axial length of 0.32 mm.

In the last experiment (Fig. 5) the measurements were no longer performed as quick as possible, but the applanation probe was kept in contact with the cornea for 7 minutes. The applanation force remained constantly at 20 units and the intraocular pressure was set at 15 cm of water column at the beginning of the experiment. The connection towards the bottle was locked. During these 7 minutes the axial length of the enucleated eye decreased from 24.7 to 24.4 mm, which means a difference of 0.3 mm.

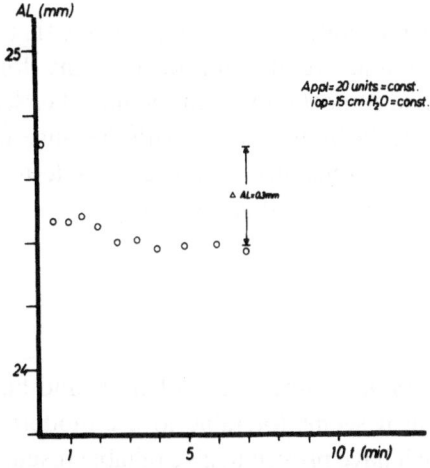

Fig. 5. Influence of applanation time on axial length when applanation power remains constant. After 7 min. of contact between transducer and cornea the axial length is decreased by 0.3 mm.

Conclusions

To summarize our results, under experimental conditions axial length measurements with contact techniques are influenced by:

1. The intraocular pressure,
2. the applanation force,
3. the time this force is applied.

Experiments have shown that this influence is already present when we alter these parameters in the range of physiological conditions. The actual amount of indentation we could produce reached 1.4 mm, but under physiological conditions it did not exceed 0.3 mm. This value has to be accepted as lying within the known variations of error even when using immersion techniques.

On the other hand our results in clinical biometry are still better using the old fashioned water bath no matter whether we use a Digital-A or B or the Kretz-instrument. We think that the patient's cooperation plays a more important role in contact techniques and considering our own hospital: we are mostly dealing with old people, who are hardly able to fixate a light properly. The slitlamp gantry is not able to angle the transducer support to compensate vertical eye movements. The patients do have difficulties in keeping the eye in an exact vertical position.

314

As a consequence of these results we are using digitized equipment with pattern recognition and we do not believe any longer that the globe indentation plays and important role in the mistakes we made, but we have come back to the old-fashioned water bath, because we feel that the hand of the examiner at the transducer is more capable to find the right direction than the same hand on the slitlamp gantry.

Note added in proof

After two more years of routine work in Ultrasound-biometry with different pieces of equipment it seems tolerable to use modern manually controlled contact probes which have proven to give reliable results in most patients.

References

Binkhorst CD, Loones LH. 1976. Intraocular lens power. Transam Acad Ophthalmol Otolaryngol 81: 70.

Buschman W. 1963. Technische Fortschritte in der ophthalmologischen Ultraschall-Diagnostik. Wiss Zbl Ernst-Moritz-Arndt-Universität, Greifswald 1: 59.

François J, Goes F. 1969. Comparative study of ultrasonic biometry of emmetropes and myopes with special regards to heredity of myopia. In: K Gitter, A Keeney, L Sarin and D Meyer (eds) Ophthalmic ultrasound. Mosby & Co., New York, p. 165.

Gernet H. 1964. Über Achsenlänge und Brechkraft emmetroper lebender Augen. Graefe's Archiv Ophthalmol 166: 424.

Lepper RD, Trier HC. 1983. Computerized ocular biometry: A newly developed compact system. In: JS Hillmann and MM Le May (eds) Ophthalmic Ultrasonography, Doc Ophthalmologica Proc Ser Vol. 38, Junk Publishers, The Hague, pp. 237–241.

Nover A, Glanschneider D. 1965. Untersuchungen über Fortpflanzungsgeschwindigkeit und Absorption des Ultraschalls im Gewebe. Graefe's Archiv Ophthalmol 168: 304.

Thijssen JM, Verhoef WA, Pasman-Scheps S, Verbeek AM. 1984. Computerized biometry and lens calculation. In: JS Hillmann and MM Le May (eds) Ophthalmic Ultrasonography, Doc Ophthalmologica Proc Ser Vol. 38, Junk Publishers, The Hague, pp. 231–235.

A clinical comparison of the Cilco A-scan and the Kretztechnik 7200 MA for pre-operative biometry

R. C. BOSANQUET

Summary

Thirty-six eyes scheduled for cataract extraction had biometry performed by the Cilco A-scan and the Kretz 7200 MA. In 28 eyes the results obtained by the two instruments differed by less than 0.5 mms. The problems encountered with using both instruments and the reasons for disparity in 8 of the eyes are discussed.

Introduction

A recent survey (Wong and Steele, 1985) of Ophthalmic Surgeons in the United Kingdom showed that 23% perform pre-operative biometry and calculate the power of the intraocular lens in order to minimise or control post-operative refractive error. Two important factors preventing more widespread use of biometry are lack of funding for ultrasound equipment and shortage of clinical time on the part of the Ophthalmologist. From the Surgeon's point of view the ideal technique for axial eye length measurement and intraocular lens power calculation should be accurate, cheap and preferably done by someone else. Hence the attraction of the dedicated A-scanners which are designed specifically for this purpose. In essence they all consist of an A-scanner which is programmed to recognise the steeply rising peak of the retinal echo. They all operate on the assumption that the visual axis will be the longest distance within the eye which is at right angles to the retina and that the retina will give rise to the first strong echo behind the lens. They are easily misled by posterior staphylomata, strong echoes from a posterior vitreous detachment or weak echoes from an irregular retina. However, they are all considerably cheaper than a diagnostic scanner with facilities for biometry incorporated and they have the advantage of being simpler to use. So far as I am aware there have been

7 Graham Park Road, Newcastle Upon Tyne NE3 4BH, United Kingdom.

J. M. Thijssen (ed.) Ultrasonography in ophthalmology.
© 1988, *Kluwer Academic Publishers, Dordrecht, ISBN 978-94-010-7083-6*

no published accounts of the accuracy of such A-scanners, nor of their advantages and limitations in practice.

I will describe our experience with just one machine, the Cilco A-scan which we have been using alongside the well established Kretz 7200 MA as well as an Ocuscan. I am aware that the Cilco has now been superseded and I look forward to seeing whether the new version is an improvement on the original.

Equipment

The probe of the Cilco A-scan incorporates a 10 MHz transducer and a built-in water bath enclosed anteriorly by a soft rubber membrane. This is placed in light contact with the patient's cornea whilst the patient's gaze is directed towards a fixation light within the probe. Whilst the transducer is on the A-scan records and displays the ten scans it considers to be optimal according to a number of in-built criteria. Acceptable scans are those with a high signal from the posterior pole, shorter measurements being rejected in favour of longer ones. The operator selects those scans which he considers to be valid. These are then averaged by the equipment and the required lens power for any required post-operative refractive error is rapidly calculated using either the SRK (Sanders and Kraff, 1980; Retzlaff, 1980) or Binkhorst (1975) formulae. One of the attractive features of this machine is the clear print-out which records all the essential data, one of the ten scans and a graph of lens implant power plotted against the calculated post-operative refractive error.

Method

Our hospital Opticians are all enthusiastic and welcomed the opportunity to become involved in biometry. They had three months to familiarize themselves with the Cilco A-scan. At first they had considerable difficulty obtaining repeatable results on elderly cataractous patients. Once they had obtained adequate expertise we examined 36 eyes of 32 patients scheduled for cataract extraction with intraocular lens implantation. Initially these were a series of consecutive patients referred from the general clinic, but later some additional myopes were included in order to encompass a reasonable span of axial eye lengths. Patients were examined on the same day by Opticians using the A-scan and by the Ophthalmologist (RCB) using the Kretz according to the well-tried technique by Ossoinig (1983). Neither operator knew the results obtained by the other.

Results

Figure 1 compares the results obtained by the two instruments. The mean difference for axial eye lengths was 0.37 mms. There was no consistency in the difference in that half the Kretz readings were shorter than those from the Cilco and vice versa. However, the larger discrepancies were all due to a longer reading from the Cilco than the Kretz. The dotted lines in the figure encompass those results where the difference was less than 0.5 mms (28 of 36 eyes; 78%).

Table 1 gives details of the 8 eyes in which the readings differed by more than 0.5 mms. In all but one the Kretz gave the shorter reading. One eye had diabetic maculopathy which probably contributed to a weak echo from the retina. Two eyes, both of the same patient, had posterior staphylomata. One patient had senile macular degeneration. The others had normal fundi. The third column was an attempt to 'back-calculate' the axial eye length knowing the final refraction and the power of the implant. However, I confess to being sceptical about these figures since they are based on the SRK formula, but the lenses were inserted by a variety of Surgeons using a number of different lenses. I am currently in the process of recalling these patients to assess their anterior chamber depth to see if back-calculation using the Binkhorst formula yields similar results.

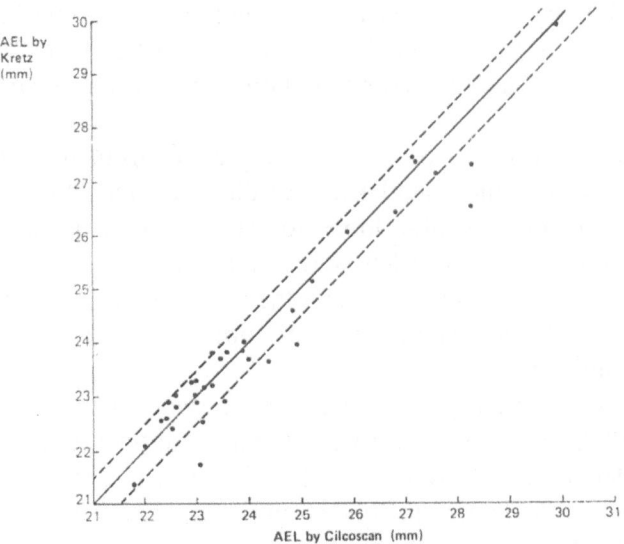

Fig. 1. Comparison of axial eye lenths measured by Cilco A-scan and Kretz 7200 MA A-scan.

Table 1. Details of eyes in which the Kretz and Cilco measurements differed by more than 0.5 mm.

Patient		AEL by Kretz	AEL by Cilco	AEL from post op. refraction	Clinical details
EC		22.54	23.10	*	
MC		23.97	24.89	24.53	Diabetic retinopathy
AD		23.83	23.26	23.71	Senile macula degeneration
JG		23.64	24.36	23.10	Normal post. pole
MM	R eye	27.30	28.31	27.90	Post. staphyloma
	L eye	26.51	28.29	*	Post. staphyloma
EH		22.92	23.56	23.07	Final vision of only 6/60 Pt. needed Yag capsulotomy and developed macular oedema
JT		21.72	23.05	20.19	Normal post. pole

* Not yet had surgery.

Discussion

In any system of axial eye length measurement there are potential sources of error. Inadvertent indentation of the cornea can occur if a water bath is not used. The Cilco assumes a sound velocity of 1550 m/sec and makes no allowance for the fact that sound travels faster through the lens (1641 m/sec) than through aqueous and vitreous (1532 m/sec). However, in this series the error thus introduced was very small (mean 0.04 mms).

By far the greatest source of inaccuracy arises from the difficulty in determining whether the sound beam is directed along the visual axis. Using the Kretz the operator looks for steeply rising peaks from the cornea, anterior and posterior lens surfaces, retina and sclera. If these are all identified and are maximal in height the sound beam can only be axial. With the Cilco's digital display it is more difficult to be certain when the alignment is optimal.

If, however, a posterior staphyloma is present it can be difficult to obtain a good A-scan with the Kretz. Without a real-time A-scan display it is even harder to centre the probe. The Cilco instrument is designed to accept the longest reading to the first strong echo, but it is not always clear whether that echo originates from the posterior vitreous face, the retina, the sclera or even orbital fat. This underlines the main drawback of this instrument: if for any reason (e.g. irregularity of the retinal surface at the posterior pole, poor patient co-operation or operator inexperience) there is difficulty in obtaining a good scan shorter measurements will be successively rejected in favour of longer ones. This explains why in 7 of the 8 patients in which the results differed by more than 0.5 mms. the Kretz reading was the shorter.

Conclusion

Having stressed the disadvantages of the Cilco A-scan I must now explain why we continue to use it. I have shown that in 78% of unselected cases of cataract patients the Kretz and Cilco A-scan agree on the axial eye length to within 0.5 mms. An error of 0.5 mms will, according to the SRK formula, result in an error of 1.25 D in the selection of intraocular lens power and of rather less than 1 D in the final refraction, so this is probably acceptable to most patients. However, out of 36 eyes we had three where there was a difference of more than 1 mm between the two methods which would result in a 2 D final refractive error − enough to spoil most Surgeons' series and sufficient to be noticed by the patient. It is extremely important therefore for the operator of the Cilco A-scan to be alert to its limitations and to recognise that inconsistent or equivocal scans may be indicative of pathology at the posterior pole and are likely to be wildly inaccurate. In our hospital our Opticians continue to use the Cilco A-scan for all routine pre-operative biometry, but when they are unhappy with their readings patients are re-examined with the Kretz 7200 MA.

References

Binkhorst RD. 1975. The Optical Design of intraocular lens implants. Ophthalmic Surg 6: 17−31.

Ossoinig KC. 1983. How to obtain maximum measuring accuracies with standardized A-Scan. In: JS Hillman and MM Le May (eds) Ophthalmic Ultrasonography, Doc Ophthalmologica Proc Ser Vol. 38, Junk, The Hague, pp. 197−216.

Retzlaff J. 1980. Posterior chamber implant power calculation: regression formulas. Am Intra-Ocular Implant Soc J 6: 268.

Sanders DR, Kraff MC. 1980. Improvement of intraocular lens power calculation using empirical data. Am Intra-Ocular Implant Soc J 6: 263.

Wong D, Steele ADMcG. 1985. A survey of intraocular lens implantation in the United Kingdom. Trans Ophthalmol Soc UK 104: 760−765.

Is ultrasonic biometry associated with keratometry reliable for evaluating refractive errors in eyes with transparent media?

D. DORO, P. BORSETTO, G. SATO AND L. CARTURAN

Summary

Thousands of satisfactory corrections of implant patients have confirmed the reliability of the regression formula technique for IOL calculation. The aim of this study was to ascertain whether ultrasonic axial length measurement combined with keratometry could be useful to predict the refractive error in 50 eyes with transparent media. On the basis of SRK formula axial length measured manually by immersion A-scan echography and K-readings were used. The results were compared to the values of cycloplegic refraction: a positive correlation was found in all examined eyes. The reliability and the application of the modified regression calculation technique for evaluating refractive errors are discussed.

Introduction

Thousands of satisfactory corrections by implant lenses have confirmed the reliability of the SRK regression formula. According to Thijssen and co-workers (1987) the regression formula approach of IOL power calculation is more accurate than the optical one. Although the SRK formula is based on the retrospective analysis of implants and was conceived for IOL calculation, to our knowledge a tentative evaluation of refraction in eyes with clear media has never been tried on the basis of SRK formula. The purpose of this paper is to assess the possible use and limits of a modified SRK formula (Retzlaff et al., 1981) in eyes with transparent media, where refraction can be easily checked by subjective and objective methods.

Patient and methods

We selected fifty eyes of forty patients whose age ranged from 20 to 50

Clinica Oculistica, Via Giustiniani 2, 35128 Padova, Italy.

J. M. Thijssen (ed.) Ultrasonography in ophthalmology.
© 1988, *Kluwer Academic Publishers, Dordrecht, ISBN 978-94-010-7083-6*

years (mean 34). All eyes had clear media and an optimally corrected visual acuity of 20/20. Cycloplegic spherical refraction ranged fron −3.25 to +4 D (mean 0.22 ± 1.76); corneal astigmatism was less than 2 D in all eyes. We obtained K-readings with a Haag-Streit Keratometer and measured the axial length with a Kretz 7200 MA Ultrasound unit using the immersion technique as advocated by Ossoinig (1983). The accuracy of the electronic measuring scale was checked prior to each axial length measurement. The patient was placed in a supine position. The 8 MHz probe was immersed into a properly adapted, (custom made), scleral shell (Fig. 1) filled with 5% methylcellulose and aligned with the visual axis of the eye. Three Polaroid pictures were taken at tissue sensitivity −20 dB with four echospikes displayed on the oscilloscope.

A ruler and a caliper were used to estimate the axial length from the pictures between the echospikes of the cornea and the retina. Axial length in microseconds was converted into millimeters by using 1548 m/sec as sound velocity. We modified the SRK formula $(P = A - 2.5L - 0.9K)$ assuming $A = 116.5$ and $P = 20$. In fact the recommended constant for most posterior chamber IOLs is 116.5 and the most used IOL power in "normal" cataractous eyes is +20 D.

Given this assumption, eyes with a refractive error should fit into the modified SRK formula $96.5 - 2.5L - 0.9K = delta$. Delta should be the differential power (from +20 D) of the IOL power to be implanted. According to Keller et al. (1985) for small spectacle corrections the corneal vertex distance may be neglected and a ratio of 1:0.75 between the posterior chamber IOL power and the differential spectacle power to emmetropize pseudophakic eyes can be employed. So, we multiplied each

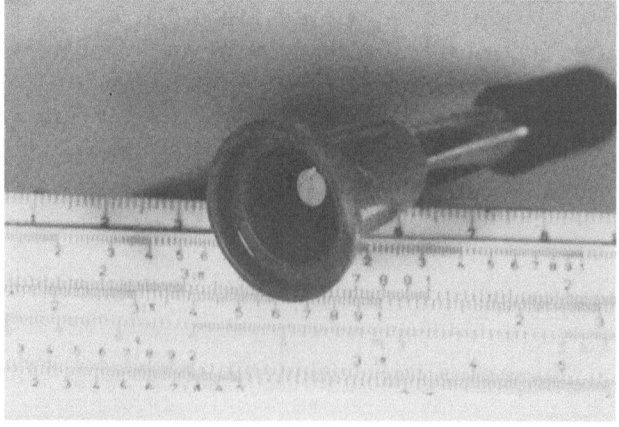

Fig. 1. Adapted scleral shell and US probe for immersion technique.

delta value by a factor of 0.75. We tried to find a correlation between the spectacle refraction and this reduced delta value in the 50 eyes. Data were processed by a computer program.

Results

The analysis of refractive errors versus reduced delta values of all eyes showed a highly significant correlation ($r = 0.93$, $p < 0.001$). The frequency distribution (Table 1) of differences between cycloplegic refraction by retinoscopy and refraction based on K-readings and ultrasound gave a mean value of (0.29 ± 0.76) D, the standard error was 0.15 D and the maximum values $+1.88$ and -1.22 respectively. The analogous frequency distribution in 26 hyperopic eyes (Table 2) gave a mean value of (0.64 ± 0.77) D, standard error of 0.21 D with maximum and minimum values of $+1.88$ and -0.55 D.

The frequency distribution in 24 myopic eyes (Table 3) was similar: mean value $= (0.08 \pm 0.5)$ D, standard error $= 0.15$ D, maximum and minimum values $= 0.52$ and -1.22 D.

Tables 2 and 3 showed a trend towards underestimation of refractive errors in both the hyperopic and the myopic eyes.

Conclusions

1. In our study a small number (50) of eyes with minor refractive errors were examined.

Table 1. Frequency distribution of differences between cycloplegic refraction by retinoscopy and refraction based on K-readings and ultrasound in 50 eyes.

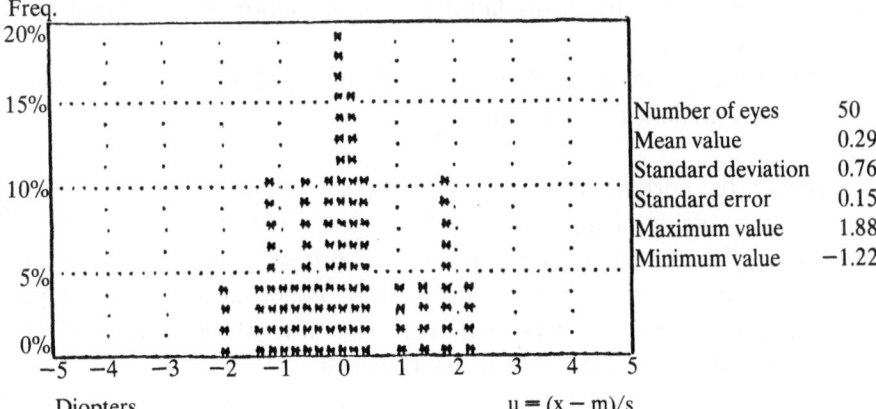

Number of eyes	50
Mean value	0.29
Standard deviation	0.76
Standard error	0.15
Maximum value	1.88
Minimum value	−1.22

Diopters $u = (x - m)/s$

Table 2. Frequency distribution of differences between cycloplegic refraction by retino-scopy and refraction based on K-readings and ultrasound in 26 *hyperopic* eyes.

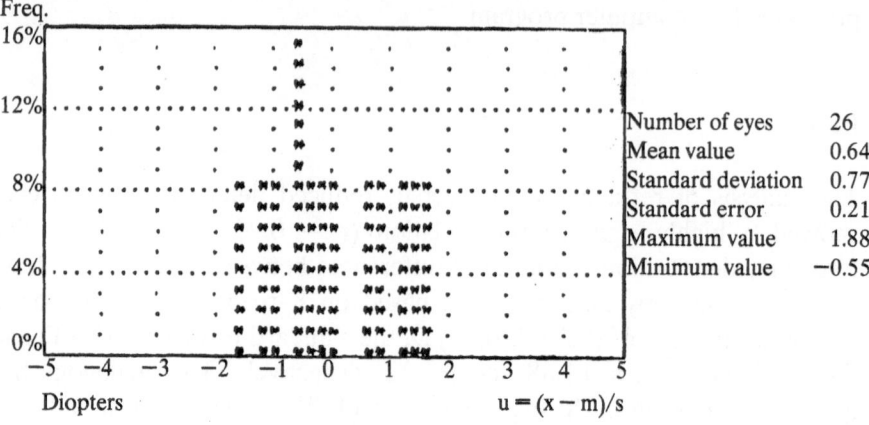

Number of eyes	26
Mean value	0.64
Standard deviation	0.77
Standard error	0.21
Maximum value	1.88
Minimum value	−0.55

Table 3. Frequency distribution of differences between cycloplegic refraction by retino-scopy and refraction based on K-readings and ultrasound in 24 *myopic* eyes.

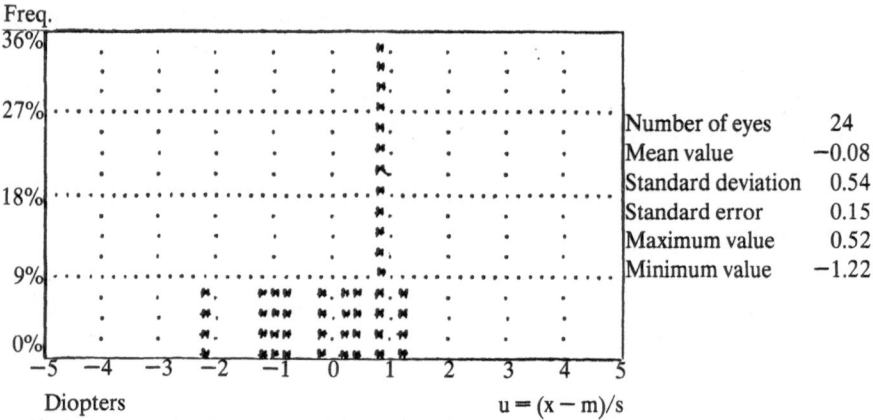

Number of eyes	24
Mean value	−0.08
Standard deviation	0.54
Standard error	0.15
Maximum value	0.52
Minimum value	−1.22

2. The regression SRK formula for IOL implantation was used to estimate the refraction.
3. The assumption of the A and P values in the SRK formula introduced small systematic errors in our study.

However, the correlation between the actual refractions and the calculated values was highly significant ($r = 0.93$, $p < 0.001$) and the mean difference of 0.29 ± 0.76 diopters between refraction by retinoscopy and refraction by keratometry and ultrasound is encouraging. As far as practical application of our modified regression formula is concerned keratometry and axial length measurement can help to estimate refraction in eyes with opaque media where retinoscopy cannot be performed and estimation of refraction may be needed.

If a larger number of examined eyes would prove the modified SRK formula reliable, or alternatively, would enable to find a new regression formula, a biometric ultrasound unit combined with a keratometer will be competitive versus other objective methods (i.e. autorefractometer) for predicting refraction.

Acknowledgements

We are indebted to Dr. Zucchetta for the computer program.

References

Keller JC. 1985. Chirurgia dell'impianto di lente in camera posteriore. In: HK Yang and OR Kline Jr (eds) Verduci Roma, pp. 11—16.

Ossoinig KC. 1983. How to obtain maximum measuring accuracies with standardized A-scan. In: JS Hillman and MM Le May (eds) Ophthalmic Ultrasonography, Junk, The Hague, pp. 197—216.

Retzlaff J, Saunders D, Kraff M. 1981. A manual of implant power calculation. American Intraocular Implant Society Symposium, pp. 17—41.

Thijssen JM, Boerrigter RM. 1984. Ultrasonic biometry for lens implantation: Fact and Fiction. SIDUO X Congress St Petersburg Beach, Fla (USA).

Ultrasonographic measurement of the posterior coats of the eye and their relation to axial length

R. GUTHOFF, R. W. BERGER[1] AND J. DRAEGER

Summary

Preceding the actual study an experiment was designed to prove the satis-factory resolution of our equipment. Then ultrasonographic measurements of axial length and thickness of the posterior coats of the eye were performed in vivo. Combining A- and B-mode ultrasound, a further separation of retina and choroidea echo was possible in about one third of the examinations.

By statistical analysis a strong negative correlation between axial length of the eye and ocular coat dimensions was established. Estimations of the volume of the posterior coats derived from these data suggested that even in eyes of different axial length the tissue volume remains rather constant.

Our results are discussed and compared with theories of axial growth under physiological and pathological conditions.

Introduction

Recently the teams of Trier (1979), Coleman (1979), Purnell (1980), and Fujioka (1982) have emphasized the development of computer supported processing of RF-ultrasound signals and have been able to differentiate multiple layers of retina and choroid.

However, during routine use it appeared that even with commercially available equipment different structures of the posterior ocular coats could be resolved. It seemed to us that there was a marked difference in the B-scan pattern of walls in myopic and hyperopic eyes and it was our intention to find a statistical correlation between axial length and ocular coat dimensions in the area of the posterior pole of the eye.

Some studies on enucleated pig eyes proved the resolution quality of our equipment. These were followed by in vivo examinations of 159 eyes

Ophthalmological Department of the University of Hamburg, FRG; [1] German Aerospace Research Establishment, DFVLR, Cologne, FRG.

J. M. Thijssen (ed.) Ultrasonography in ophthalmology.
© 1988, *Kluwer Academic Publishers, Dordrecht, ISBN 978-94-010-7083-6*

in 95 patients, which comprised an axial length measurement (Kretz, 7200 MA at 10 MHz) and an investigation of the posterior ocular walls with a focused 15-MHz-B-scan probe (Cooper, Ultrascan).

Results

Values of the overall thickness of ocular coats (ranging from 0.75 mm in highly myopic to 2.34 mm in hyperopic eyes, mean value 1.55 mm) were obtained in all patients, in many cases a further differentiation of the posterior pole echo was possible. By statistical analysis a strong inverse correlation between axial length and ocular coat thickness was established ($r = -0.77$, $p < 0.001$).

From axial length and thickness data we derived calculations of the coat volume of the posterior half of the globe, which, for the sake of simplification, was assumed to be spherical. While the absolute amount of wall material was about 1600 mm^3 over the whole range of refractions the percentage was found to vary from 12% in the most myopic globe to 50% in the most hyperopic. After rearrangement of the equations there was evidence for a constant tissue volume regardless of the varying axial length parameters in myopic and hyperopic eyes.

This is in good agreement with Lindner's (1939) theory of the development of myopia. He postulated that only a pathological expansion of tissue is responsible for the enlargement of the myopic eye. It also fits in the results of Luyckx (1967) and Rivara (1968) who found correlations between scleral rigidity and ocular volume.

Accepting some simplification in the process of calculating the ocular coat volume, our measurements suggest that there is a constant tissue volume of approximately 1600 mm^3 for the posterior half of the globe, which corresponds to a portion varying from about 12% to 50% of the overall posterior volume depending upon the axial refraction of the eye.

Reference

Coleman DJ, Lizzi, FL. 1979. In vivo choroidal thickness measurement. Am J Ophthalmol 88: 369—375.

Decker D, Trier HG, Lepper RD, Reuter R. 1979. Das Projekt 'Rechnergestützte Gewebsdifferenzierung' der Arbeitsgemeinschaft Bonn/Stuttgart. I. and II. In: Gernet (ed) Diagnostica ultrasonica in Ophthalmologia, Remy, Münster, pp. 00.

Fujioka C, Kobayashi Y, Emi K, Yokoyama M. 1983. The biometry of each thickness of the retina, choroid and sclera by ultrasound and Fourier analysis, I., II., III. Acta Soc Ophthal Jap 86: 1801—1803 and 87: 70—78.

Lindner, K. 1939. Neue Gedanken über die Entstehung der Kurzsichtigkeit. Klin Mbl Augenheilk 103: 582.

Luyckx J. 1967. Relation entre le coefficient de rigidité et la longueur de l'oeil mesurée par échographie ultrasonique. Ophthalmologica 155: 355—366.

Purnell EW. 1980. Ultrasonic biometry of the posterior ocular coats. Trans Am Ophthal Soc 78: 1027—1078.

Rivara A, Zingirian M. 1968. Volume du bulbe et rigidité sclérale. Ophthalmologica 156: 394—398.

Post surgery depth of anterior chamber after extracapsular cataract extraction with IOL: influence on definitive correction

F. L. CATANIA AND M. T. PADOIN

Summary

The authors examine the lens implantation cases operated on during eighteen months in his department.

He compares the foreseen theoretical power of the Binkhorst formula with the actual necessary power calculated after some months. The influence of post operative astigmatism on the final correction and post surgery anterior chamber depth variability are discussed as well. In all cases the IOL was implanted in the posterior chamber. The biometries were done in immersion with A-mode equipment (Kretz Technik 7200 MA).

Visual acuity after ECCE with IOL not only depends on correct biometry and ophthalmometry so that a formula yields the exact IOL value to be implanted, but on anterior chamber post surgery depth and post surgery dioptric power of corneal meridians also.

We examined 140 eyes operated on with ECCE + IOL in posterior chamber in our department during 18 months. In this group are absent:

— surgery and out follow-up patients
— corneal oedema, uveitis, hyphema cases
— cases with troubled vitreous and retinal pathology.

Presurgery biometry of eyes was performed with the immersion technique using a Kretz Technik 7200 MA equipment. The calculation of IOL values was performed following the Binkhorst formula, that considers A.C. depth after surgery of 4 mm.

Figure 1 shows the power of glasses that must be added before the most ametropic meridian of the implanted eye, after having implanted an IOL with the exact calculated power (this has not always been done). It is obvious that in spite of biometry and ophthalmometry care mistakes were

Civil Hospital S. Maria dei Battuti, Department of Ophthalmology, Conegliano Veneto (Treviso), Italy.

J. M. Thijssen (ed.) Ultrasonography in ophthalmology.
© 1988, Kluwer Academic Publishers, Dordrecht, ISBN 978-94-010-7083-6

332

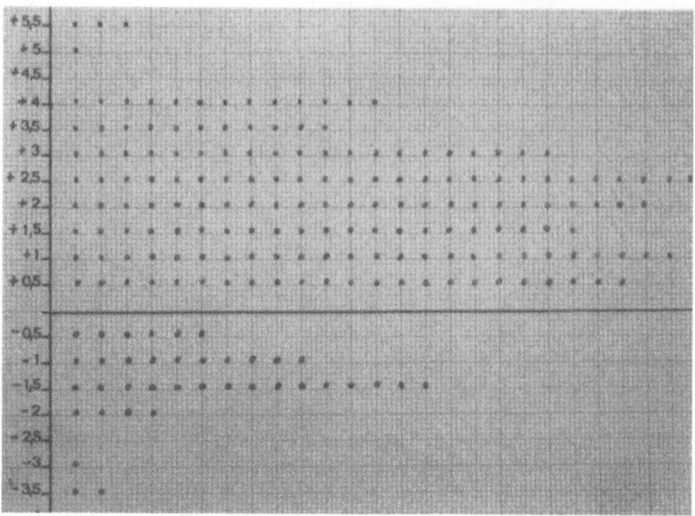

Fig. 1. Frequency histogram: Dioptric power of glasses that must be added before the most ametropic meridian of the implanted eye.

often serious. The influence of ophthalmometric values becomes clear with the following example:

— a bulbus 34 μs long with corneal power 43 D needs a + 11.08 D IOL
— a bulbus 34 μs long with corneal power 43.25 D needs a + 10.8 IOL
  (an almost 0.3 D difference).

$$\frac{1336 \times (4 \times 7.84 - 26.3)}{(26.3 - 4) \times (4 \times 7.84 - 4)} = 11.08 \text{ D}$$

$$\frac{1336 \times (4 \times 7.80 - 26.3)}{(26.3 - 4) \times (4 \times 7.80 - 4)} = 10.8 \text{ D}$$

Considering that the ophthalmometer might not be adequately calibrated and that ophthalmometric values are often subjective, the IOL calculation may not be exact. In addition the ophthalmometric values frequently change in relative and absolute aspect after surgery. Therefore, a very important aspect is the post surgery depth of the anterior chamber. We have done echobiometry of A.C. in fifty pseudophakic eyes of the reported group (distance between posterior surface of cornea and IOL anterior surface).

As Fig. 2 shows, the values range from 2.85 mm to 4.6 mm. If calculation is executed with the Binkhorst formula, changing only this parameter, the difference in the result is as follows

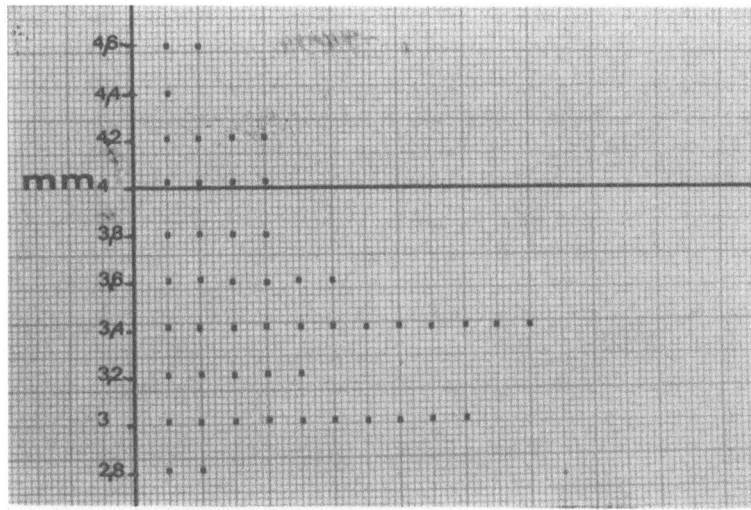

Fig. 2. Frequency histogram: Post-operative A.C. depth, values range from 2.85 mm to 4.6 mm.

$$\frac{1336 \times (4 \times 7.5 - 24)}{(24 - 4) \times (4 \times 7.5 - 4)} = 15.4\,D$$

$$\frac{1336 \times (4 \times 7.5 - 24)}{(24 - 3.8) \times (4 \times 7.5 - 3.8)} = 15.14\,D$$

Conclusion

Care and meticulousness in doing bulbus biometry and in searching for other data to calculate IOL value are no doubt useful. In this way big mistakes may be avoided (myopic and hyperopic eyes) but cannot guarantee a precise final result.

The role of echography in adult glaucoma

A. REIBALDI[1], T. AVITABILE AND M. G. UVA

Summary

The use of echography is not common in the investigation and diagnosis of adult glaucoma; in this study however, we present both the value of echography in different forms of glaucoma and its routine use in clinical practice to achieve an early and correct diagnosis. In confirmation of this the authors present case-reports of the last 10 years from which, based on the different role according to the different types of glaucoma, it is possible to identify the following groups:

(a) glaucoma where echography is *fundamental*; phacolytic glaucoma, some forms of secondary glaucoma (to ocular tumours, orbital vascular malformations, Graves' orbitopathy), glaucoma with opaque media.
(b) glaucoma where echography is *important*: narrow angle glaucoma, acute glaucoma, phacomorphic and phacotopic glaucoma, absolute glaucoma, malignant glaucoma, post-operative course;
(c) glaucoma where echography is *accessory*: chronic simple glaucoma, unilateral glaucoma, low tension glaucoma.

Introduction

In recent years, the diagnosis of glaucoma has been steadily improving, adding to the present clinical investigations up-to-date instrumental techniques such as: computerized visual field and tonography, optic disc stereophotography and computerized biometry of the same, ERG and VEP pattern, etc.

Ocular echography, on the contrary, despite its increasing use, has not won a wide and codified interest in this specific field, although the information available with this method is known to be important (Reibaldi and Avitabile 1986).

Clinica Oculista, University of Catania, Catania, Italy.

J. M. Thijssen (ed.) Ultrasonography in ophthalmology.
© 1988, *Kluwer Academic Publishers, Dordrecht, ISBN 978-94-010-7083-6*

In our opinion it is possible to differentiate the echographic possibilities, in relation to the different types of glaucoma in adult subjects, in the following groups:

(1) Glaucoma where echography is FUNDAMENTAL
(2) Glaucoma where echography is IMPORTANT
(3) Glaucoma where echography is ACCESSORY

Aim of the present study is to analyze in detail each group evidencing advantages and limits of the ultrasonographic investigation, in the light of 10 years-experience at the Glaucoma and Echography Centres of the Eye Clinic of Bari University.

(1) We deem that, in adult subjects, glaucomas where echography is FUNDAMENTAL are:

(A) phacolytic glaucoma.
(B) glaucoma secondary to ocular and orbital tumours, to vascular orbital malformations, Graves' ophthalmopathy etc.
(C) glaucoma with opaque media.

(A) *Phacolytic glaucoma.* Everybody knows the clinical feature of phacolytic glaucoma represented essentially by conspicuous increase of intraocular pressure (I.O.P.), open angle, hypermature cataract etc. (Flocks et al., 1955, Moro et al., 1972, 1973, 1982, etc.).

By echography, it is often possible to show abnormal relations between the posterior surface of the lens and the anterior vitreous. (Reibaldi et al., 1985). In these cases with contact B-scan we can recognize:

— lens thickening (normally the lens is not evident, or in the best case it is possible to see only the posterior cortical surface).
— presence of retro-lental vitreous opacities, with medium reflectivity, due to the involvement in the process of the vitreous at the back of the lens.

In standardized A-scan, by using Ossoinig's scleral shells for echobiometry, we have noted:

— change in anterior chamber depth;
— lens thickening, with in-out spikes irregularity, related to structural modifications of the lens.
— a series of spikes of medium reflectivity starting from the posterior surface of the lens and spreading into the vitreous for some microseconds.

We have noted the above features in 9 out of the 14 cases of Phacolytic glaucoma observed in our 5 year-case report (the length of this report is shorter because this particular study was started just 5 years ago). Echography has allowed us to plan surgery foreseeing an anterior and retro-pupillar vitrectomy to limit the intra- and post-surgical complications in addition to cataract extraction. In confirmation of the above we have noted:

(1) The onset, after 2 days, of a membrane, partially occupying the pupillary foramen in 1 case where vitrectomy was not performed because echographically was negative.

(2) A good functional result also for the normalization of the I.O.P. in all cases treated with vitrectomy. In our opinion, this is due particularly to the vitrectomy which removed the lens material residues floating in the anterior vitreous, and causing residual increased I.O.P.

(B) *Secondary glaucoma*. Echography is fundamental in the following 4 types of glaucoma secondary also:

Ocular tumours: even with transparent media, echography, and above all standardized A-scan, gives the possibility, not only to recognize a neo-plastic lesion, but also to detect its nature, even if within certain limits. We pass over the echographic features since they are very well known (Ossoinig 1969, Gallenga et al., 1971, Reibaldi, 1976).

Our case report includes the following 7 cases:

— 1 patient who had already had an operation for glaucoma presenting a residual increased I.O.P. and a fundus which couldn't be visualised. Our echographic diagnosis of choroidal melanoma was histologically confirmed after enucleation.

— 2 subjects using miotic drugs which made observation of the peripheral fundus difficult. In these cases a melanoma and a metastatic tumour were diagnosed respectively and both confirmed by subsequent investigation.

— 4 patients with perfectly transparent media where echography together with other investigations, was useful to confirm the clinical diagnosis.

Orbital vascular malformations: echography is important especially when the objective symptomatology of the malformations is not indicative enough.

The carotid-cavernous fistula is echographically detectable as a low reflecting mass, capsulated, soft, with spontaneous movements (pathog-

338

nomonic features allowing us the differential diagnosis from other orbital pathology) for which the inner spikes look blurred since presenting vertical movements (Ossoinig 1979).

3 cases with similar glaucoma were observed by us.

Orbital tumours: even if rarely causing an increased I.O.P. (Rossi, 1981), they can be easily detected and echographically differentiated as for ocular tumours (Ossoinig, 1979).

In our case report there were 2 patients treated for several months with common antiglaucoma drugs, who, owing to persisting increased I.O.P., were transferred to our Eye Clinic.

Objectively they did not present exophthalmos, but only a very slight episcleral venous congestion. The echographic examination showed two rather big carcinomas starting from the ethmoidal cells. The surgical operation confirmed our diagnosis in both cases.

Graves' ophthalmopathy: echographic examination includes the accurate defining of extra-ocular muscle thickening even in the absence of exophthalmos. This is always present, according to Ossoinig (1982) and, in our opinion it is, the most cases, one of the cause of the I.O.P. increasing. In 6 observed cases, where an open angle glaucoma had been diagnosed (3 with slight bilateral exophthalmos, 1 with unilateral exophthalmos, and 2 patients with absence of exophthalmos) and the thyroidopathy had not been previously diagnosed, the echobiometry detected a thickening of extraocular muscles typical of Graves' disease. It allowed us to diagnose in these cases "a glaucoma secondary to thyroidopathy". Further specific tests (FT3, FT4, TSH, TRH for TSH) confirmed our echographic diagnosis.

Table 1 summarizes our case report concerning the secondary glaucoma:

Table 1.

7 cases of ocular tumours.
3 cases of orbital vascular malformations.
2 cases of orbital tumours.
6 cases of Graves' ophthalmopathy.

(C) *Glaucoma with opaque media.* There are a number of possible causes of media opacity, but in most cases, the cause is cataract.

It is obvious that in subjects presenting glaucoma plus cataract echography plays a fundamental role. In our case report we detected 7 vitreous haemorrhages, 2 primary retinal detachment and 1 secondary retinal detachment.

We should add 3 cases respectively with localized melanoma, a "corolla" shaped melanoma with orbital metastasis, and a metastatic carcinoma. In these cases the glaucoma was absolute, confirming Duke Elder's study (1969).

Table 2 summarizes the above said cases:

Table 2.

7 cases of vitreous haemorrhage:	Primary
2 cases of primary retinal detachment:	open angle
1 case of secondary retinal detachment:	glaucoma
1 case of localized melanoma	
1 case of "corolla" shaped melanoma:	absolute
1 case with orbital metastasis:	glaucoma
1 case of metastatic carcinoma.	

Another cause of media opacity is vitreous haemorrhage, found especially in neovascuolar glaucomas and, above all, in diabetic subjects.

In our case report we noticed 5 cases of proliferative retinopathy, 3 cases of vitreous haemorrhage and vitreo-retinal traction, 1 case of vitreo-retinal traction with retinal detachment (see the following table).

Table 3.

5 cases of proliferative retinopathy
3 cases of vitreous, haemorrhage and vitreo-retinal traction
1 case of vitreo-retinal traction with retinal detachment.

It is obvious that to know such pathology is extremely relevant to the therapy.

(2) In our opinion, echography is IMPORTANT in the following types of glaucoma

(A) Glaucoma with reduction of the anterior chamber depth.

(B) Post operative course.

(A) *Glaucoma with reduction of the anterior chamber depth* (narrow angle glaucoma, acute glaucoma, phacomorphic and phacotopic glaucoma); in this group the parameters which can be echographically explored are:

- anterior chamber depth;
- lens thickness;
- lens position;
- lens position relative to the other structures of the eye;
- anterior-posterior eye-ball axis length.

Such parameters can be obtained with standardized A-scan with the immersion method using Ossoinig's sceral shells.

Cennamo et al. (1985) using this technique has shown:

- a lens thickness increasing of about 1.2 mm in subjects aged from 20 to 80 years;
- the lens thickening in a normal eye has not a linear, but a curvilinear course, especially increasing from 70 to 80 years;
- the lens thickening curve in patients with narrow angle glaucoma has values superior to the normal ones; in this case too, the course is curvilinear, with a maximal increase from 55 to 70 years.

Finally, the useful clinical information we obtain by echobiometry in such types of glaucomas are:

- lens thickness, especially related to antero-posterior eye-ball axis (highly hypermetropic eyes).
- differentiation of phacomorphic glaucoma, due to the lens thickening, from the phacotopic one, due to the lens advancement, and, therefore, the possibility to plan appropriate surgery.

In our report, we have treated 7 cases of acute attack of glaucoma with only lens extraction after a Yag-laser iridotomy, and in 6 of them, we have obtained an I.O.P. normalization, while in 1 case presenting an increase of I.O.P. some days after the surgical operation, it was controlled by Phospholine Iodide 0.125% instillation twice daily.

(B) *Postoperative course.* Among post surgical complications in an anti-glaucomatous operation, we point out above all choroidal detachment and malignant glaucoma.

Echography plays an important role where these complications are associated to a cornea oedema, hyphaema, cataract, miosis; vitreous haemorrhages, which hinder the visualisation of posterior structures. With standardized A-scan, choroidal detachment appears as a pathognomonic bifid spike, with maximum reflectivity, followed by a series of spikes with more or less low reflectivity. The same show the nature of the subchoroidal fluid (serous, haemorrhagic, coagulated) and prognosticate if and when it will be absorbed (Reibaldi et al., 1984).

We can obtain topographical information about an eventual sclerotomy by B-scan (Coleman et al., 1977), where the choroidal detachment presents with a pathognomonic picture, represented by a particular angle between detached choroid and sclera, (Poujol, 1981) due to its attachment to the vortex veins. In malignant glaucoma, which is one of the rarest but most dreadful complications in glaucoma surgery, there is the formation of aqueous humor pockets, visible sometimes also by biomicroscopy (Simmons, 1972). Doro et al. (1984) have shown by a clinical-experimental study that A-scan standardized echography is useful, especially if there is opacity of the media, to detect and localize these aqueous pockets appearing by a medium-low reflectivity echo, in the vitreous chamber, due to the slight difference between the acoustic impedance of the vitreal thickened surface and the aqueous humour.

This is confirmed by the spike disappearance when a diathermy perforation is performed to empty the pockets, while they appear, experimentally, on injection of aqueous humour into the rabbit vitreous chamber.

(3) We have considered ACCESSORY the role of echography in Chronic simple glaucoma. In 1977 Bellone et al. have defined secondary the use of echography in this type of glaucoma.

Several Authors, however, and Ossoinig (1979) above all, speaking about echography and glaucoma, have shown B-scan use in detecting the glaucomatous cup. In our case report, we deemed its role as accessory because with transparent media we obviously prefer other investigations, in order to better evaluate the cup (ophthalmoscopic, photography, computerized analysis of the optic disc etc.) (Reibaldi et al., 1986). In case of opaque media, it is more important for us to detect other types of possible pathology, than to investigate the cup, which is evident only when it reaches certain dimensions. Further accessory parameters given by echography are:

— eye-ball axis length/corneal diameter ratio, which results are increased if compared with normal subjects. Such dimensions, genetically transmitted, would predispose to glaucoma (Leighton et al., 1971),
— a relationship between posterior chamber dimension and I.O.P., to explain the aetiology of unilateral glaucoma (Machekhin, 1972).
— an increase of vitreous chamber in the low tension glaucoma (Tomlinson et al., 1972).

Conclusions

Echography has not traditionally been included among the techniques for investigating glaucoma.

Based on our experience and after a careful study of the literature about this subject, we stress the possibilities of echography in the diagnosis of glaucoma and have presented its different role in the different types of glaucoma. It is FUNDAMENTAL because it gives indispensable information in: phacolytic glaucoma, in secondary glaucoma (to ocular and orbital neoformations, to carotid-cavernous fistula, to Graves' orbitopathy), in glaucoma with opaque media.

It is IMPORTANT because it gives useful but not indispensable diagnostic clues in: glaucoma with reduction of the anterior chamber depth (acute glaucoma, narrow angle glaucoma, phacotopic and phacomorphic glaucomas) in which it gives us above all information about lens dimension and position, and in the post-surgical course, to diagnose a choroidal detachment or a malignant glaucoma.

It is ACCESSORY because it gives us secondary information, which usually does not substantially modify the diagnosis in: chronic simple glaucoma, in unilateral glaucoma and in low tension glaucoma.

References

Bellone G, Rossi PL. 1977. L'ecografia nel glaucoma cronico semplice. LVIII Congr, S.O.I., pp. 313—352.

Cennamo G, Rosa N. 1985. Ecografia e glaucoma. Acta XIX Congr S.O.M., 21—32, Capri.

Coleman DJ, Lizzi FL, Jack RL. 1977. Ultrasonography of the eye and orbit. Philadelphia, Lea & Febiger.

Doro D, Perrone S, Steidler P, D'Ermo F. 1984. L'ecografia nel glaucoma maligno: la nostra esperienza clinica e sperimentale. Acta VIII Congr Naz S.I.S.U.M., Clin Ocul e Patol Ocul Suppl Vol. 5, pp. 30—32.

Duke Elder S. 1969. System of Ophthalmology. Vol. 9, Kimpton, London, p. 553.

Flocks M, Littwin C, Zimmermann L. 1955. Phacolytic glaucoma. Arch Ophthal 54: 37—45.

Gallenga R, Bellone G, Gallenga PE, Pasquarelli A. 1971. Ultrasonografia clinica dell'occhio e dell'orbita. In: Recenti acquisizioni di semeiotica oculare. Acta S.O.I., pp. 161.

Leighton DA, Tomlinson A. 1971. Relationship between ocular dimension and the effects of provocative tests. Br J Ophthalmol 55: 607.

Machekhin A. 1972. Ultrasonic biometry in unilateral glaucoma. Invest Ophth 5: 7—11.

Moro F, Cavallaro N. 1972. Glaucoma facolitico. Acta LIV Congr S.O.I. Roma, pp. 370—394.

Moro F, Sanfilippo S, Cavallaro N. 1973. Glaucome phacolytique. Recherches sur l'ultrastructure de trabeculum. Bull Soc Ophthalm Franc 86: 128.

Moro F, Cavallaro N. 1981. Glaucoma facolitico (contributo clinico). Clin Ocul e Pat Ocul 3: 86—90.

Ossoinig KC. 1971. Basics on echographic tissue differentiation: I Experimental and clinical examinations of the influence of system parameters on the diagnostic value of echograms. In: J Bock and KC Ossoinig (eds) Ultrasonographia Medica (Proceedings of the First World Congress on ultrasonic diagnostics in Medicine and S.I.D.U.O. III, Wien 1969) Verlog Wiener Med Akademie. Vol. I, pp. 155—168.

Ossoinig KC. 1979. Standardized echography: Basic principles. clinical applications and results. Int Ophthalm Clinics 194: 127—285.

Ossoinig KC. 1982. Advance in diagnostic ultrasound. Acta XXIV Int Congress of Ophthalmol, San Francisco, pp. 89—114.

Poujol J. 1981. A characteristic echographic sign of choroidal detachment. In: JM Thijssen and AM Verbeek (eds) The appearance of the angle of junction with the ocular wall. Ultrasonography in Ophthalmology, Docum Ophthalmol Proc Series, Vol. 29, Junk, The Hague, pp. 265—267.

Reibaldi A, Montrone F, Ranieri G. 1976. Semeiotica clinica dei tumori endobulbari. X Congress S.O.M., Brindisi, pp. 215—221.

Reibaldi A, Lorusso VV, Delle Noci N. 1981. Eight years of A- and B-Scan ultrasonography in tumoral diagnostic of the globe and orbit. In: JM Thijssen and AM Verbeek (eds) Ultrasonography in Ophthalmology, Docum Ophthalmol Proc Series, Vol. 29, Junk, The Hague, pp. 323—326.

Reibaldi A. 1982. Biometric ultrasound in the diagnosis and follow up of congenital glaucoma. Ann of Ophthalmol 8: 707—708.

Reibaldi A, Avitabile T, Guerriero S. 1984. L'ecografia nella patologia della coroide. VIII Nat Congress S.I.S.U.M., Clin Ocul c Pat Ocul Suppl Vol. 5, 6, pp. 19—22.

Reibaldi A, Montrone F, Avitabile T. 1985. L'ecografia ed il glaucoma facolitico. I Congress S.I.E.O., Ferrara.

Reibaldi A, Avitabile T. 1986. Ecografia e glaucoma. II Meeting Associazione Italiana Studio del Glaucoma (AISG), Rapallo.

Reibaldi A, Bellizzi M, Uva MG. 1986. Our trends in early diagnosis of open angle glaucoma. X International Glaucoma Congress. Hollywood Flo., USA.

Rossi A. 1981. Clinica dei tumori dell'occhio e dell'orbita. LXI Congr S.O.I., Roma.

Sampaolesi R. 1974. Glaucoma. Hedica Panamericana, Buenos Aires.

Simmons RJ. 1972. Malignant glaucoma. Br J Ophthal 56: 263—272.

Tomlinson A, Leighton DA. 1972. Ocular dimensions in low tension glaucoma compared with open angle glaucoma and the normal. Br J Ophthal 56: 97—105.

Tomlinson A, Leighton DA. 1974. Ocular dimensions and the heredity of open angle glaucoma. Br J Ophthal 58: 68—74.

Oculometric features of high myopia, around the age of 35. A 10-year follow-up

H. C. FLEDELIUS, E. GOLDSCHMIDT AND M. STUBGAARD

Summary

Our concept of complication risks in high myopia is probably strongly biased from (1) what the retinal surgeon tells us, and (2) statistics of visual handicap, social blindness etc. Evidently focus is on the heavy end of the spectrum in clinical reports thus founded. With the aim of drawing a valid epidemiological picture, the present longitudinal study has a quite different approach. Fourteen-year-olds with high myopia have been re-examined with 10 year intervals. With 29 available (out of 39) the oculometry status was presented at the SIDUO VII conference in 1978. Recently, 25 have been seen again, now at the age of 34. In most cases myopia has been fairly stable, and the changes in ultrasound measurements have been small, accordingly. The results are discussed, with reference also to high myopia in general.

Introduction

In Goldschmidt's thesis 'On the etiology of high myopia' (1968) myopia was reported in 9.5% of 9,243 Copenhagen schoolchildren aged 13—14 years. High myopia — of at least 6 diopters — was encountered in 39 subjects, bilaterally in 23, or in one eye only (n = 16). In six of the latter, the less myopic eye came close to the −6 D limit.

For the 39 with high myopia, a prospective study was planned, with an intended follow-up every 10th year, the exceptional feature being an unselected group from the outset. This should enable us to make an epidemiologically valid analysis of the ophthalmic (and social) risks of high myopia. The risk is easily overestimated when evaluated from hospital materials, with retinal (or other) complications having led to inclusion.

The loaded prognosis derived herefrom is reflected for instance by the

Eye Department, County Hospital, 3400 Hillerød, Denmark.

J. M. Thijssen (ed.) Ultrasonography in ophthalmology.
© 1988, *Kluwer Academic Publishers, Dordrecht, ISBN 978-94-010-7083-6*

higher insurance pays generally demanded from the highly myopic individual. Probably this is not fair to all. On clinical grounds we do know that high myopia may indeed be pathological, but in other cases we are probably facing physiological variants with a much lower morbidity risk. A longitudinal study might clarify this.

Out of the 39, we succeeded in examining 29 at the ten-year follow-up. On that occasion ultrasound eye measurements were added to the examination scheme. Previously, a report on oculometry findings was given at the Münster SIDUO VII conference (Fledelius, 1979). A more detailed presentation was published by Goldschmidt et al. in 1981.

Now aged 35 years, 27 from our group were able to attend for the present 20-year follow-up, with all but two having attended also on the former occasion. This gives us a sample of 25 with repeated ultrasound oculometry. In the following, emphasis will be on the oculometry results. In this context, the age homogeneity should be stressed. This eliminates the influence of age otherwise seen in oculometry samples, with bearing on anterior eye segment structures in particular.

Material and methods

The material has been outlined above.

A thorough history was taken, with the aim of analysing the influence of the refractive state on education, occupation, sport, and other free-time activities.

The clinical examinations (done by EG) comprised: Best corrected visual acuity of both eyes, with glasses, contact lenses, or both; Topcon refractometry; light retinoscopy and subjective determination of refraction; slit lamp evaluation and applanation tonometry; direct ophthalmoscopy and fundus photography. Exophthalmometry and corneal thickness measurements as performed earlier were not done this time.

Corneal curvature radius was measured by Haag-Streit keratometry.

Axial ultrasound oculometry was performed by a Kretz Technik 7000 apparatus and an Ultrasonolux 10 MHz transducer, coupled to the eye by a Methocel-filled contactglass (Fledelius, 1976). Due to the inter-equipment variation to be expected, we desisted from using more recent oculometry equipment, in order to make the results as "longitudinal" as possible. The same subjects thus had repeated measurements performed by the same examiner (HCF) using the very same technique and equipment. Careful water calibrations ensured that the apparatus characteristics still made it suitable and ready for use. Lens power estimates were done by way of a Texas 58 computer with the Binkhorst program for intraocular lens calculation. We decided to express lens power as the calculated power of a thin lens placed at the site of the anterior lens surface, in a hypothetical aphakic situation, and resulting in the refractive value the eye actually had.

Many parameters being suitable for parametric statistical evaluation, the customary calculations of mean values with standard deviations, regression analyses, t-tests, etc. have been performed, however, with non-parametric evaluations added in cases where this was proper. Computer programming was performed by MS, according to SAS system manual.

Results

The material is presented in the regression plot of 54 eyes (from 17 females and 10 males) shown in Fig. 1, with refraction and axial length as variables. The regression line is given by $y = -0.345x + 23.23$ ($r = -0.83$).

In the following the material will be divided in (a) high myopia (<-6 D, 47 eyes) and so-called low myopia, comprising 7 fellow eyes with low degree myopia or even emmetropia; and (b) the high myopia group will be divided by sex, in 31 female and 16 male eyes. Many results will be based on all 27 subjects, while the sections dealing with *changes* from the age of 24 to 35 comprise only the 50 eyes with repeated measurements.

Table 1 shows refractive values and oculometry results in the above subgroups. Again it is confirmed that high myopia is primarily axial, with no significant differences pertaining to anterior segment structures when compared to low myopia.

The higher refractive value of males as compared to females is not

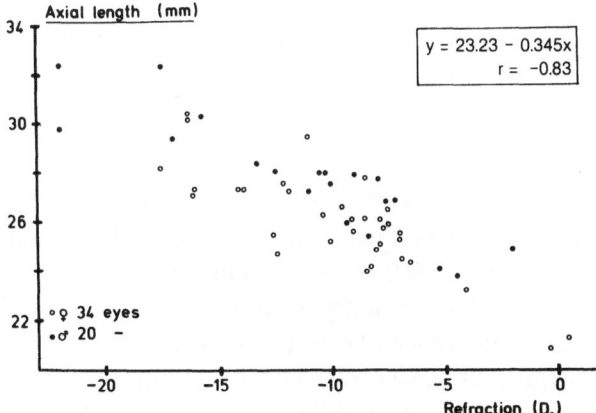

Fig. 1. Refraction (on abscissa) and axial length (on ordinate) of the 54 eyes actually re-examined, with regression line and correlation coefficient indicated at top.

Table 1. Refraction and oculometry recordings given as mean value and SD (at top), median value, and range (at bottom) in four subgroups of the present sample. To the left, the 54 eyes (n = 27) are divided according to the −6 diopter limit. The 47 eyes with high myopia are further divided by sex (right; range omitted).

	High myopia (47 eyes)	Low myopia (7 eyes)	High myopia	
			females (31 eyes)	males (16 eyes)
Refraction (D.)	−11.0 (3.90) −10.0 (−6.5 to −22)	−2.7 (2.27) −3.7 (0.7 to −5.3)	−10.5 (3.35) −9.0	−12.1 (4.75) −10.4
Corn. radius (mm)	7.73 (0.30) 7.68 (7.15—8.35)	7.76 (0.31) 7.84 (7.15—8.15)	7.63 (0.29) 7.55	7.94 (0.21) 7.75
Ant. chamber depth (mm)	3.68 (0.29) 3.70 (3.3—4.4)	3.64 (0.24) 3.70 (3.3—4.0)	3.68 (0.33) 3.70	3.70 (0.20) 3.70
Lens thickness (mm)	4.09 (0.25) 4.1 (3.6—4.6)	3.96 (0.26) 4.0 (3.6—4.4)	4.14 (0.25) 4.10	4.01 (0.18) 4.0
Vitr. length (mm)	19.30 (1.66) 20.2 (16.6—24.8)	16.66 (1.35) 17.2 (14.2—17.9)	18.72 (1.39) 18.4	20.44 (1.59) 20.1
Axial length (mm)	21.10 (1.74) 27.0 (24.5—32.4)	24.26 (1.45) 24.9 (22.0—25.9)	26.53 (1.53) 26.2	28.14 (1.66) 28.0
Lens power equivalent (D.)	19.91 (2.07) 20.0 (16.3—25.6)	19.0 (2.22) 19.6 (14.3—20.8)	20.0 (2.10) 20.0	19.76 (2.07) 19.9

significant statistically. The axial length (and vitreous length) of males is however significantly longer than in females (p < 0.01), and further we find a flatter cornea (p < 0.01) and a thinner lens (p < 0.05) in males. Those are the general oculometry features related to sex, here to be demonstrated also in the group of extreme myopia.

Seventy-nine percent having changed one diopter or less during the later ten-year period, refractive stability was encountered in most eyes. The median refractive change was 0.5 D towards myopia (range −1.7 D (less myopic) to 8 D (more myopic)). In five eyes myopia had worsened by more than 2 diopters. The marginal 8-diopter change appeared in a male eye, now with -22 D, only to continue the marked progression (7 D) of his first ten-year period.

From the above, only slight longitudinal changes in ultrasound measurements are to be expected. Obviously, the sample will be marked by the majority of cases with quite stable refraction. In such cases, deviating recordings might as well be due to measurement errors as to actual changes in size, and methodological errors might even blur in the few cases where changes are probable. For instance, it may be hard to obtain a well-defined steep echo-start from the backwall of a very long eye. A sloping posterior eyewall may lead to selection of skew soundbeam directions, with associated fluctuations in vitreous and axial length recordings.

Anyhow, significant associations could be demonstrated between axial length change (on y-axis) and refractive change (on x-axis) over the present ten-year period, up to the age of 35, with a regression line of $y = 0.19x - 0.022$ ($r = 0.59$, highly significant). The median and mean axial length change in high myopia was -0.1 and 0.1 mm respectively (range -0.6 to 2.1 mm, with the cases of apparent eye shortening probably being explained by method factors, cf. above). In consistency with the axial length results we found $y = 0.162x - 0.105$ ($r - 0.53$) with 10-year change of vitreous length as dependent variable and refractive change on x-axis. Changes in anterior chamber depth and lens thickness proved insignificant for refractive change.

Positive correlations between axial length on the one hand, and corneal curvature ($r = 0.38$) or anterior chamber depth ($r = 0.39$) could be demonstrated. Ten years earlier, only the first of the two associations was significant. On that occasion anterior chamber deepening with increasing axial length only came close to significance, a result in better accord with earlier reports claiming that from a certain eye size the anterior chamber depth no longer keeps pace with the elongating posterior eye segment (cf. Delmarcelle et al., 1976). We have no valid explanation for this slight variance in results, except that the two recording sets shared only 25 subjects, while correlations were calculated from the full samples comprising also a few 'singletons'. Small samples being sensitive, this is probably enough to explain the apparent inconsistency.

Discussion

Above, oculometric features have been discussed at some length already. Let it here be added only that we have investigated an age interval characterized by a certain stability, also clinically. By and large, the eyes have retained their visual acuity. This statement is valid in particular for the leading eye of the subject, with maintenance of social vision. So far we have not encountered progressing posterior staphyloma, and there were no cases of retinal detachment or glaucoma. Hopefully, we (and our myopia group) can keep the spirit so that we might return in another ten years with a report of what is to happen next. Obviously, we come nearer to age levels where complications are liable to develop.

References

Delmarcelle Y, Francois J, Goes F, Collignon-Brach J, Luyckx-Bacus J, Verbraeken H. 1976. Biometrie Oculaire Clinique. Masson, Paris, pp. 280—82.

Fledelius HC. 1976. Prematurity and the eye (thesis). Acta Ophthalmol (Copenh). Suppl 128.

Fledelius HC. 1979. Oculometry in high myopia in a representative sample of young adults aged 24. In: H Gernet (ed) Diagnostic Ultrasonography in Ophthalmology. Remy, Münster, pp. 195—197.

Goldschmidt E. 1968. On the etiology of myopia (thesis). Acta Ophthalmol (Copenh), Suppl 98.

Goldschmidt E, Fledelius HC, Erlin Larsen F. 1981. Clinical features in high myopia, A 10-year follow-up. In: JM Thijssen and AM Verbeek (eds), Ultrasonography in Ophthalmology, Doc Ophthal Proc Series, Vol. 28, Junk, The Hague, pp. 233—44.

Foetal ocular echobiometry: possibilities and limits

L. FALCO[1], G. CASCIO[2], P. E. GALLENGA[3], A. POLIZZI[4],
L. PISSARELLO[4], A. PANDIMIGLIO[5], G. PAGANO[6],
R. FORCUCCI[7], M. VALENZANO[8] AND M. ZINGIRIAN[4]

Summary

The Authors present a multicentre echographic study of growth of the foetal eye. The foetal eye transverse diameter was measured by means of B-scan echography, from the 14th to the 39th week of uncomplicated pregnancies. A curve of normal foetal eye growth was drawn.

Introduction

The possibility to demonstrate and measure echographically orbital and ocular structures in the foetus has been reported by several authors (Bots et al., 1981; Lannirubeto and Tajani, 1981; Seanty et al., 1982; Falco et al., 1983; Valenzo et al., 1983; Falco et al., 1984).

In particular, the measurement of external and internal interorbital diameters, useful for evaluating eyeball diameter indirectly (Valenzo et al., 1983), and a growth curve of the ocular transverse diameter, were reported (Falco et al., 1984). The present research, utilizing the cooperation of obstetricians and ophthalmologists in four centres, permitted the collection of a large amount of biometric data on the foetal eye.

Material and methods

747 pregnant women were examined in Obstetrics Centres for routine echographic control during a period of eight months. The women included in the study had a history of regular menses, no abortion, no malformed foetuses and no systemic and/or metabolic diseases. They were examined echographically from the 14th to 39th week of pregnancy. The biometric parameters of the foetuses (biparietal diameter, skull circumference, abdominal diameter and femur length) were normal.

University Eye Clinics of [1] Florence, [2] Palermo, [3] Chieti, [4] Genoa and University Clinics of Obstetrics and Gynaecology of [5] Florence, [6] Palermo, [7] Chieti, and [8] Genoa, Italy.

J. M. Thijssen (ed.) Ultrasonography in ophthalmology.
© 1988, *Kluwer Academic Publishers, Dordrecht, ISBN 978-94-010-7083-6*

352

The echobiometry of the foetal eye was performed by linear (ALOKA SS D 250; TOSHIBA SAL 20 A) and sectorial (COMBISON 320; COMBISON 202 R; Kretz-Technik) B-mode real-time echography, with a 3.5 MHz probe frequency and speed of 1600 m/sec (advised by the European Committee on Ultrasound in Obstetrics).

Biometric data were obtained by means of transverse scans of the foetal head, which is usually aligned along an oblique axis in relation to the mother's abdomen. In this way, it is possible to measure the transverse diameter of the foetal eyeball, which is usually spherical. To obtain more precise measurements of this diameter, it is necessary that the ocular walls are clearly distinguished from the orbital walls and that the image of the foetal lens is recognizable (14th week of pregnancy).

In general, it is possible to visualize only one eye, the one nearer to the mother's anterior abdominal wall. The study protocol also included periodic measurement of the foetal eye in the same patients and ocular biometry of the neonatal eye: these are presently in progress. The bio-metric data were statistically analyzed by means of the average and the measurement interval, in which there is a 95% possibility that the measure-ment of the transverse diameter of the foetal eye is not pathological.

Results

Preliminary results permitted the construction of a growth curve of the transverse diameter of the foetal eyeball (see Fig. 1). The increase in the transverse diameter is in agreement with other reports.

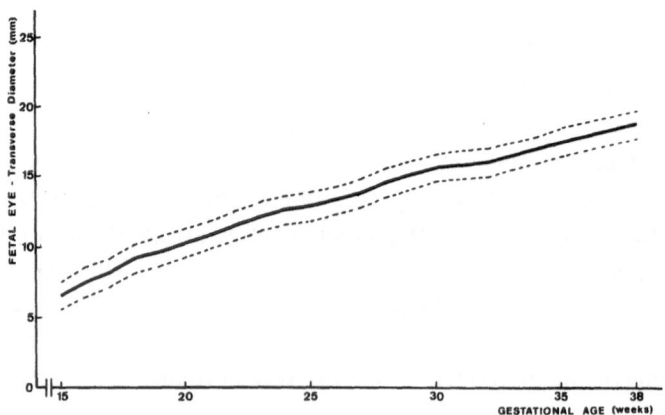

Fig. 1. Transverse diameter of the foetal eye vs. gestational age (solid line), 95 percent confidence interval (dashed lines).

Discussion

The aim of this study was the production of a growth curve of the foetal eyeball, the diameter of which is a parameter used in the screening of prenatal ocular diseases which are accompanied by biometric alterations of the eyeball (for example congenital glaucoma).

Presently, it is only possible to detect alterations when they deviate greatly from the average. The limits of the research are in relation to the technical difficulties in performing biometry and the difficulties of organizing a multicentre study.

It is sometimes difficult to visualize the ocular structure, both in the very early gestational period, because of the small dimensions of the eye and the difficulty in differentiating the ocular from the orbital wall, and also in the latest period, due to the position of the foetal head and the decreased amount of amniotic fluid.

Some imprecision in the measurements was caused by the limits of resolution of the echographic instruments which were lower than in those used in ophthalmology; by the slight elliptical deformation of the image that sectorial scanning echographic instruments can produce and by the incorrect positioning of the markers. There was also some difficulty in organizing the collaboration between the different centers, which are rather far apart and between two conceptually different specialities.

Conclusion

The present multicentre study, a collaboration between obstetricians and ophthalmologists, permitted the collection of a good amount of biometric data on the foetal eyeball. The growth curve of which shows that its diameter increases regularly during pregnancy.

References

Bots R, Nijhuis J, Martin C. 1981. Human foetal eye movements: detection in utero by Ultrasound. Early Human Development 5: 87.

Falco L, Pandimiglio A, Bartolomei MP, Nardi M. 1983. Nuovo parametro di ecobiometria fatale: misurazione del bulbo oculare. Ultr Ost Gin 3—4: 212—216.

Falco L, Pandimiglio A, Bartolomei MP, Carelli F, Nardi M. 1984. Curva di accrescimento del bulbo oculare fetale: Determinazione ecografica in gravidanza. Clinica Oculistica, p. 6.

354

Falco L, Nardi M, Passani F, Bartolomei M, Mazzeo V. 1987. Ultrasonic measurements of foetal eyeball diameter. In: KC Ossoinig (ed) Ophthalmic Echography Doc Ophthal Proc Ser, Vol. 48. Martinus Nijhoff/Junk, Dordrecht, pp. 93—99.

Ianniruberto A, Tajani A. 1981. Lo studio ecografica dei movimenti ocularidel feto umano. VI Congr Naz SISUM, Firenze.

Jeanty P, Dramaix-Wilmet M, VanGansbeke D, VanRegemorter N, Rodesh F. 1982. Foetal ocular biometry by Ultrasound, Ultrasound 143: 513—516.

Valenzano M, Costanini S, Carta E, Punto PF, Ragni N, Balestra V. 1983. Valutazione preliminare su due nuovi parametri ecografica: i diametri interorbitari fetali. Corso Internazionale di aggiornamento in Medicina fetale, Genova, pp. 481—488.

Valenzano M, Constantini S, Carta E, Venturini P, Ragni N. 1983. Crescita dei diametri interorbitari fetali e loro correlazioni con i parametri cefalici convenzionali. VIII Riuione Gruppo di Studio e di Ricera in Medicina Foetale, Milano, pp. 185—193.

The reduction of error in intraocular lens power calculation

J. S. HILLMAN

Summary

The final accuracy of the power of an implant lens is dependent on the accuracy with which the keratometry and the ultrasonic biometry have been performed. The various sources of measurement errors are discussed and suggestions for improving either the equipment, or its employment are given. The presence of an adequate A-mode display is strongly advocated. The merits of the various available lens power calculation methods are discussed.

Introduction

The intraocular lens (I.O.L.) has been accepted for the correction of aphakia because of the high quality of postoperative vision without demands upon the patient. Biometry and the implantation of I.O.Ls of selected power allow the surgeon to exercise a high degree of control over the postoperative refraction and to obtain the best refractive result for each individual patient. This is the standard management in the U.S.A. and it is becoming so in Europe as well. Surveys carried out by the U.K. Intraocular Implant Society have indicated that in 1984 25.4% of (responding) U.K. surgeons carried out biometry to determine I.O.L. power whilst in 1985 56.0% were using biometry and half of these surgeons measured in all their cases.

The benefits of I.O.L. calculation have been confirmed in a number of studies (Table 1) which indicate the high level of control over postoperative refraction. With the use of standard power I.O.Ls one can expect 80% to be within ± 2 D and 70% to be within ± 1 D of emmetropia whilst with calculation this can be improved to 99% within ± 2 D and 94% within ± 1 D of a chosen refraction (Hillman, 1982). Without calculation a

Department of Ophthalmology, St. James's University Hospital, Leeds LS9 7TF England.

J. M. Thijssen (ed.) Ultrasonography in ophthalmology.
© 1988, *Kluwer Academic Publishers, Dordrecht, ISBN 978-94-010-7083-6*

number of eyes show an unexpected postoperative high ametropia. This is inevitable because of the multifactorial nature of the refractive power of the eye, which is the product of the optical power of the cornea, the power and position of the natural lens and the axial length of the eye. Any of these factors may be abnormal and may be compensated or compounded by an abnormality in another compartment.

It is important to appreciate the limitations of biometric instruments and techniques and the potential sources of error in order to minimise them.

Keratometry

Keratometry is an important potential source of error that is often overlooked because of its apparent simplicity. An inaccuracy of 0.1 mm will be responsible for 0.5 D error in I.O.L. power calculation. Greater accuracy of measurement is required than that needed for contact lens fitting and keratometers must have their calibration checked against steel calibration balls. As the corneal surface is not that of a simple sphere, care must be taken to ensure measurements are made from central cornea by accurate symmetrical positioning of the target mires on the cornea. The autokeratometer gives more consistent results than simple manually-operated optical keratometers.

Axial length

The measurement of axial length has been given more attention because of its apparent complexity but the development of clinical echobiometers specifically for I.O.L. calculation has simplified the procedure. An inaccuracy of 0.1 mm, however, will be responsible for 0.25 D error in I.O.L. power calculation. Alignment along the optic axis is essential as off-axis alignment will give short measurement and correct alignment is indicated by sharp vertical echoes from the cornea, lens surfaces and vitreo-retinal interface (Fig. 1). For this reason, biometers which give a digital axial length measurement without a display of the scan are more liable to give inaccurate measurements.

The axial length measurement of the aphakic eye for secondary I.O.L. implantation is complicated by the absence of the lens echoes for scan alignment. In this situation the operator must select the longest measurement which is obtained consistently with sharp corneal and scleral echoes. The accuracy of echobiometers is increased by low system sensitivity which ensures that all signals are at the same phase of oscillation.

Table 1. Results of a number of studies to show the accuracy of calculation of intraocular lens power.

Author		n	± 1.0 D	± 2.0 D
Binkhorst	(1978)	26	81%	100%
Jaffe	(1978)	200	50%	85%
Kraff et al.	(1978)	100	72%	93%
Johns	(1979)	108	61%	92%
Lindstrom et al.	(1979)	100	52%	82%
Hoffer	(1980)	63	86%	95%
Retzlaff	(1980)	176	66%	95.4%
Sanders and Kraff	(1980)	924	79%	95.2%
Hillman	(1981)	100	94%	99%
Shammas	(1982)	500	78.8%	90%
Shammas	(1982)	100	95%	100%
Sanders and Kraff	(1982)	200	82%	98%

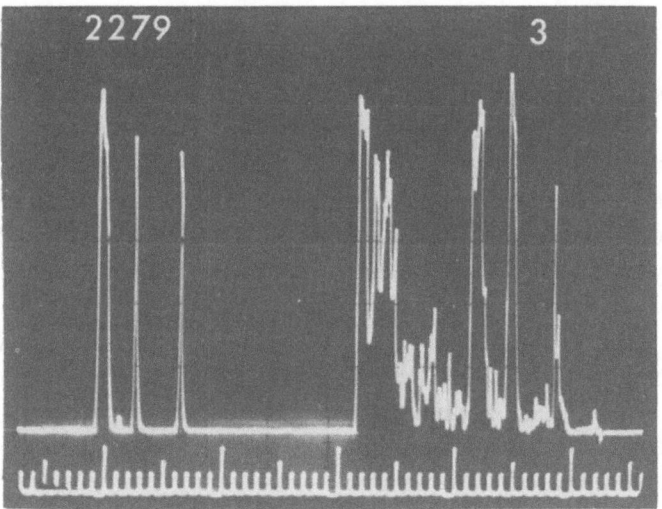

Fig. 1. On-axis scan indicated by clear sharp echo peaks from the cornea, lens surfaces and vitreo-retinal interface.

When applying the ultrasound probe to the cornea, care must be taken to minimise globe indentation. This is not a problem with instruments such as the Kretz 7200 MA which are used with a scleral contact lens water-bath containing water or methylcellulose to eliminate direct probe-eye contact. A number of direct-contact instruments employ a small probe which can be mounted in a slit-lamp tonometer mount which is set at 10 mmHg pressure whilst others have a special spring-controlled mount to standardise the applied force. It should be remembered, however, that such controlling devices can be overcome by rough use and the transducer should make the lightest possible contact with the cornea. The precise point of corneal contact is indicated by the appearance of the scan on the display oscilloscope screen. In some patients with poor fixation a position of slight upward gaze makes it impossible to obtain an axial scan with the probe fixed horizontally in a mount and the probe should then be removed from the mount and controlled with the fingers.

Measurements may be taken off the scan in several ways. With the Kretz 7200 MA reference is made to Polaroid photographs carrying a calibration scale which is set by the operator and Thijssen and Deutman (1981) and Ossoinig (1984) have stressed the greater accuracy of peak to peak measurements over baseline measurements. A number of workers have added electronic gates to the Kretz 7200 MA to simplify measurement (Thijssen et al., 1984) and others have devised their own systems (Lepper and Trier, 1984). Most of the many instruments dedicated to I.O.L. biometry incorporate electronic gates but they differ regarding the limits of scan quality acceptability and these automatic systems are not "foolproof". The electronic gates should be adjusted so that the cardinal echoes for measurement are at the front edge of each gate. Figure 2 demonstrates a potential source of error when an electronic system accepts a low amplitude artefact echo instead of the subsequent corneal echo. The electronic engineering design criteria of instruments differ regarding the amplitude below which an echo will be disregarded as insignificant and not taken for measurement. This information is not usually volunteered, but it can be determined by the operator by moving the gates on a scan with a range of echoes of different amplitudes.

The results presented in Table 1 illustrate the improvements which have been made with the development of I.O.L. biometry and calculation in recent years but in addition some degree of training an experience is important in the use of keratometers and echobiometers if consistently accurate results are to be obtained.

Formulae

The geometrical optical formulae require a value for the postoperative anterior chamber depth (A.C.D.). This must be an estimate as it does not bear a constant relationship to the preoperative depth. It does, however, vary according to the axial length of the eye, being shallower in the small hypermetropic eye and deeper in the long myopic eye. In the Binkhorst module calculation is improved by multiplying the theoretical A.C.D. for

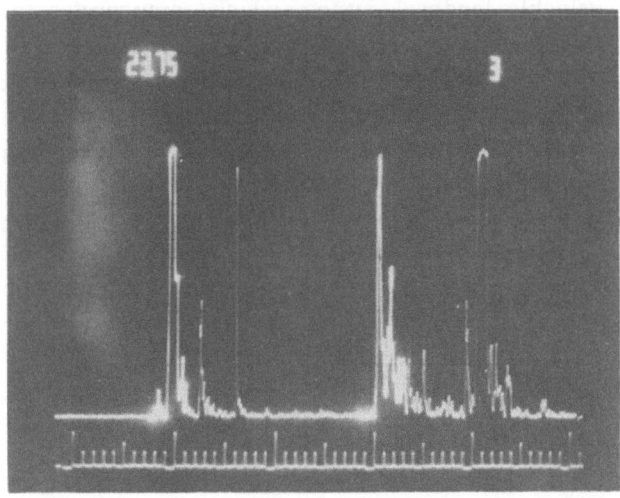

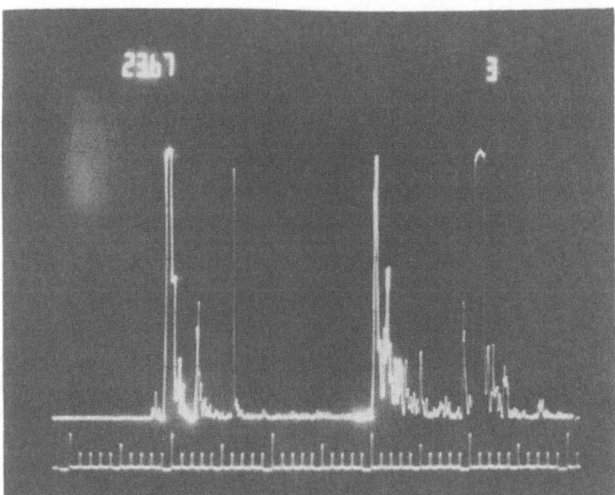

Fig. 2. Example of a potential source of error when an electronic gate accepts a low amplitude artefact echo instead of the following corneal echo. This is corrected by adjusting the first gate so that the corneal echo is the first echo in the gate.

the style of I.O.L. by the ratio of the axial length to 23.45 (mean axial length).

$$\frac{\text{modified}}{\text{A.C.D.}} = \frac{\text{theoretical}}{\text{A.C.D.}} \times \frac{\text{axial length}}{23.45}$$

The mathematical regression SRK formula does not require a value for the A.C.D. and it incorporates the valuable feature of an A-constant which can be personalised for each individual surgeon and style and make of I.O.L.

This is a valuable feedback system which compensates for consistent errors of measurement or technique. The same feedback must be applied when a geometrical optical formula is used by a review of results and a 'fudge factor' applied if necessary.

Opinions differ regarding the relative merits of the geometrical optical and regression formulae and Fig. 3 compares the results of calculation of I.O.L. power using the Binkhorst and SRK formulae. It can be seen that the Binkhorst formula tends to give a stronger power I.O.L. for the short eye and this difference is reduced by the use of the modified A.C.D.

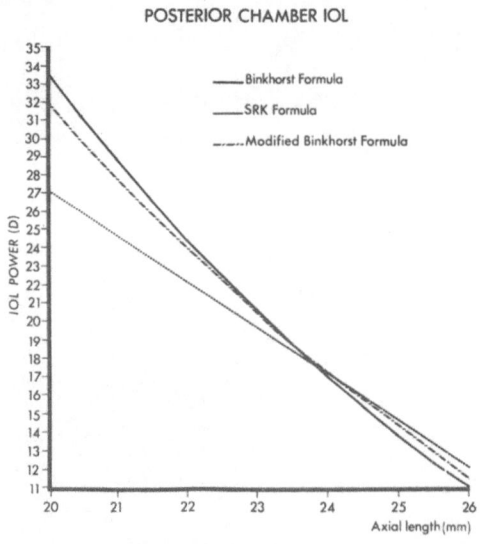

POSTERIOR CHAMBER IOL

Fig. 3. Comparison of the results of calculations of posterior chamber intraocular lens powers for emmetropia using the Binkhorst and SRK formulae and the modification of the Binkhorst formula to adjust the anterior chamber depth according to the axial length.

Table 2 presents the axial lengths of 100 consecutive eyes measured for I.O.L. power calculation and shows that 94% eyes lie between 21 mm and 25 mm and 68% between 22 mm and 24 mm. In practice, the difference between the formulae is not great. Whichever systems of measurement and calculation are used, it is important to keep the results under constant review. Eyes in which there have been significant errors should be re-measured. Surgery should not significantly change the mean corneal curvature. On echobiometry, scan axis alignment is indicated by a descending cascade of echoes from the I.O.L. which behaves as a round intraocular foreign body and produces reverberating echoes (Fig. 4).

The goals of I.O.L. power calculation differ with each individual patient. Theoretical problems of aniseikonia can be controlled by limiting anisometropia (Hillman and Hawkswell, 1985) without the specific calculation

Table 2. Distribution of axial lengths in 100 eyes measured consecutively for intraocular lens power calculation.

Axial length (mm)	Number
20.0—21.0	4
21.1—22.0	14
22.1—23.0	37
23.1—24.0	31
24.1—25.0	12
25.1—26.0	2

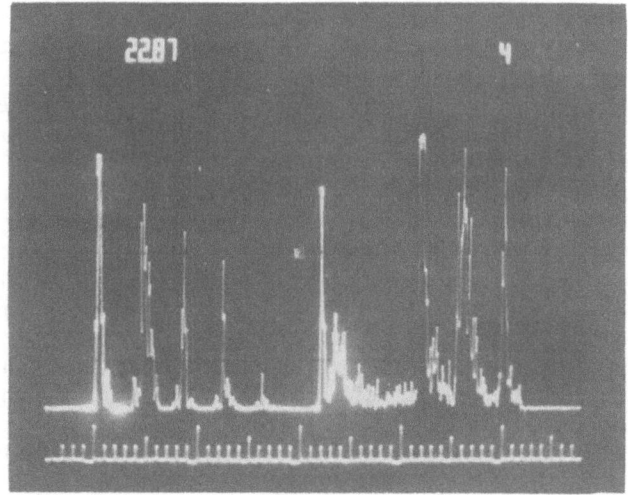

Fig. 4. On echobiometry of an eye containing an intraocular lens, the lens appears as a descending cascade of echoes from reverberation as with a round intraocular foreign body.

of iseikonic I.O.L. power. Low myopia is generally considered to be preferable to emmetropia or hypermetropia because of the benefits for near vision. The control of postoperative astigmatism by careful suture tension and the selective cutting of sutures allows the creation of myopic astigmatism to give pseudophakic pseudo-accommodation (Huber, 1981). In this situation the patient uses the emmetropic meridian for distance and the myopic meridian for near, so reducing the dependence upon spectacles.

Biometry and the calculation of I.O.L. power are now so well established that there is no justification for leaving the patient's postoperative refraction to chance.

362

References

Binkhorst RD. 1978. Biometric A-scan ultrasonography and intraocular lens power calculation. In: JM Emery (ed) Current concepts in cataract surgery. Mosby, St Louis, pp. 175—182.

Hillman JS. 1982. The selection of intraocular lens power by calculation and by reference to the refraction. Trans Ophthal Soc U.K. 102: 495—497.

Hillman JS, Hawkswell A. 1985. The control of aniseikonia after intraocular lens implantation. Trans Ophthal Soc U.K. 104: 582—585.

Hoffer KJ. 1980. The biometry of 7500 cataractous eyes. Amer J Ophthalmol 90: 360—368.

Huber C. 1981. Myopic astigmatism as a substitute for accommodation in pseudophakia. Docum Ophthalmol 52: 123.

Jaffe NS. 1979. The changing scene of intraocular implant lens surgery. Amer J Ophthalmol 88: 819—828.

Johns GE. 1979. Clinical evaluation of the DBR A-scan unit. Amer Intraoc Implant Soc J 5: 213—216.

Kraff MC, Sanders DR, Lieberman HL. 1978. Determination of intraocular lens power: a comparison with and without ultrasound. Ophthal Surg 9: 81—84.

Lepper R-D, Trier HG. 1984. Computerised ocular biometry: a newly developed compact system. In: JS Hillman and MM Le May (eds) Ophthalmic ultrasonography. Doc Ophthal Proc Series 38, Junk, The Hague, pp. 237—241.

Lepper R-D, Trier HG. 1984. Refraction after intraocular lens implantation: results with a computerised system for ultrasonic biometry and for implant lens power calculation. In: JS Hillman and MM Le May (eds) Ophthalmic ultrasonography. Doc Ophthal Proc Series 38, Junk, The Hague, pp. 243—248.

Lindstrom RL, Lindstrom CW, Harris CW. 1979. Accuracy of lens implant power determination using A-scan. Contact and Intraocular lens Med J 5: 61—66.

Ossoinig KC. 1984. How to obtain maximum measuring accuracies with standardised A-scan. In: JS Hillman and MM Le May (eds) Ophthalmic ultrasonography. Doc Ophthal Proc Series 38, Junk, The Hague, pp. 197—216.

Retzlaff J. 1980. A new intraocular lens calculation formula Am Intra-ocular Implant Soc J 6: 148—152.

Sanders DR, Kraff MC. 1980. Improvement of intraocular lens power calculation using empirical data. Am Intra-ocular Implant Soc J 6: 263—267.

Sanders DR, Kraff MC. 1982. A comparison of the Digital Biometric Ruler-300 and Echo-oculometer-3000: a report of 200 cases. Am Intra-ocular Implant Soc J 8: 365—369.

Shammas HJF. 1982. Axial length measurement and its relation to intraocular lens power calculation. Am Intra-ocular Implant Soc J 8: 346—349.

Shammas HJF. 1982. The fudged formula for intraocular lens power calculations. Am Intra-ocular Implant Soc J 8: 350—352.

Thijssen JM, Deutman AF. 1981. Predictive value of calculated dioptric power of pre-pupillary implant leses. In: JM Thijssen and AM Verbeck (eds) Ultrasonography in Ophthalmology. Doc Ophthal Proc 29, Junk, The Hague, pp. 239—244.

Thijssen JM, Verhoef WA, Pasman-Scheps F, Verbeek AM. 1984. Computerised biometry and lens calculation. In: JS Hillman and MM Le May (eds) Ophthalmic ultrasonography. Doc Ophthal Proc 38, Junk, The Hague, pp. 231—235.

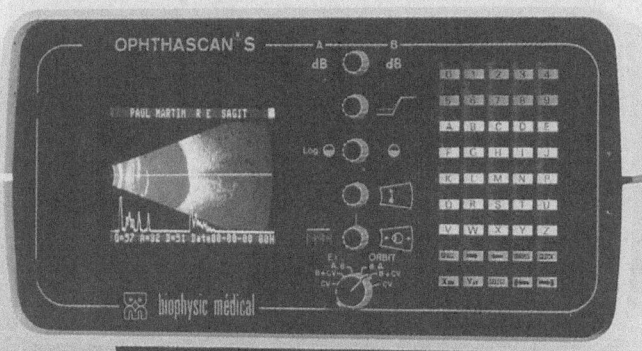
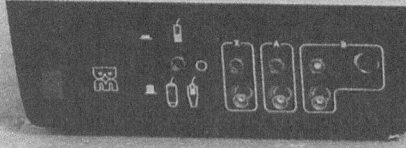
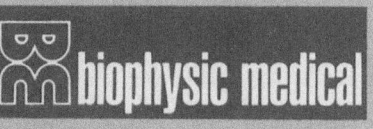

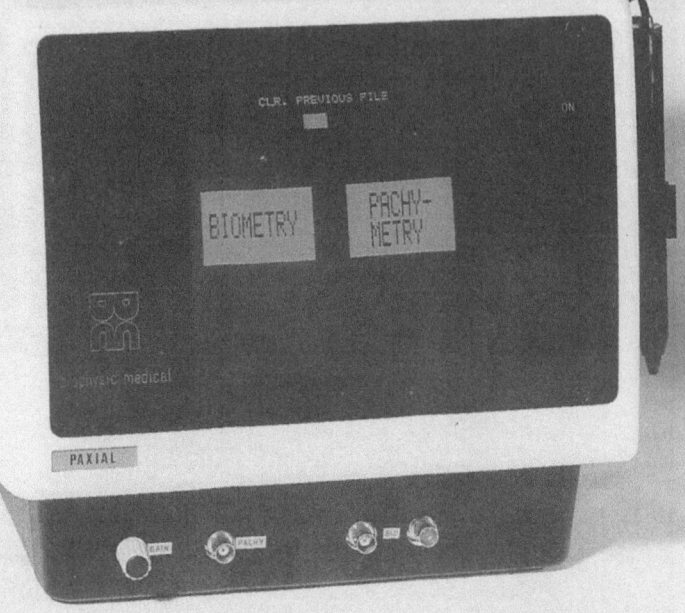
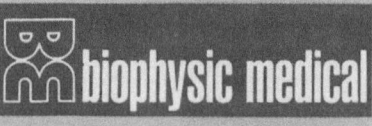

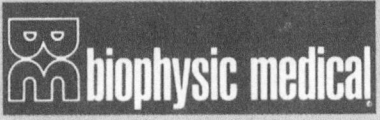

Authors index

368

Documenta Ophthalmologica Proceedings Series

16. H.-J. Merté, ed.,
Genesis of Glaucoma. 1978. ISBN 90–6193–159–2
17. A.F. Deutman, ed.,
Neurogenetics and Neuro-Ophthalmology. 1977. ISBN 90–6193–159–2
18. O. Hockwin and W.B. Rathbun, eds.,
Progress in Anterior Eye Segment Research and Practice. 1979. ISBN 90–6193–158–4
19. E.L. Greve, ed.,
The Third International Visual Field Symposium, Tokyo 1978. 1979. ISBN 90–6193–160–6
20. J. Francois, S.I. Brown and M. Itoi, eds.,
Proceedings of the Symposium of the International Society for Corneal Research. 1979. ISBN 90–6193–157–6
21. J. François, E. Maumenäe and I. Esente, eds.,
First International Congress on Cataract Surgery. 1979. ISBN 90– 6193–162–2
22. E.L. Greve, ed.,
Glaucoma Symposium Amsterdam. Diagnosis and Therapy. 1980. ISBN 90–6193–164–9
23. E. Schmöger and J.H. Kelsey, eds.,
Visual Electrodiagnosis in Systematic Diseases. Proceedings of the 17th I.S.C.E.V. Symposium, Erfurt June 5–10, 1979. 1980. ISBN 90–6193–163–0
24. A. Hamburg, ed.,
Symposium on Uveal Melanomas. 1980. ISBN 90–6193–722–1
25. H. Zauberman, ed.,
Proceedings of the Conference on Subretinal Space, Jerusalem October 14–19, 1979. 1981. ISBN 90–6193–721–3
26. E.L. Greve and G. Verriest, eds.,
Fourth International Visual Field Symposium, Bristol April 13–16, 1980. 1981. ISBN 90–6193–165–7
27. H. Spekreijse and P.A. Apkarian, eds.,
Visual Pathways. Electrophysiology and Pathology. 18th I.S.C.E.V. Symposium, Amsterdam May 18–22, 1980. 1981. ISBN 90–6193–723–X
28. H.C. Fledelius, P.H. Alsbirk and E. Goldschmidt, eds.,
Third International Conference on Myopia, Copenhagen August 24– 27, 1980. 1981. ISBN 90–6193–725–6
29. J.M. Thijssen, ed.,
Ultrasonography in Ophthalmology, 8th SIDUO Congress, Nijmegen, The Netherlands, September 21–25, 1980. 1981. ISBN 90–6193–724–8
30. L. Maffei, ed.,
Pathophysiology of the Visual System, Pisa Italy, December 12–15, 1980. 1981. ISBN 90–6193–726–4
31. G. Niemeyer and C. Huber, eds.,
Techniques in Clinical Electrophysilogy of Vision. Proceedings of the 19th I.S.C.E.V. Symposium, Horgen–Zurich, June 1981. 1982. ISBN 90–6193–727–2
32. A.Th.M. van Balen and W.A. Houtman, ed.,
Strabismus Symposium. 1982. ISBN 90–6193–728–0
33. G. Verriest, ed.,
Colour Vision Deficiencies VI. 1982. ISBN 90–6193–729–9
34. A. Roucoux and M. Crommelinck, eds.,
Physiological and Pathological Aspects of Eye Movements. 1982. ISBN 90–6193–730–2
35. E.L. Greve and A. Heyl, eds.,
Fifth International Visual Field Symposium. 1983. ISBN 90–6193– 731–0
36. R. Birngruber and V.-P, Gabel, eds.,
Laser Treatment and Photocoagulation of the Eye. 1984. ISBN 90– 6193–732–9
37. H.E.J.W. Kolder, ed.,
Slow Potentials and Microprocessor Applications. 1983. ISBN 90– 6193–733–7
38. J.S. Hillman and M.M. Le May, eds.,
Ophthalmic Ultrasonography. 1984. ISBN 90–6193–734–5
39. G. Verriest, ed.,
Colour Vision Deficiencies VII. 1984. ISBN 90–6193–735–3
40. J.R. Heckenlively, ed.,

Pattern Electroretinogram, Circulatory Disturbances of the Visual System and Pattern–Evoked Responses. 21st ISCEV Symposium. 1984. ISBN 90–6193–503–2

41. E.C. Campos, ed.,
    Sensory Evaluation of Strabismus and Amblyopia in a Natural Environment. In honour of Professor Bruno Bagolini. 1984. ISBN 90–6193–508–3

42. A. Heyl and E.L. Greve, eds.,
    Sixth International Visual Field Symposium. 1985. ISBN 90–6193– 254–5

43. E.L. Greve, W. Leydhecker and C. Raitta, eds.,
    Second European Glaucoma Symposium Helsinki, May 1984. 1985. ISBN 90–6193–526–1

44. P.C. Maudgal and L. Missotten, eds.,
    Herpetic Eye Diseases 1985. ISBN 90–6193–527–X

45. B. Jay, ed.,
    Detection and Measurement of Visual Impairment in Pre–Verbal Children. 1986 ISBN 0–89838–789–2

46. G. Verriest, ed.,
    Colour Vision Deficiencies VIII. 1987. ISBN 0–89838–801–5

47. P.L. Emiliani, ed.,
    Development of Electronic Aids for the Visually Impaired. 1986. ISBN 0–89838–805–8

49. E.L. Greve and A. Heijl, eds.,
    Seventh International Visual Field Symposium, Amsterdam, September 1986. 1987. ISBN 0–89838–882–1

50. D. BenEzra, S.J. Ryan, B.M. Glaser and R.P. Murphy, eds.,
    Ocular Circulation and Neovascularization. 1987. ISBN 0–89838– 892–9

51. J.M. Thyssen, ed.,
    Ultrasonography in ophthalmology 11. 1988. pp. x + 368. ISBN 0– 89838–378–1